Clinical Signs in Small Animal Medicine

Michael Schaer
University of Florida, College of Veterinary Medicine, USA

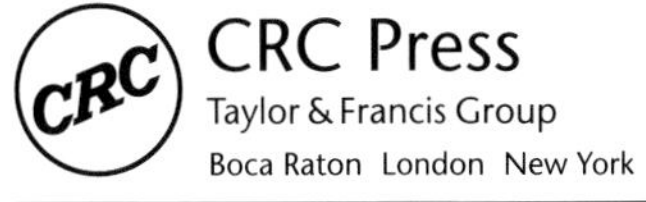

CRC Press is an imprint of the
Taylor & Francis Group, an **informa** business

CRC Press
Taylor & Francis Group
6000 Broken Sound Parkway NW, Suite 300
Boca Raton, FL 33487-2742

Printed and bound in India by Replika Press Pvt. Ltd.

Printed on acid-free paper
Version Date: 20160607

International Standard Book Number-13: 978-1-4987-6684-5 (Paperback)

Visit the Taylor & Francis Web site at
http://www.taylorandfrancis.com

and the CRC Press Web site at
http://www.crcpress.com

Contents

Preface

This 2nd edition of *Clinical Signs in Small Animal Medicine* is written to share the visual experiences of the author spanning the period from 2007 to 2015. It continues with its primary basis of instruction that "one picture is worth 1,000 words". It has served my students well and the same is intended for my veterinary colleagues who are outside the boundaries of my classroom. Quoting one of my graduates from the University of Florida (UF) Class of 1980: "Dr. Schaer, the other day a dog walked into my clinic with the exact physical abnormalities of one of the dogs you showed me during your student slide rounds, and I nailed that diagnosis strictly because of the impression that image left in my memory bank 25 many years ago." Because of this and similar feedbacks that have confirmed the effectiveness of the visual teaching method, I have continued that exercise right to the present day – 40 years later. It stimulated me to publish the 1st edition of *Clinical Signs in Small Animal Medicine* in 2007 and continued to motivate me to compose this second edition.

Having progressed into the digital age of photography after the year 2000, assembling my clinical images has been a lot more efficient. Nobody was more delighted for this than my wife, MJ, who had scanned nearly 30,000 slide images into digital format. In order to maintain my organized filing system, I have disciplined myself to download any new images from my camera on the same night that the pictures are taken and to label them for reference to be used at a later date. These images are then edited and stored in an alphabetically arranged computer folder system until such time as they are needed for my lectures, publications, or for a colleague who needs them for his/her academic development. The images are captured as they appeared through the author's lens on a chance basis as they came to the clinics. Thus the background for the 'photobiography' of my wonderful clinical experiences from 1971 to 2015. To complement the images and legends, I have added phrases from my "Uncle Mikey's Maxims" and "Clinical Pearls" lectures that will add just the right amount of take-home messages for you to dwell on for the remaining parts of your career. These basically represent my clinical philosophy of medicine. I hope that you find them of value.

The reader will note that these first two editions do not represent every possible clinical disorder and their various types of presentations – an impossible objective for sure. However, if used together, both volumes complement the deficiencies of the other because much effort was made to avoid repeating any images that appear in any one textbook. The topics, on the other hand, will be duplicated in order to cover the various forms of the disorder that are not represented in the other edition.

It would be unfair to take credit for all of the images in this textbook. Those acquired through the radiology section image library at The University of Florida College of Veterinary Medicine (UFCVM) have been an important source of information throughout this textbook. It is through the expertise of the radiology staff and faculty that the images have been made available in our hospital digital imaging library for other faculty members to access. I thank them immensely for all of their wonderful efforts, which occur daily at UFCVM. The same gratitude extends to my small animal medicine and surgery colleagues, clinical pathology, and pathology faculty members, house officers, and alumni who have shared their specimens and images with me during my career at Florida. It has been through their assistance that clinicians such as me have been able to take each valuable piece of clinical information and use it as a valuable teaching tool.

The period spanning 2012 to 2015 at Florida offered a new experience for me. Those of you who have known me over the years have seen me in the role as a small animal internist, but a few years ago, I was given the most fortuitous opportunity to make the section of Emergency and Critical Care (ECC) my new home. This transition has been an amazingly exciting experience for me because it immersed me directly into a group of highly intelligent colleagues who patiently accepted my internist kind of thinking and found that our efforts complemented each other for the unified outcome of enhanced patient care. Besides, they made each day a new learning opportunity for me. So to my ECC colleagues – I thank you.

To all of my house officers, students, support staff, administrators, and colleagues at UF, I extend my continued gratitude for your support toward providing me with so many wonderful moments during my career as a faculty member. I am a seeker of constant inspiration, and it was you who energized me on a daily basis to be the best doctor and teacher that I could be. As I continue with this last lap of my career, I pledge my constant efforts to further the missions of education and quality medicine at The University of Florida.

In closing, my failure to recognize the staff at CRC would be an unforgiveable sin, for it is they who have made all my publishing efforts possible. The expertise of Kate Nardoni, Jill Northcott, Peter Beynon, and Paul Bennett will unfold as you read the *Clinical Signs* textbooks, and because of this, I am forever grateful.

Michael Schaer

Abbreviations

ACTH adrenocorticotropic hormone
ADH antidiuretic hormone
BUN blood urea nitrogen
CPR cardiopulmonary resuscitation
CRT capillary refill time
CSF cerebrospinal fluid
CT computed tomography
DI diabetes insipidus
DIC disseminated intravascular coagulation
DMSA dimercaptosuccinic acid
DOCP desoxycorticosterone pivalate
ECF extracellular fluid
ECG electrocardiogram
FeLV feline leukemia virus
FIV feline immunodeficiency virus
GABA gamma-aminobutyric acid
GH growth hormone
GI gastrointestinal
H&E hematoxylin and eosin (stain)
ICU intensive care unit
IGF insulin-like growth factor
IMHA immune-mediated hemolytic anemia
ITP immune thrombocytopenia
LRS lactated Ringer's solution
MRI magnetic resonance imaging
NSAID nonsteroidal anti-inflammatory drug
PAS periodic acid–Schiff (stain)
PCO_2 partial pressure of carbon dioxide
PCV packed cell colume
PD polydipsia
PICC peripherally inserted central catheter
PPD pyschogenic polydipsia
PTH parathyroid hormone
PU polyuria
RBC red blood cell
SCC squamous cell carcinoma
SG specific gravity
TCO_2 total carbon dioxide
TP total protein
TSH thyroid-stimulating hormone
WBC white blood cell

Dedication

To all of my patients, pet owners, students, and house officers, I thank you for the true inspiration you have given me. Unfortunately, the height of any clinician's 'bone pile' bespeaks of years of painful experiences and the everlasting stings of mistakes. Forgive me for those that I have committed, but rest assured that I have done everything possible to make sure they are not repeated. Thank you all for allowing me to honestly say that "If I had to do my career all over again, I would follow in the paths that you have guided me".

Introduction

The knowledge explosion has done much to advance the science of veterinary medicine. This manuscript will attempt to fill in the large gap left behind despite the high technology that we use – this being the Art of Veterinary Medicine. After 40 plus years of practice, I would like to share some of the painful lessons of the past and present, otherwise known as "Uncle Mikey's Maxims".

1. Treat for the treatable

This very important statement forms the basis of the optimistic approach to the sick patient. Many clinicians will periodically find themselves confronted with a very distressed or moribund patient during the 'off-hours' when important diagnostic facilities and personnel are unavailable. The patient is dying, you don't know the diagnosis, yet something must be done to stabilize the animal until certain definitive answers are known. Another scenario occurs when the work up must be limited for any number of reasons. The answer – 'treat for the treatable'. This is clearly illustrated in the situation where a puppy is examined for an acute onset of dyspnea. The history rules out chest trauma but the physical examination findings include an oral commissure ulceration and moist rales heard especially over the dorsal caudal lung lobes. Without using any diagnostic tests, the clinician begins immediate treatment for neurogenic pulmonary edema resulting from an electric cord bite and saves the puppy's life. This is only one of many examples where it is important to 'treat for the treatable before the treatable becomes nontreatable'.

2. Assumptions lead to trouble; therefore don't assume

Perhaps we can extract this lesson from many that we have already learned in everyday life. The main reason for being aware of this common judgment error with our patients is that assumptions can sometimes lead to misdiagnosis and perhaps even the animal's demise. Why assume that a sick, polydipsic, polyuric, middle-aged female dog does not have a pyometra just because the recently recorded signalment of the new patient record denotes previous neutering? Isn't it best to verify this fact verbally with the owner in order to turn an assumption into a certainty, or obtain an abdominal radiograph anyway?

3. Always interpret clinical information within the context of the patient's presentation

Today's veterinarian has access to various forms of advanced medical technology, and in the majority of instances our patients benefit from the data that is generated. Sometimes, however, clinicians become overly dependent on the laboratory tests and diagnostic instrumentation and come to accept the results at face value without interpreting the information within the context of the patient's presentation or weighing the test results against the degree of evidence-based medicine available. This can result not only in misdiagnosis and in mistreatment of the patient, but also it can lead to added expense and emotional distress for the client as well. This situation can result from sample collection errors, laboratory or instrument errors, or the clinician's unfamiliarity with certain clinical disorders. There are a few instances in the text where images are used in more than one chapter. This is because of their pertinence in the respective chapters.

4. Avoid tunnel vision

This all too frequent human mistake might very well qualify for being the main pitfall of the diagnostician. This is a trap that constantly awaits each of us, and its avoidance requires the utmost vigilance and discipline. It is so easy to focus our minds on an obvious problem while simultaneously losing sight of the rest of the animal. Take, for example, the middle-aged Poodle that is examined for rapid-onset cataracts and the clinician who either forgets to inquire about the presence of polydipsia and polyuria or fails to weigh the significance of these important historical facts, which might contribute to the diagnosis of diabetes mellitus.

5. Treat your patient, not just its disease

These words of caution are closely related to the tunnel vision problem. The emphasis here, however, is therapeutics, not diagnostics. All medications should be adjusted according to each patient's individual needs and the clinical setting in which they are required. It would be unwise to treat an abscess with aminoglycoside antibiotic injections if the animal who owns the abscess has chronic renal insufficiency and a serum creatinine level of 6 mg/dl (530 µmol/l).

6. Avoid overmedicating

This error in medical management usually occurs as a result of the clinician's good intentions to do something helpful. The several problems that result from this practice include toxic drug reactions, excess expense, and sometimes interference with the correct interpretation of laboratory test results and the patient's progress.

It is only after many years of practice, studying, and objective thinking that the clinician would hopefully learn when not to use certain medications that he/she might have used with reflex reaction in the past.

7. Be honest with yourself

We have all been anointed with these words of wisdom before. In medicine, there is a special place for this advice in our day-to-day practice situations because our patients' lives depend on our objectivity. Perhaps the best judge and jury of them all is the necropsy.

8. Don't postpone today's urgencies until tomorrow

This advice is easily accepted when you think that the main consequence might be a 'no tomorrow' for the patient. Diagnostic and therapeutic delays might occur because we are fatigued at the end of a busy day, the patient presents during the off-hours emergency period, or the patient's arrival conflicts with other commitments. Although we might not consciously mean to be neglectful, our subconscious desires might deter us from our professional obligations. Why should a dyspneic animal with severe pleural effusion be forced to agonize overnight until its diagnosis becomes a convenience for his doctor on the following day? Let us never forget that 'our patients can die waiting'.

9. Think that common things occur commonly
Remembering this will help you to Treat for the Treatable, especially when certain logistics or restraints impede an expedient diagnosis. This is illustrated in the middle-aged dog that presents during a 3-day holiday weekend (a time when most laboratories are closed) with a peracute onset of weakness, anemia, icterus, hemoglobinuria, and hemoglobinemia. Here it is important to recognize that these signs are compatible with an acute hemolytic event, and that autoimmune hemolytic anemia is the most common disease in this type of clinical setting. This line of reasoning allows for the immediate treatment of the treatable until proven otherwise.

10. Look closely at your patient; it will usually tell you what is wrong
The essence of the seasoned diagnostician is having the ability to (1) first recognize that the animal is sick, (2) then be able to localize the exact source of the problem, and (3) plan an initial judicious therapeutic strategy while the diagnostic test results are pending. Obviously one cannot proceed to steps 2 and 3 unless step 1 is realized. This is illustrated in the case of the anorectic and depressed cat that is sick because of pyothorax. This patient cannot be appropriately helped until the clinician first recognizes that the cat has an abnormal respiratory pattern.

This is also illustrated in the dog that postures with an arched back from spinal radicular pain, and the examining clinician misinterprets the signs as abdominal in origin or perhaps even fails to recognize the abnormal posture.

11. Never let your patient die without the benefit of the silver bullet (steroids)
Most of us tend to find this token bit of philosophy humorous or perhaps potentially dangerous. Although there are many diseases that can worsen as a result of repeated doses of glucocorticoid drugs, there are few (if any) that will progress to the patient's demise from one or two doses of this medication. This is not to imply that the indiscriminate use of glucocorticoid drugs is recommended; it is rather a reminder that animals can die of certain disorders such as nonseptic meningitis, autoimmune thrombocytopenia, immune-mediated hemolytic anemia, and acute adrenocortical insufficiency if they do not receive glucocorticoid treatment. Certain empirical therapeutic judgments have their place in medicine, especially when we are practicing under various economic, emotional, and diagnostic constraints.

12. When you hear hoof beats look for horses, but don't forget about the zebras
We can effectively practice medicine by remembering that common diseases occur commonly. However, there are those occasional situations when that extra amount of knowledge or index of clinical suspicion will facilitate the diagnosis of a not so common disease and consequently lead to the patient's cure.

Take, for instance, the dog from Portugal that presents with moderate anemia, fluctuating fever, hyperglobulinemia, and splenomegaly. How many of you can suspect that the zebra in this scenario is leishmaniasis?

13. Never sell the basics short
There is no substitute for the thorough history and physical examination. When the clinical hypothesis cannot be substantiated, go back to 'square one' beginning with the basics. As Sir William Osler taught: 'Trying to practice medicine without a strong foundation is like navigating a ship without a compass in uncharted waters'.

14. If you don't think it, you won't find it
This is easily illustrated in the mature vomiting cat with acute pancreatitis. All too often the clinician will think of many other etiologies, but if he/she doesn't consider acute pancreatitis in the differential diagnosis, the condition will easily be missed.

15. Never let a biological specimen go to waste
How many times have we admitted a sick patient only to find 8–24 hours later (when the laboratory results become available) that the animal is a ketoacidotic diabetic? Imagine how beneficial it would have been if we had tested that patient's urine, which was available on the cage floor, soon after admission. The same applies to other biological specimens such as feces, sputum, etc.

16. Disaster lurks whenever a patient's problem is 'routine'
The incident that taught me this painful lesson involved a 2-year-old Poodle that went into fulminating anaphylaxis immediately following its yearly vaccination. The patient died. Same for my own kitten that died during a 'routine' spay under a surgeon's supervision at the Teaching Hospital. How about the endoscope that perforated a cat's stomach during 'routine' gastroscopy under the purview of an experienced endoscopist or the cat that arrests during a bronchial lavage? The saga continues...........

17. If it's not getting worse, give it a chance to get better
Although this is the 'quick serve' period in our society, there are many medical disorders that simply will not commit themselves to our quick-fix mentality. Take, for instance, the patient with hemorrhagic pancreatitis who might very well require up to 4–5 weeks of a rather stormy convalescence. This insight is essential before calling certain disorders nontreatable.

18. Don't stray too far from the patient – the diagnosis will eventually appear
A lot of different conditions can fall into this situation. Take, for instance, the dog with waxing/waning episodes of restlessness, hyperventilation, and peripheral vasodilatation that might someday be explained when its pheochromocytoma is diagnosed. Remaining close to the patient and the pet owner will often give you that important opportunity to go back to square one and perhaps eventually realize the true diagnosis. If these measures fail to diagnose the patient - REFER IT.

19. Don't give your patient a disease it doesn't deserve to have
Think about it. It is you and the patient, with you having the power to apply any label to the signs that you detect. Now stop and ask yourself if you are satisfied with the accuracy of your interpretation and the logic of your mental processing. Quoting Dr. Peter Mere Latham:

'Truth in all of its kinds is most difficult to win, and truth in medicine is the most difficult of all.'

20. Don't let technology make you decerebrate
With the availability of advanced medical technology, transtelephonics, and e-mail, how easy it is for clinicians to let go of their basic skills and leave the

diagnosing and prescribing to those who haven't even looked at the patient. To keep your skills sharp you must use them. Only then will your patient benefit the most.

21. The necropsy is the clinician's trial by jury

The necropsy is often the pinnacle in the search for truth in medicine, for it usually holds the definitive answers for the patient's maladies. Although it might yield the pain of a misdiagnosis, let it be the source of a lesson well learned and one that best not be repeated.

22. The wisdom of experience should never be ignored

Let the fear of aging be offset by the confidence gained from knowing. It is the result of an enormous data processing punctuated by the corrected mistakes of the past. Let the wisdom be complemented with evidence-based medicine to maximize the benefit to our patients.

23. The diagnostician should always ask him/herself these two questions: where am I with this patient, and where am I going?

These two questions will function as a system of checks and balances during the management of any given patient and hopefully avoid the pitfalls of blind pursuit in search of a diagnosis.

24. If the patient isn't going where you expect it to be going, then go back to square one

So often the outcome of a misdiagnosis could have been avoided with a heightened awareness by the clinician in charge. Seek not the false comfort brought about with tunnel vision by allowing each new day to call for a complete reassessment of the clinical findings at hand.

25. In order to successfully treat a cat, you must think like a cat

The cat is such a unique creature who takes great offense when we mistakenly handle them as 'small dogs'. You must respect their independence while simultaneously provide them with the utmost of tender loving care. Always try to deal with them on their terms! Failing to remember this will be an experience not to be forgotten.

26. Avoid the pitfalls of the red herring

Laboratory errors will cost you and the owner time and expense if you pursue nonsensical results. When in doubt, repeat the test or speak with the lab technician.

27. If they can't afford a 'caddy', then offer them a 'chevy'

All too frequently the most expensive tests and treatments are not the sole means of an optimistic outcome.

28. Know thy patient

It is essential that you remember all historical and clinical details about your patient so that no vital information is forgotten. This includes a physical examination done with the patient out of the cage on each day of hospitalization.

29. Nobody wants to pay a big bill for a dead animal
This especially applies to the emergency doctor who frequently has situations and issues that need immediate attention. Bottom line is to get compensated as soon as possible or be prepared to suck-up the loss.

30. What matters is not so much what you say to a concerned client, but how they perceive what you said
The absence of eye contact, the pressures of ongoing catastrophes, and the mounting build up of fatigue all contribute to the misunderstandings that might end up before an ethics review board. Never forget that your pet owners demand compassion and respect – always.

31. Diagnostic cloudiness will soon be replaced by clear skies – be patient
The difficult to diagnosis patient can lead to frustrations and sometimes wrong decisions. If it is not a life-threatening problem, give the disorder time to unveil or refer the patient to a specialist, if possible.

32. Better that the dying patient expire in the hospital than during the car ride home
This is to avoid the horror that this can cause the pet owner who has no idea what to expect. Such memories last forever, especially in the mind of the child.

33. You must have cognition to be a competent clinician
This is an essential requirement, especially in emergency medicine where time is critical to the patient's outcome.

34. To prognose you must first be able to diagnose
Giving the wrong diagnosis will certainly cause a domino effect on all subsequent actions for your patient. Better to know why a certain action must be taken rather than to regret that it was taken.

35. The toaster effect
Just as bread will pop up in the toaster when it is ready, so will your sick patients rise and eat when they reach the turning point for recovery.

36. To cut is to see; to see is to do; to do is to cure
The diagnostic lap is still a valid procedure for obtaining a definitive diagnosis.

Clinical pearls: practice tips or reflections about many clinical situations

After 25 years of practice, a clinician can come to the clear conclusion that the practice of medicine consists of a fine blend of both the art and the science. Perhaps it might be rather bold to state that at times the value of the art might even surpass that of the science, even in the academic environment. The main objective of this gathering of thoughts is to share some of the lessons that I have learned over the years with the hope that you will walk away with a few PEARLS that will benefit your sick patients. For the sake of simplicity, thoughts have been categorized according to organ system and will be presented in short and simple phrases. First, a bit of philosophy on the art of diagnosis from R. Kreisburg MD:

'To make the correct diagnosis, we need the right choices.
To consider the right choices, we need the right information.
To obtain the right information, we need to ask the right questions.
Asking the right questions is the hallmark of clinical expertise.'

Note: Excerpts from the 'Pearls' listed below have been deliberately repeated in the relevant chapters to which they relate.

Patient evaluation

- Pallor can be caused by hypoxia, shock, anemia, and an epinephrine injection.
- Anemic pallor plus icterus causes a yellow hue.
- Pink mucous membranes plus icterus causes a more orange color.
- Massive generalized lymphadenopathy usually means lymphoma.
- If it looks, smells, and tastes (?) like pus, then it must be pus.
- Chest plus abdominal fluid accumulation commonly depicts a bad disease. Common causes: neoplasia, heart failure, diffuse inflammation, hypoproteinemia.
- Septic shock: hypotension, hypothermia, thrombocytopenia.
- Skin turgor difficult to assess with cachexia and obesity.

- Sudden facial hemorrhagic lymphedema swelling, hemorrhagic oral mucosa, subdued mentation – think eastern diamondback rattlesnake envenomation (in Florida).
- Various causes of hyperventilation: cardiorespiratory, pyrexia, brain disease, Cushing's, metabolic acidosis, anxiety, pain, shock, anemia.
- Fever plus immune-mediated disease – appetite can persist.
- Fever plus sepsis – anorexia.
- Nasal crustiness, scleral injection, muddy mucous membranes – think uremia.
- On palpation: "Touch but don't squeeze the Charmin".
- Take the patient out of the cage and look at it!
- If something just "ain't" right – think neuro.
- Look under the tongue in any vomiting cat (and dog).
- Watch those hindlimbs for the earliest sign of weakness.
- The Big 6: PCV and TP, BUN, glucose, urinalysis, chest/abdominal radiographs.
- After therapeutic paracentesis, go back and repeat abdominal palpation so you don't pass the mass.
- Have you been palpating each mammary gland?
- A lump is a lump until you stick it.
- It's all in the history.
- Don't just look at it (a lump) – stick it!
- Heat stroke >109.4°F (43.0°C) – look out for DIC.
- If the patient is eating and drinking without excess fluid losses, then it doesn't need intravenous fluids.
- Every sick and trauma patient should have chest and abdominal radiographs on initial work up.
- 'The toaster effect'. The patient will be standing with returned appetite when it is well.

Urogenital

- Rule out pyometra in any sick intact female.
- "Never let the sun set on a pyo." (Garvey, M).
- Murky urine can be caused by pus, chyle, or crystals.
- Bilateral renomegaly means very serious disease: lymphoma, hydronephrosis, pyonephrosis, granuloma, inflammation, subcapsular edema, polycystic.
- In cats with chronic kidney disease: one big kidney plus one small kidney can mean one fibrotic and one compensatory hypertrophic with fibrosis.
- Hematuria without stranguria – consider coagulopathy or renal bleed; however, recent renal bleed plus clots in the urinary outflow can cause stranguria.
- Male dog plus stranguria – must radiograph to rule out obstructive uropathy.
- Cessation of polyuria in sick patient – consider oliguria/anuria – a bad sign.
- Oliguric renal failure – hyperkalemia common.
- High output chronic kidney disease – normo- or hypokalemia common.
- Emphysematous cystitis – rule out diabetes mellitus.
- PD plus PU plus isosthenuria – consider chronic kidney disease, even with normal BUN and creatinine, but watch out for Cushing's.
- Be careful when performing 'cystocentesis' with a pyometra – look before your stick!

- Prostate trends: carcinoma – asymmetrical, hard, mid or caudal pelvis; BPH – symmetrical, firm, anterior displacement.
- Empty urine line: anuria, recent emptying, obstruction.
- Always assess urine SG before starting fluid therapy.
- BPH: passive penile bleed, normal urination, normal dog.
- Detecting urethral pathology in female dog – do a rectal examination.
- Prostate inflammation → 'prostatic shuffle' during ambulation.
- For oliguria, try dopamine at 3–5 µg/kg/minute.

Fluids and electrolytes

- SC fluid administration – isotonic, 18 gauge needle, gravity flow.
- Metabolic alkalosis plus hypokalemia common with upper GI obstructions.
- 0.9% NaCl plus KCl – best for upper GI obstructions.
- TCO_2 >40 mEq/L is always metabolic alkalosis (usually with hypokalemia).
- TCO_2 <10 mEq/L – usually means severe metabolic acidosis.
- Potassium penicillin contains 1.7 mEq K+/million units – take heed when bolusing.
- Treatment of hypocalcemia when intravenous not an option: add 2.5 ml/kg 10% calcium gluconate to 150 ml 0.9% NaCl – give subcutaneously q12h (for adult sized cat). Discontinue if inflammation occurs.
- When giving subcutaneous fluids avoid hypokalemia – add 3.5 mEq KCl/150 ml lactated Ringer's solution – give subcutaneously (for adult sized cat).
- All intravenous maintenance fluids should contain 7–10 mEq/KCl/250 ml; exceptions: oliguria and untreated addisonian.
- To make up 2.5% dextrose solution increments, add 12.5 ml D-50-W to 250 ml of isotonic crystalloid fluid or add 50 ml of D-50-W to a liter of isotonic crystalloid (lactated Ringer's solution, NaCl).
- Rehydrate before inducing diuresis; check urine SG first.
- Volume load with isotonic crystalloid.
- Avoid detrimental tissue edema by restricting excess fluids with severe pulmonary, brain, and general trauma.
- Intraosseous cannulas can be life saving.
- Dextrose given intravenously at doses >0.5 g/kg/hour might cause glycosuria.

Gastrointestinal

- GI obstructions – main sign is vomiting.
- Acute excruciating abdominal pain (like never before seen!) – consider bowel infarction and intestinal volvulus.
- Causes of coffee ground vomitus: gastric ulcers (primary/secondary), uremic gastritis.
- Melena causes: upper GI lesion, thrombocytopenia.
- Occult blood loss – think GI.
- Melena detection – "Let your finger do the walking".
- Black stools: upper GI bleed, thrombocytopenia, swallowing blood, 'Pepto-bismol' (bismuth subsalicylate), iron, charcoal.
- Elevated BUN plus normal creatinine – consider upper GI bleed, especially if kidney can concentrate urine.

- Bile in vomitus signifies pyloric patency.
- The lower the obstruction, the more feculent the vomitus.
- Sudden mental depression 2–3 days post enterotomy – rule out dehiscence and sepsis.
- Never let the sun set on a linear foreign body intestinal obstruction.
- Diffuse inflammatory bowel disease can often be diagnosed with distal colon biopsy.
- Sepsis can cause cholangiostasis.
- Gas in the gallbladder is bad and is a surgical disease.
- Bilirubinuria in cats signifies liver disease.
- J-tube feeding for managing the prolonged period of *nil per os* in pancreatitis can be beneficial.
- Look for pancreatic pathology when the right kidney is easily visible on a radiograph.
- For benign ptyalism administer diphenoxylate/atropine (Lomotil) 0.25 mg/kg q12h. Add minocycline q12h to treat accompanying perioral dermatitis.

Cardiorespiratory

- Many die without ever showing open-mouth breathing.
- Watch for the exaggerated abdominal component.
- Cardiomegaly does not always cause tall ECG complexes.
- A standing lead II ECG is satisfactory for rate, rhythm, and interval measurements.
- Do not use beta-blockers until pulmonary edema resolves.
- Muffled chest sounds: fluid, mass, air, obesity, deep chested, 'plugged ears'.
- Diffuse muffling – usually chest fluid.
- Dorsal muffling – air or mass in chest.
- Coughing cats: allergic bronchitis, flukes, lungworms, heartworms, hair or foreign body in trachea, tumor.
- Sudden-onset diffuse pulmonary infiltrates – think acute respiratory disease syndrome.
- Cats with heart disease rarely cough.
- Bacterial pneumonia plus leukopenia (bone marrow associated) – causes minimal radiographic infiltrates.
- Heartworm treated dog at discharge: dispense prednisone and furosemide for the earliest signs of pulmonary thromboembolism.
- Echocardiogram for diagnosing vegetative endocarditis.
- Ketamine (3–5 mg [total] intravenously) for a dyspneic cat can allow 'survival' radiographs.
- Remember – good side UP when radiographing dyspneic patient.
- Digoxin intoxication can cause any cardiac arrhythmia.
- Aspiration pneumonia can be worse when H2 blockers are used due to altered GI microflora.
- Only pulmonary edema can clear from the lungs after 36–48 hours.
- Dyspneic patients find it difficult to sleep because they know they are dying.

Neoplasia

- Cutaneous mast cell tumors can mimic any type of skin growth.
- Assume any firm mammary nodule as carcinoma until proven otherwise.
- Mammary tumors – don't stick it, cut it.

- Don't miss lymphangitic inflammatory mammary carcinoma.
- Nasal disease can do anything.
- Copious mucoid nasal discharge, think nasal adenocarcinoma.
- Try gastric biopsy forceps for nasal biopsy.
- Closed mouth nasal cavity radiographs are useless.
- Cancer can cause an elevated temperature and WBC count.

Drugs

- Observe for drug interactions.
- Do not use theophylline with ciprofloxacin – causes theophylline overdose.
- Best avoid intravenous route for thiamine (better intramuscularly) and vitamin K_1 (better subcutaneously).
- Rehydrate prior to using aminoglycosides.
- Prednisone for craniomandibular osteopathy.
- Cimetidine enhances metronidazole-induced neurotoxicity.
- Aspiration pneumonia worse when H2 blockers in use.
- Oral tetracycline can cause fever in cats.
- Follow all oral doxycycline and clindamycin tablets/capsules with water to swallow.
- Chloramphenicol is still a darn good antimicrobial.

Hematology

- Unclotted blood in clot tube – consider coagulopathy.
- Massive splenomegaly – splenic torsion, lymphoma, myeloproliferative or mast cell splenic neoplastic infiltrate.
- Thrombocytopenia plus anemia – causes pale petechiae!
- Fleas plus thrombocytopenia – cause 'lots of' lumbosacral petechiae.
- Low WBCs, low RBCs, low platelets – rule out bone marrow suppression.
- Fulminant hemolysis: anemia, hemoglobinemia, hemoglobinuria, weakness, depression, +/- vomiting; then icterus.
- Bone marrow derived leukopenic animals don't make pus!
- Keep IMHA and ITP patients on long-term every other day maintenance prednisone for 9–12 months to avoid relapse.
- Try danazol (Danocrine) with prednisone for refractory IMHA and ITP.
- Observe for autoagglutination and spherocytes in IMHA.
- Newly acquired bleeding – think anticoagulant rodenticide intoxication.
- A normal bleeding time ensures adequate platelet hemostasis, a normal platelet count does not.
- Owners can use urine dipsticks to detect hemeprotein for early signs of recurrent hemolysis.

Endocrine

- Hypercholesterolemia plus elevated creatine kinase – rule out hypothyroidism; hypocholesterolemia – rule out Addison's disease.
- U-100 syringe (or 1.0 ml tuberculin syringe) should be used for U-100 insulin.

- Do not forget K+ when treating diabetic ketoacidosis.
- Oliguric diabetics have marked hyperglycemia.
- IV fluids alone can lower blood glucose by as much as 50–60% during correction of dehydration.
- Glycosuria can occur with diabetes, proximal renal tubular disease, stress, IV dextrose.
- Marked hyperglycemia with minimal glycosuria – consider oliguria/anuria.
- Morning marked glycosuria and afternoon diminished glycosuria – typifies transient insulin response (need split dose).
- Can use soiled urine to detect glycosuria.
- Hyperglycemia can sometimes be detected in tears using urine glucose test reagent pads.
- Blood glucose meters not very accurate at the high and low ends of the scale.
- Assess the eclampsia dog for hypoglycemia.
- Try mannitol for severe hypoglycemic encephalopathy.
- When fludrocortisone acetate (Florinef) does not work well, use desoxycorticosterone pivalate (DOCP) and prednisone.
- The hypocalcemic cat has not read the book of clinical signs.
- Keep an eye out for the atypical addisonian.
- If you have a diabetic dog with Cushing's disease that is receiving both insulin and mitotane (o'p'-DDD; Lysodren), and the dog becomes weak and depressed, remember this:
  - If the dog is mitotane toxic, **its appetite will have been absent that day** and vomiting may or may not have occurred.
  - If dog is insulin overdosed, it **very likely will have eaten that morning**. Coma and seizures can be present.
  - If dog has both hypoglycemia and mitotane toxicity, any combination of all of the above can occur, and this is where '**treat for the treatable**' comes in if laboratory tests are unavailable and where treatment would call for both dextrose and glucocorticoid.

Neurology

- Rapid onset lower motor neuron paralysis – think ticks, organophosphate, botulism, polyradiculoneuropathy, metronidazole, coral snake.
- Cats with dilated pupils and blank stare – think thiamine.
- Coma: diffuse cerebral, brainstem, but don't forget metabolic.

Intoxication

- Ethylene glycol sometimes fluoresces under Wood's lamp.
- Dimercaptosuccinic acid (DMSA, succimer) – an oral treatment for lead poisoning.
- Unexplainable radiodense particles in the bowel – think lead.
- 4-methylpyrazole for antifreeze intoxication; avoids hangovers (dogs require lower dosages than cats; veterinary product currently unavailable).
- Newer anticoagulant rodenticides – treat with oral K_1 for 4–6 weeks.
- Newly acquired bleeding – think anticoagulant rodenticide intoxication.

Patient management

- Old dogs are poorly tolerant to tranquilization.
- Avoid sedating acutely ill patients unless absolutely necessary.
- Don't sedate at the end of day and leave the animal overnight without IV fluid support, especially old patients.
- Increased spontaneity might pre-empt death.
- Heparinized syringe might contain as much as 200 units heparin – too much for puppies and kittens.
- Traumatic ear flush can cause inner ear and vestibular disease.
- Cats hate atropine drops – causes marked salivation; use ointment instead.
- Some pathologic bladders can leak after cystocentesis.
- Do not forget thiamine in cats.
- Glycerine suppositories for patients with pelvic fractures or constipation will be most appreciated!
- Ketamine (3 mg total dose intravenously) can adequately restrain the sick cat with urethral obstruction.
- Take care with subcutaneous fluids – dogs are not cats and they like to slough!
- Manual expression of a male dog's bladder is hazardous to its health – it can rupture.
- Subcutaneous fluid administration – stay behind the scapula and in front of the wing of the ilium. Use 18 gauge needle and 50 ml/site (adult cat).
- Don't forget glucose for the babies.
- Imipenem for life-threatening infections.
- A clean cat is a happy cat.
- No Fleet enemas for obstipation, unless you want to treat a good case of hypocalcemia.
- When is the last time you hugged your patients?
- A dynamic duo: good science and experience.
- Heat lamp and rubbing alcohol = one **hot** dog.
- Nothing is routine.
- If client can not afford a "Cadillac", there is nothing wrong with a "Chevy".
- Body bandage in cats cause pseudoparalysis.
- Rapid abdominocentesis is effective and safe for chronic ascites, except when it is caused by chronic liver disease, when simultaneous IV plasma or albumin infusion is recommended.
- Best avoid intravenous B_1 and K_1 – give subcutaneously or intramuscularly.
- Never kill'em based on cytology results.

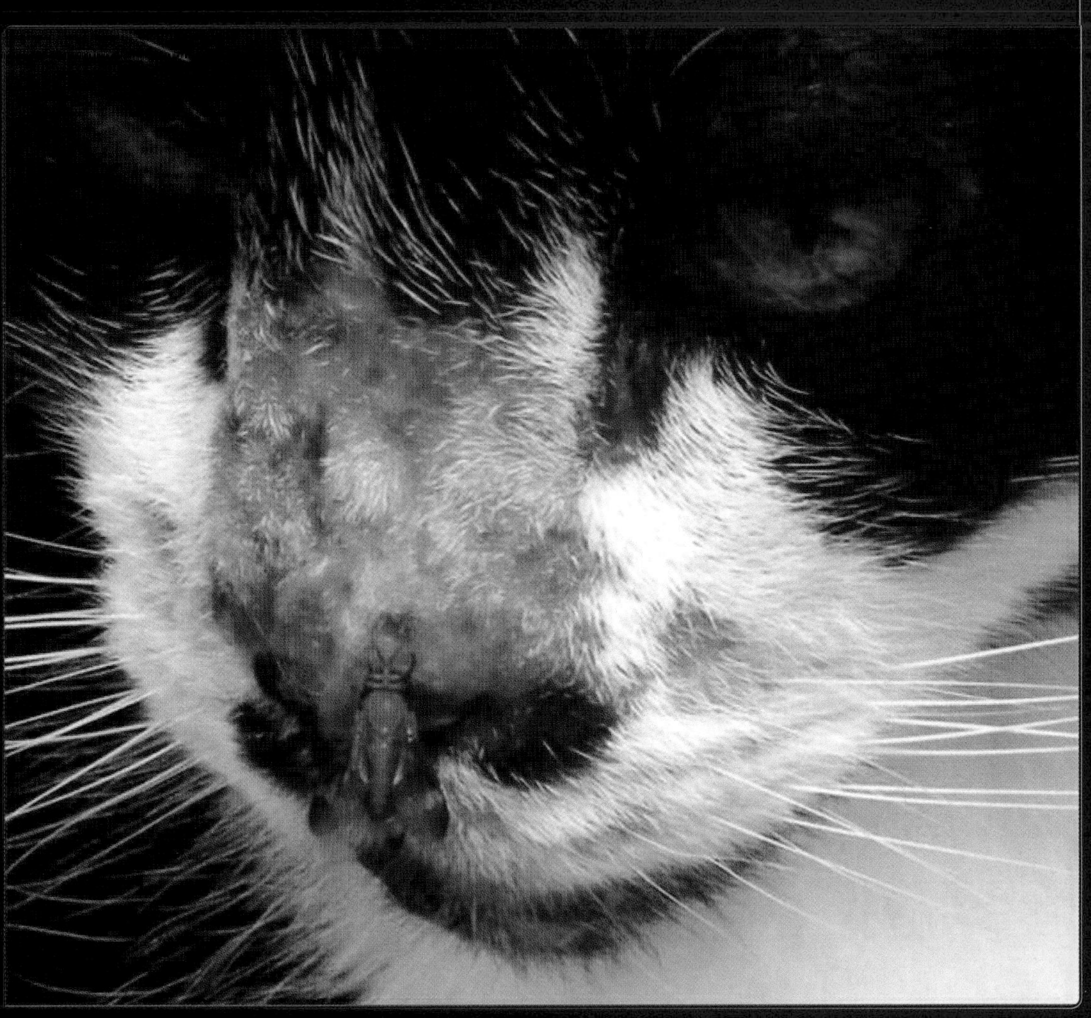

▲ This cat has hypersensitivity of its nasal planum caused by insect bites.

1

Dermatologic disorders

DERMATOLOGY is derived from the Greek term *derma*, meaning skin, and *logos*, meaning study or speech, word, or reason. It is an essential discipline for the practitioner because of the high incidence of skin disease that one can encounter daily in practice. These disorders can occur as primary lesions or syndromes or they can be a reflection of some other internal disease process in the body. Adherence to the essentials of obtaining a full history and doing a complete physical examination will be most helpful in determining the cause of the dermatologic disorder. Perhaps the most common group of skin diseases involve hypersensitivity states, but other important conditions might be associated with autoimmune disorders, infectious diseases, neoplasia, nutritional disorders, and various metabolic and endocrine conditions. The diagnostic methodology of skin diseases, after taking a full history and conducting a physical examination, includes general tests such as a complete blood count, serum biochemistry profile, immune or infectious disease serology, skin hypersensitivity testing, and biopsy. The advantages of these tests are that they are readily available to the practitioner and noninvasive for the patient. In many instances the classic appearance of certain lesions will allow for a minimal diagnostic evaluation, thus saving the owner a substantial amount of expense.

1 Dermatologic disorders

- A lump is a lump until you stick it.
- Don't look at it, stick it.
- Skin turgor is difficult to assess with obesity and cachexia.
- Excessive SC fluids cause skin slough.

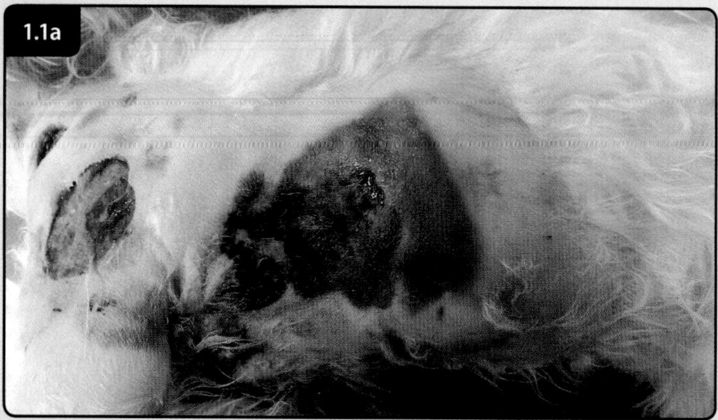

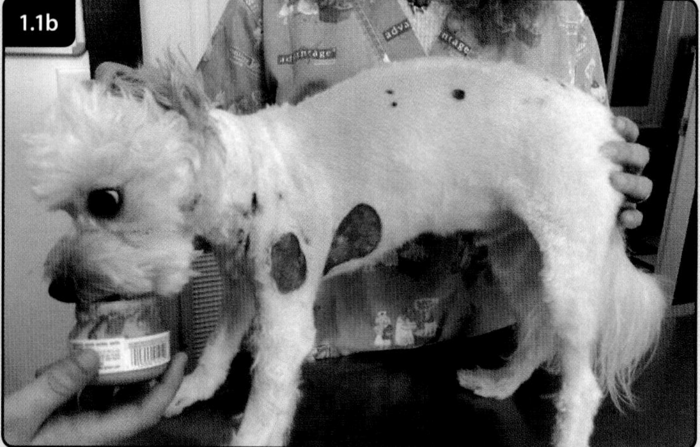

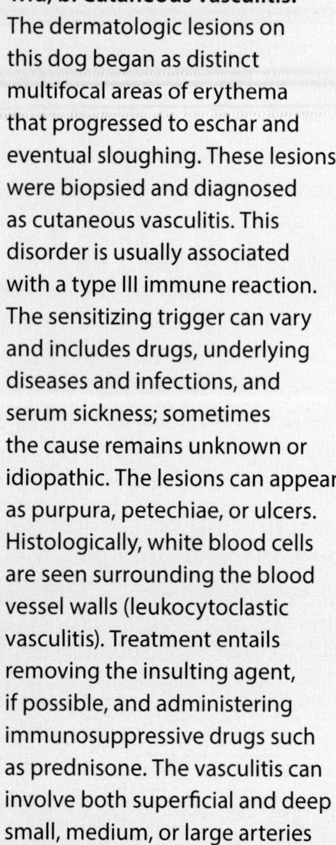

1.1a, b. Cutaneous vasculitis. The dermatologic lesions on this dog began as distinct multifocal areas of erythema that progressed to eschar and eventual sloughing. These lesions were biopsied and diagnosed as cutaneous vasculitis. This disorder is usually associated with a type III immune reaction. The sensitizing trigger can vary and includes drugs, underlying diseases and infections, and serum sickness; sometimes the cause remains unknown or idiopathic. The lesions can appear as purpura, petechiae, or ulcers. Histologically, white blood cells are seen surrounding the blood vessel walls (leukocytoclastic vasculitis). Treatment entails removing the insulting agent, if possible, and administering immunosuppressive drugs such as prednisone. The vasculitis can involve both superficial and deep small, medium, or large arteries and arterioles.

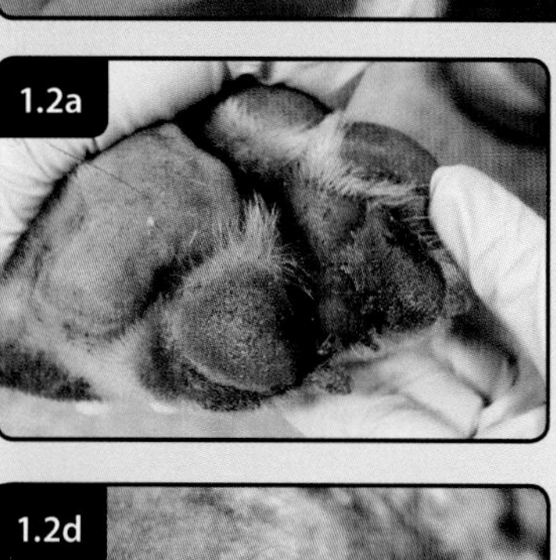

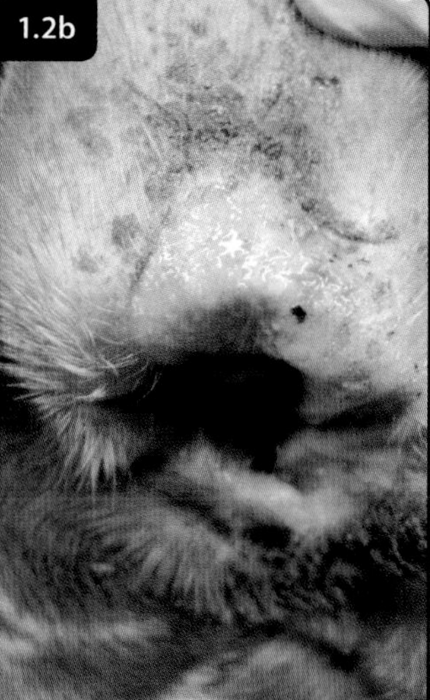

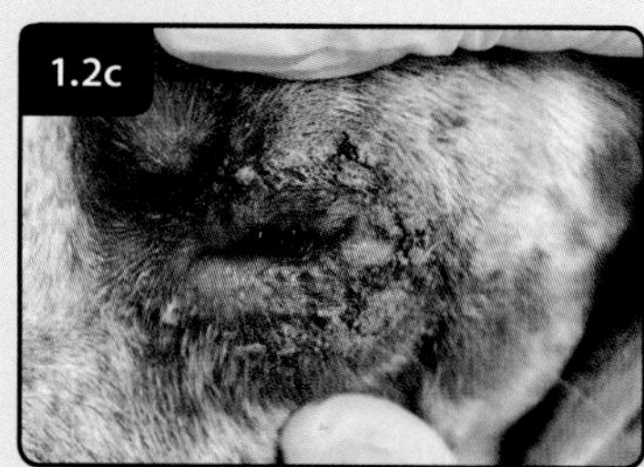

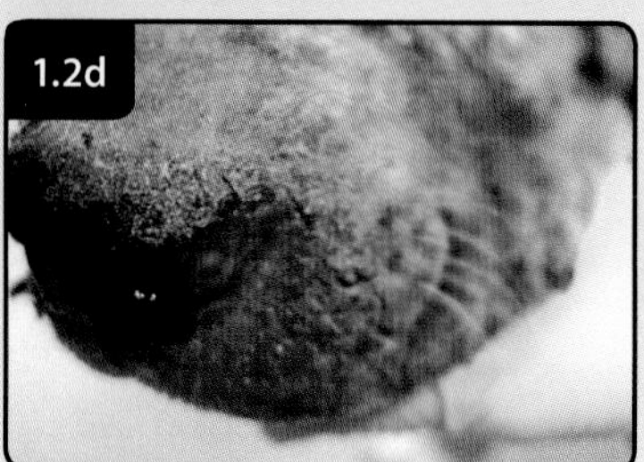

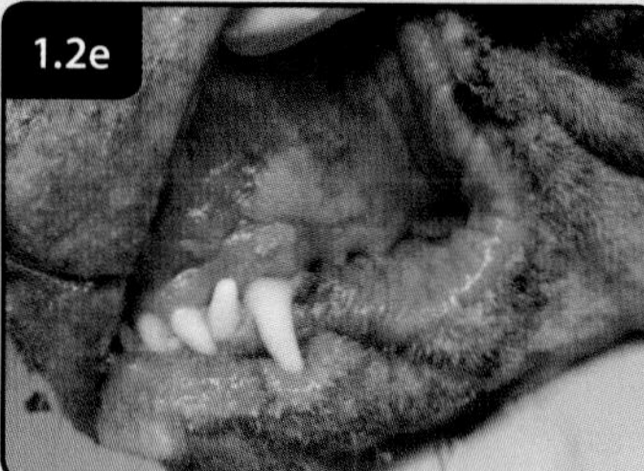

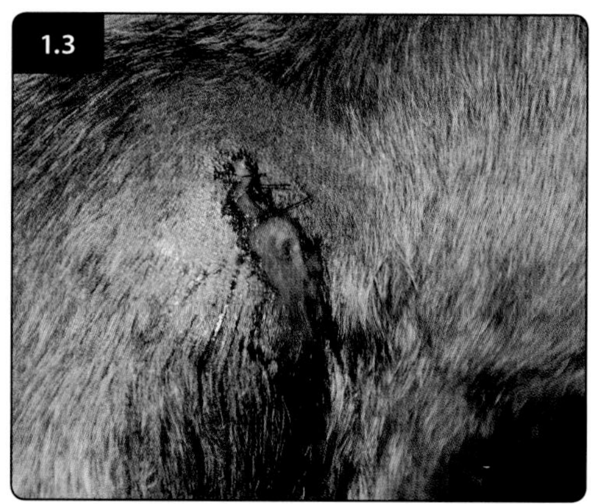

1.3. Atypical mycobacterial infection. Shown is a chronic draining skin wound that had not responded to wound care and antibiotics. This scenario should prompt consideration of atypical mycobacterial infection, which requires special growth media for optimal culture conditions. Diagnosis requires obtaining deep tissue sampling. Once diagnosed these infections require months of continuous treatment and re-evaluation for the possibility of having to alter the antimicrobial treatment because of resistant bacterial strains. Recurrent infection is possible, especially if immunosuppression is present.

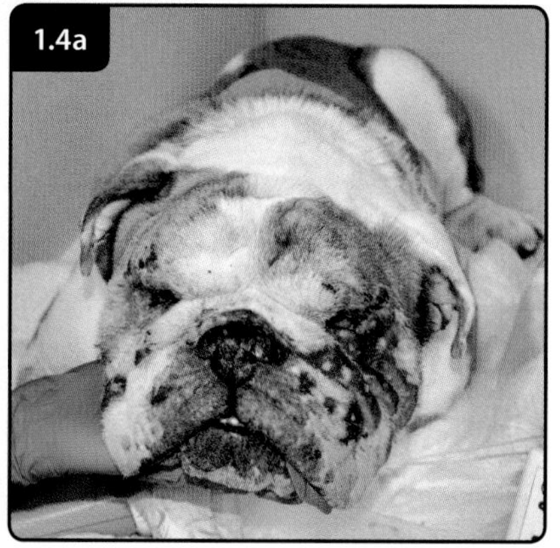

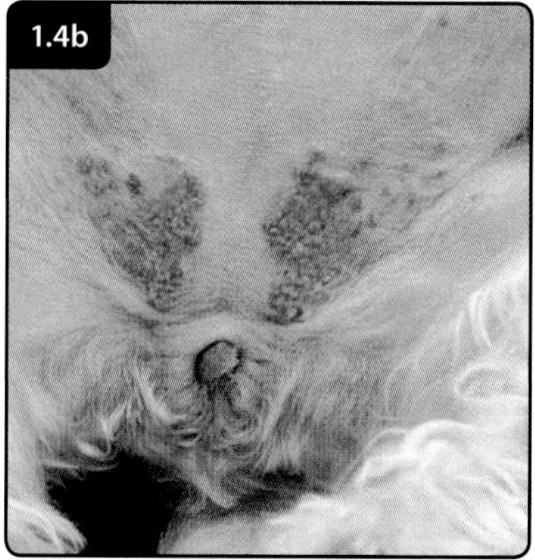

1.4a, b. Calcinosis cutis. This dermatologic condition is commonly associated with Cushing's disease and, more rarely, with other medical disorders. Various forms occur, which can appear as moist inflamed skin lesions or as a dry form that is not inflamed. A yellow colored mineralized deposit in the superficial forms is typical. There is no specific treatment other than treatment of the underlying condition. Most cases will resolve once the hypercortisolism is resolved.

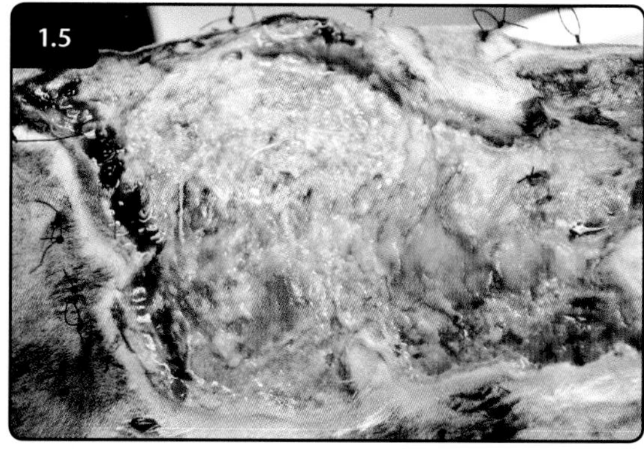

1.5. Heat pad-induced skin burns. Thermal skin injuries can be very extensive, as illustrated in this dog's lesion. It is usually acquired when prostrate animals are covered with heat emitting devices such as heat pads and hot water bags. The earliest signs are erythema, soon followed by a hardening texture to the skin often accompanied by eschar formation, which eventually fissures and causes the draining of tissue fluid. Treatment entails good client communication, meticulous wound care, antibiotics following culture and sensitivity testing of the wound, and successive surgical wound closure procedures over several months. Predisposing in-hospital practices should be corrected.

◀ **1.2a–e. Drug-induced vasculitis.** This dog developed diffuse superficial ulcerations involving its ears, oral mucosa, periocular skin, nose, and digits. Note the mucocutaneous localization, which would be typical of immune system involvement. The cause was the drug prazosin, which had to be discontinued and replaced by another drug with similar action.

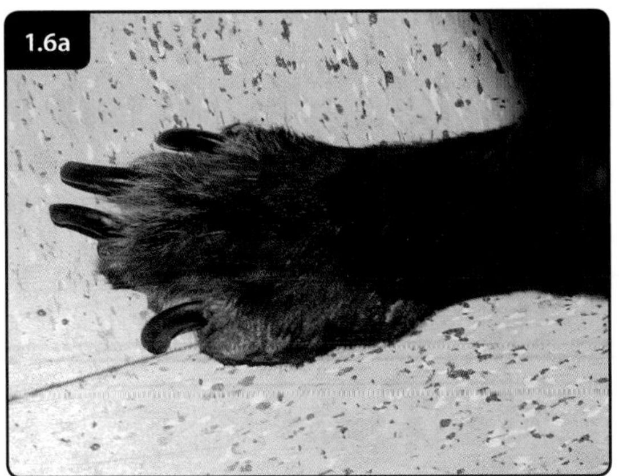

1.6a–c. Hepatic cutaneous syndrome. This complicated skin abnormality is also called superficial necrolytic dermatitis and is thought to result from amino acid and other nutrient deficiencies due to underlying liver disease or glucagonoma (pancreatic alpha cell carcinoma). The proliferation of the palmar and volar skin is very characteristic. Skin lesions also appeared on this dog's prepuce. The underlying cause in this particular dog was metastatic glucagonoma. The hyperglucagonemia also caused insulin resistance and diabetes mellitus. Treatment of the skin condition involved intravenous amino acid administration, while surgical therapeutic measures were undertaken to treat the underlying disease.

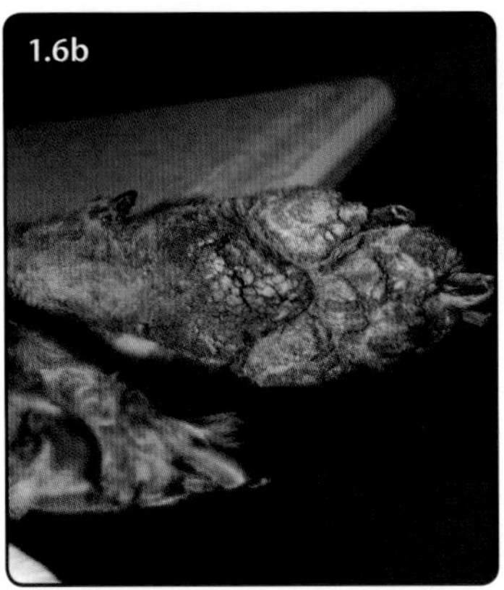

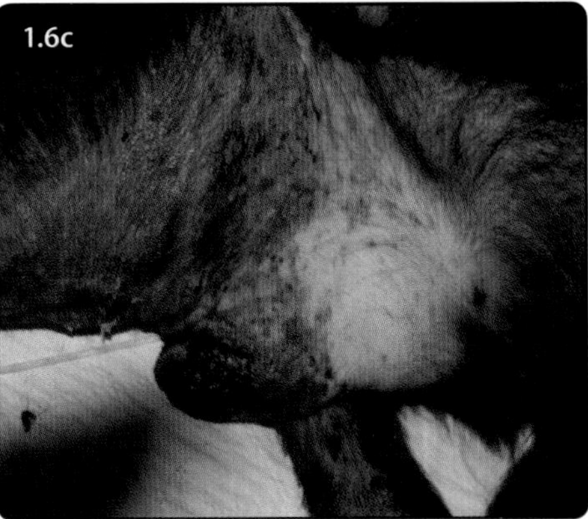

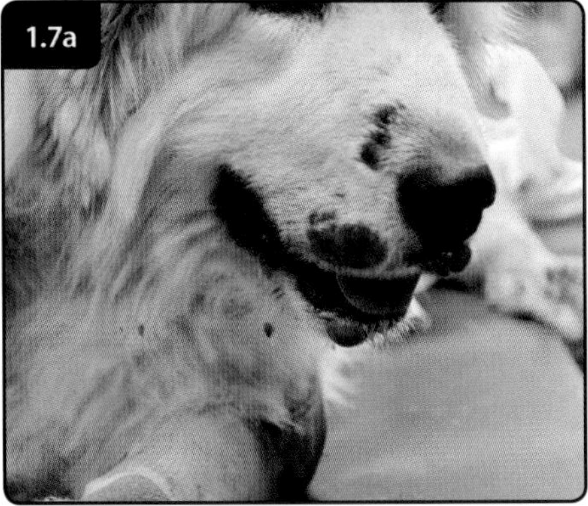

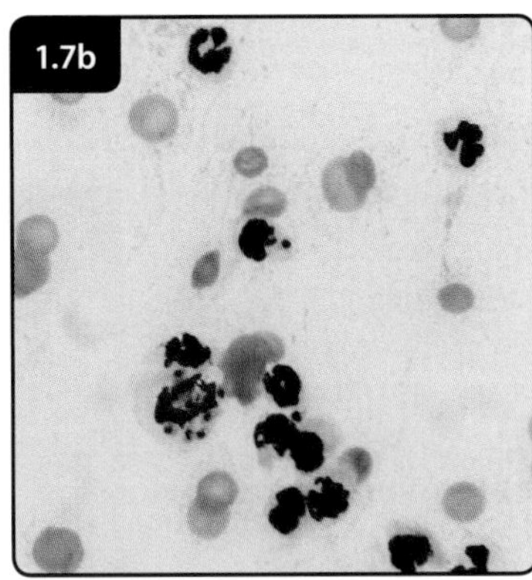

1.7a, b. Cutaneous leishmaniasis. This dog has cutaneous leishmaniasis. This was an unexpected diagnosis in a dog that lives exclusively in Florida where the disease is not indigenous. This protozoal disease can involve the skin and also occur as a systemic disease, the latter being more indigenous to the Mediterranean region of the world. The cutaneous and visceral forms are commonly found in Brazil. The *Phlebotomus* fly is the vector and the dog serves as a reservoir host. The amastigotes can be found in circulating mononuclear phagocytic cells, as shown in Figure 1.7b. Diagnosis is made by identifying the amastigotes in macrophages on bone marrow aspiration cytology examination. Skin biopsy allows for identification of the promastigotes. Treatment often involves organic antimonial drugs and the prognosis is guarded.

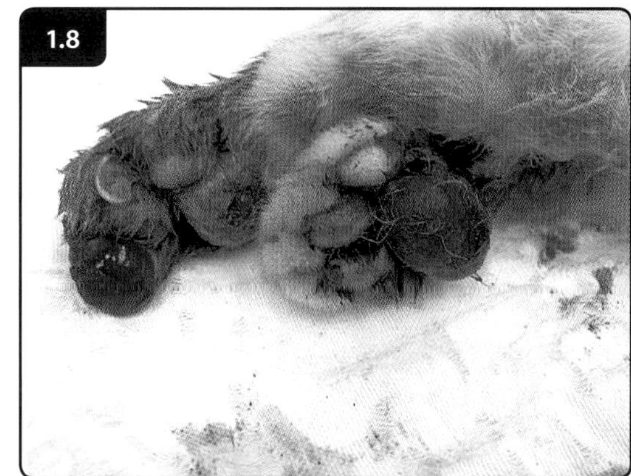

1.8. Feline lymphocytic–plasmacytic pododermatitis. This condition affects cats and has no known proven etiology. It can cause marked debilitation, especially when it advances to the extent shown in this cat. Treatment is palliative and rarely surgical.

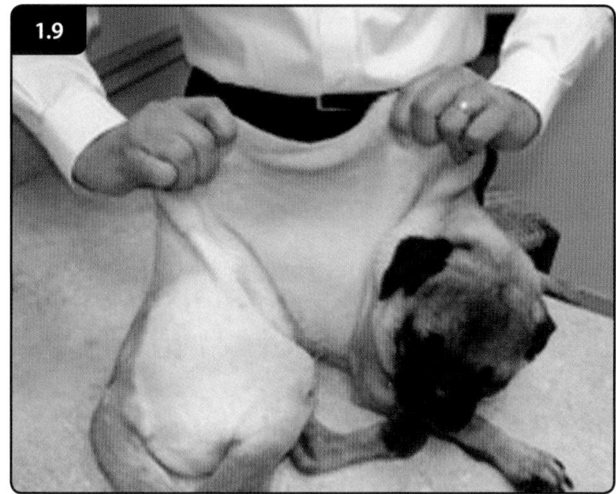

1.9. Cutaneous hyperelastic syndrome. The skin in affected dogs and cats is characteristically hyperelastic and it is quite friable. This is a congenital connective tissue disorder and bears some resemblance to Ehlers–Danlos syndrome in humans. Because of the high occurrence of skin lacerations in these patients, prophylactic control strategies must be implemented. Paw or claw coverings or the declaw procedure (in dire situations) will help prevent self-mutilation associated with simple skin scratching.

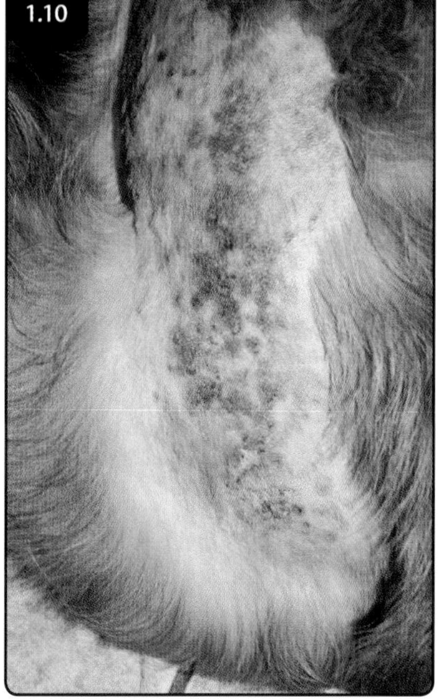

1.10. Acute skin hypersensitivity. The skin reaction shown on this Golden Retriever occurred over hours and was accompanied by pruritus. This type of acute papular dermatitis along the lumbar area was very likely a hypersensitivity reaction that could have been caused by a mosquito swarm, which was common during that particular summer. Treatment consists of clipping the skin, gentle cleansing, and short-term (7 days) glucocorticoid and antihistamine drugs. Removing the fur is very conducive to healing.

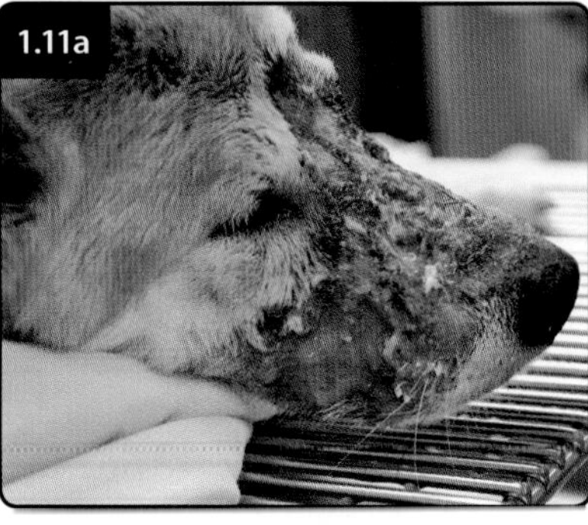

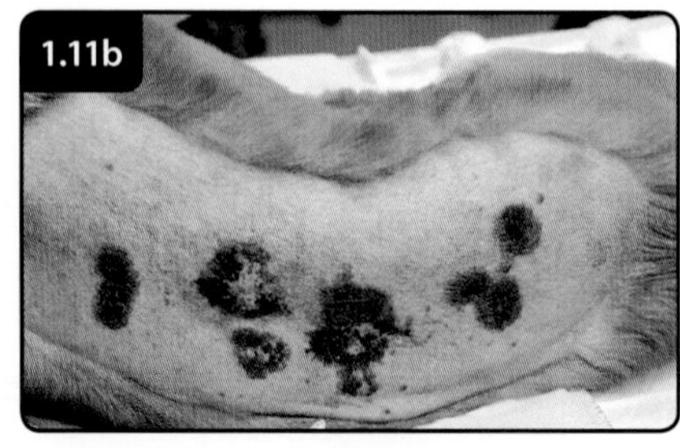

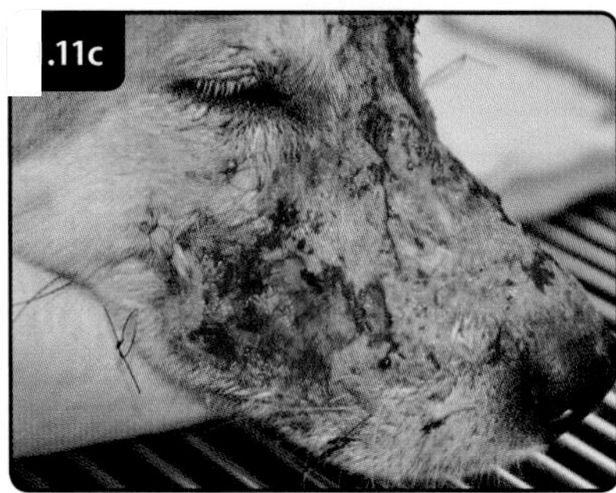

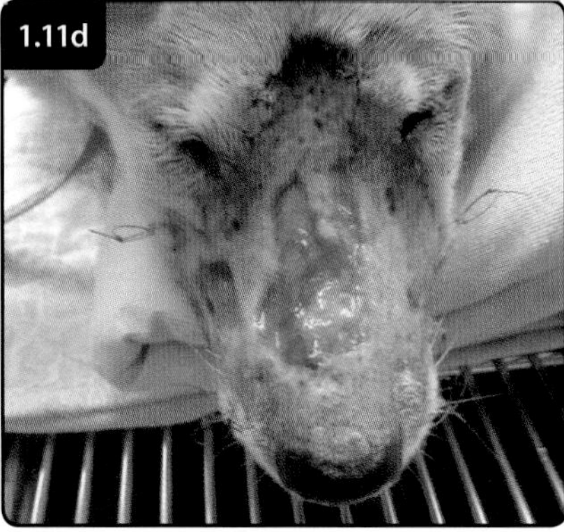

1.11a–d. Necrotizing skin disease. This dog initially presented with erythema and eventually sloughed its facial skin. Biopsies showed it as a necrotizing skin lesion with many bacterial cocci that were cultured as *Streptococcus*. The rapidly progressive nature of this disease was clinically comparable to the necrotizing fasciitis skin disease that occurs in humans. Figures 1.11a, b show the acute stage and Figures 1.11c, d show the healing period 3 weeks into treatment, which consisted of antibiotics and wound care. Figure 1.11b shows a vasculitis type of lesion that suggested an immune-mediated component in the disease process. Glucocorticoid drugs were added after the first month after the healing process ceased. The condition improved immediately and then healed completely.

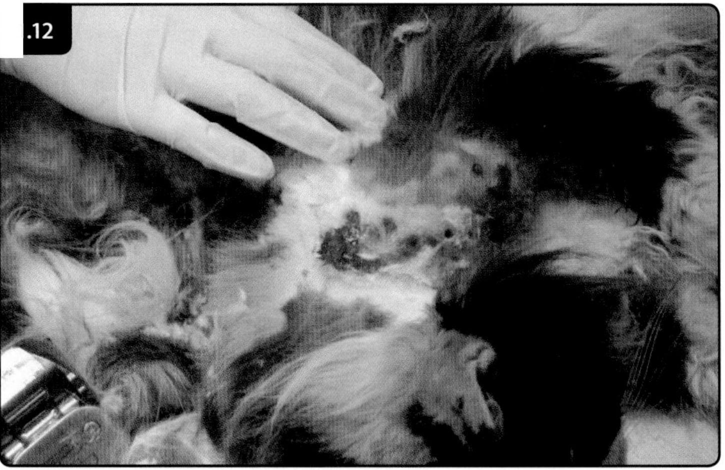

1.12. *Nocardia* skin infection. The skin lesions in this cat were characterized as multiple fistulae that drained a suppurative exudate. Biopsies and bacterial culture were necessary to identify the *Nocardia* bacteria. *Nocardia* is an aerobic filamentous organism that is acid-fast positive. Surgery might facilitate cure while antibiotic (sulfa drugs) treatment must be extended for many months and sometimes for as long as a year.

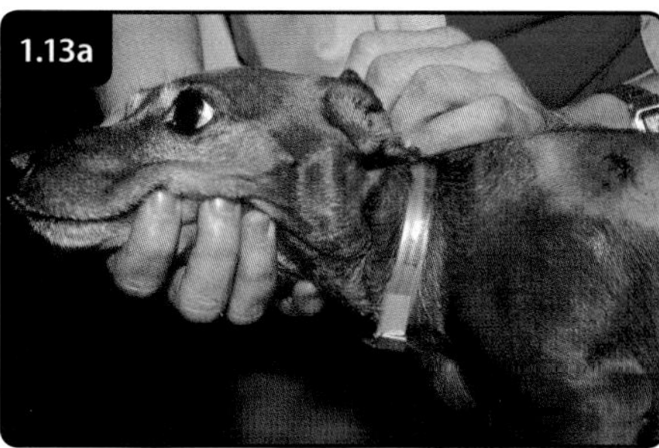

1.13a

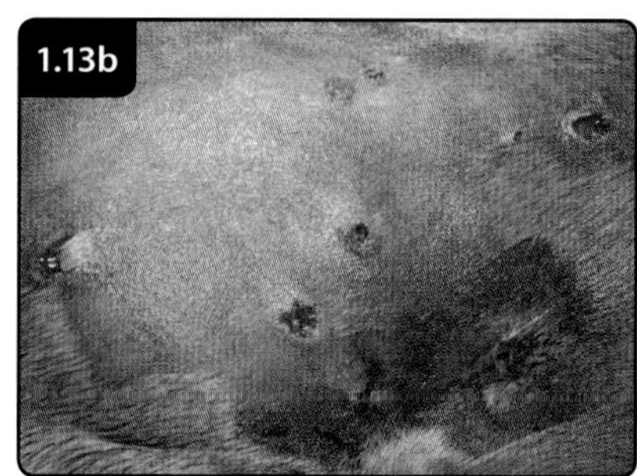

1.13b

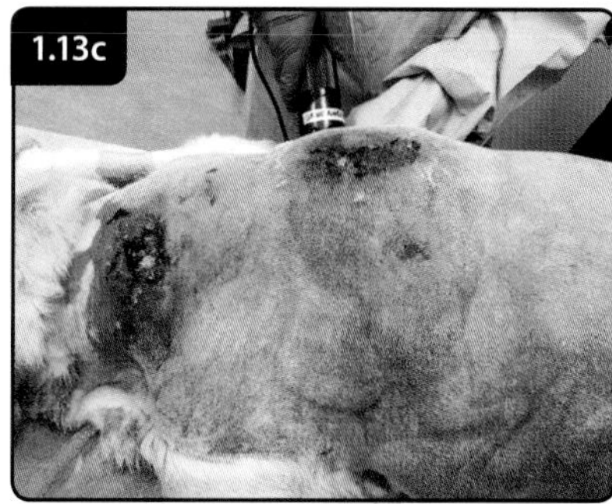

1.13c

1.13a–c. Nodular panniculitis. These three dogs represent nodular panniculitis, which is characterized by fever, lethargy, decreased appetite, and skin lesions consisting of nodules that eventually ulcerate and drain. The fluid can be oily, representing the underlying subcutaneous fat inflammation. This can be demonstrated with a touch impression smear of the draining nodule. Neutrophils are also present. The cause is idiopathic but there might be some immune-mediated component. This condition has been found to be responsive to long-term glucocorticoid treatment.

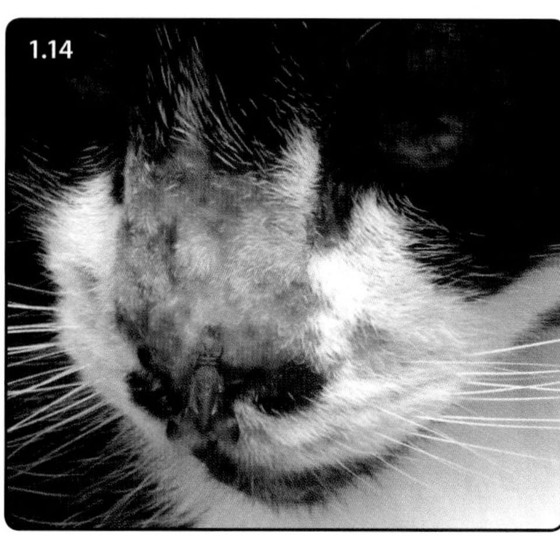

1.14

1.14. Hypersensitivity. This cat has a typical hypersensitivity response to mosquito bites. Although such a reaction involves mosquito bites, this particular cat was sensitive to the biting fly, as shown in the image. The lesions typically involve the nose and consist of an acute dermatitis. Treatment consists of using insect repellents, reducing environmental exposure by keeping the cat inside during the darker hours, and administering glucocorticoid drugs for the inflamed nasal tissue.

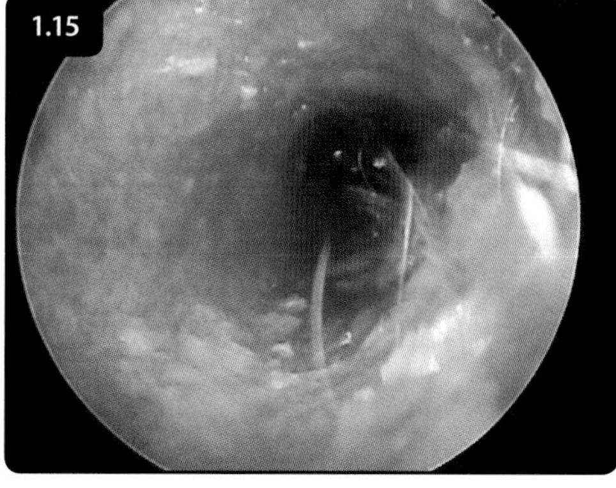

1.15

1.15. Bacterial otitis externa. Otitis can have many causes including hypersensitivity, primary infection, or infection secondary to impaired ear canal drainage. This otoscopic image in a Golden Retriever dog shows marked acute inflammation caused by *Pseudomonas aeruginosa* infection, which likely occurred secondary to the dog's swimming and maintaining a moist environment in the deep ear canal that was conducive to bacterial proliferation. Treatment consisted of 6 weeks of fluoroquinolone antimicrobial administration, and topical application of combined antibacterial/anti-inflammatory ear ointments, and Tris-EDTA application into the ear canal. Surgery would be indicated in cases that have an obstructed vertical ear canal.

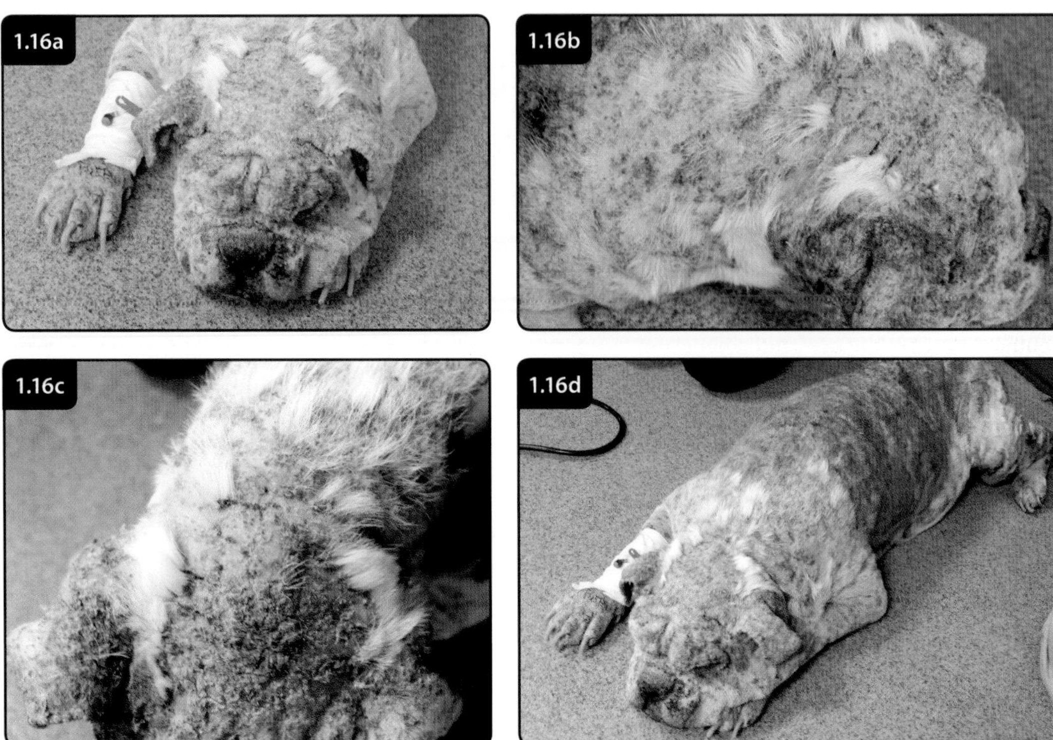

1.16a–d. Pemphigus foliaceus. Pemphigus foliaceus is one of the autoimmune skin diseases found in the dog and cat. It is a pustular and crusting dermatitis involving the face and trunk (as shown). The foot pads and nail beds can also be involved. Neutrophils, eosinophils, acanthocytes, and keratinocytes can be seen on cytology. Biopsy is confirmatory. Treatment requires immunosuppressive doses of glucocorticoids, which often have to be administered long term. Other immunosuppressive drugs such as cyclosporine, tacrolimus, and azathioprine can also be used to hopefully reduce the amount of glucocorticoids required, thus avoiding their many side-effects.

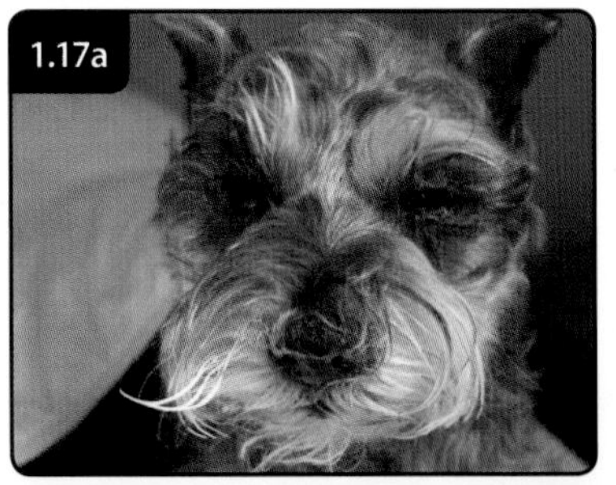

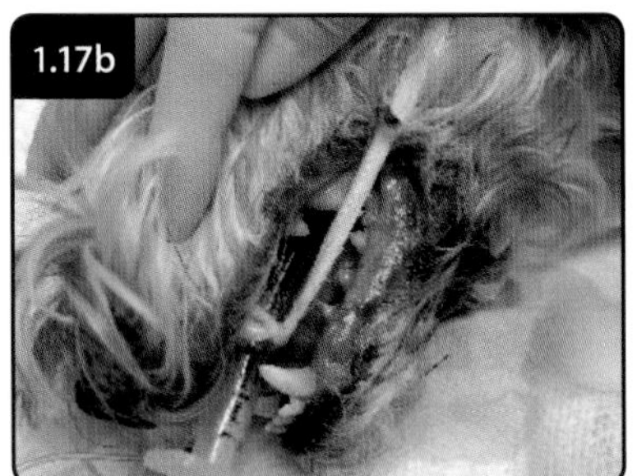

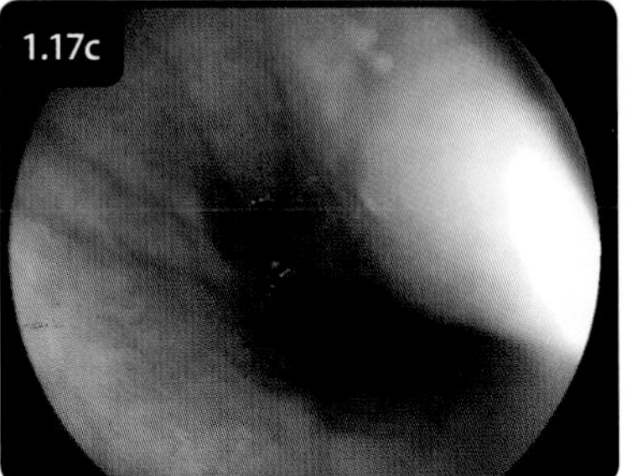

1.17a–c. Pemphigus vulgaris. This Schnauzer shows the typical mucocutaneous ulcerations associated with this autoimmune skin disease. The dog additionally showed signs of regurgitation and esophageal reflux, which prompted an esophagoscopy procedure that identified esophageal ulcers. Diagnosis is suspected on clinical features and cytology (acanthocytes) and biopsy. Treatment entails long-term high-dose glucocorticoid drugs that often cause unpleasant side-effects. This patient also required H2 histamine blocking drugs and sucralfate for its esophagitis. The prognosis is guarded because of the potential for long-term debilitation.

1.18. Impetigo. As illustrated in this figure, impetigo is a superficial pyoderma that commonly occurs on the ventral abdominal skin of young dogs. *Staphylococcus pseudintermedius* is a common pathogen. Superficial single or several pustules typify this condition. In most cases impetigo occurs as the sole condition, but in others it might be accompanied by other conditions such as skin parasites or fungal infections. In the Southern states of the USA, and other warm areas of the world, fire ant bites can precede infection. Isolated and limited infections can often resolve with good nutrition and basic skin hygiene using medicated shampoos. Sometimes oral antibiotic treatment is required for 2–4 weeks. Prognosis is good in most cases.

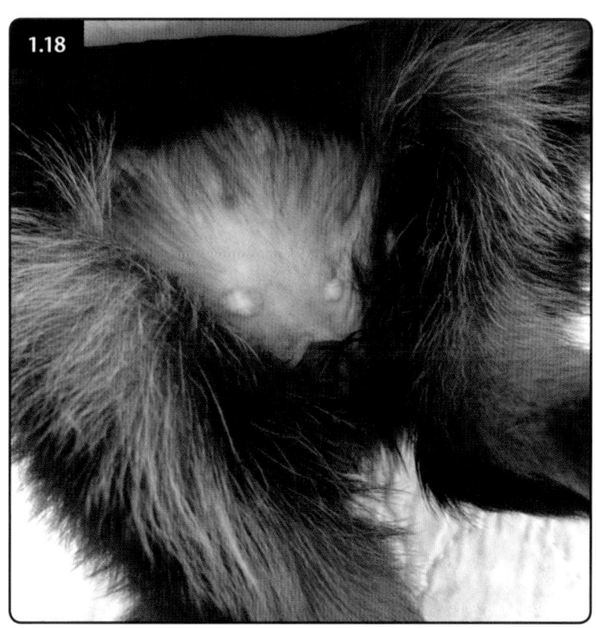
1.18

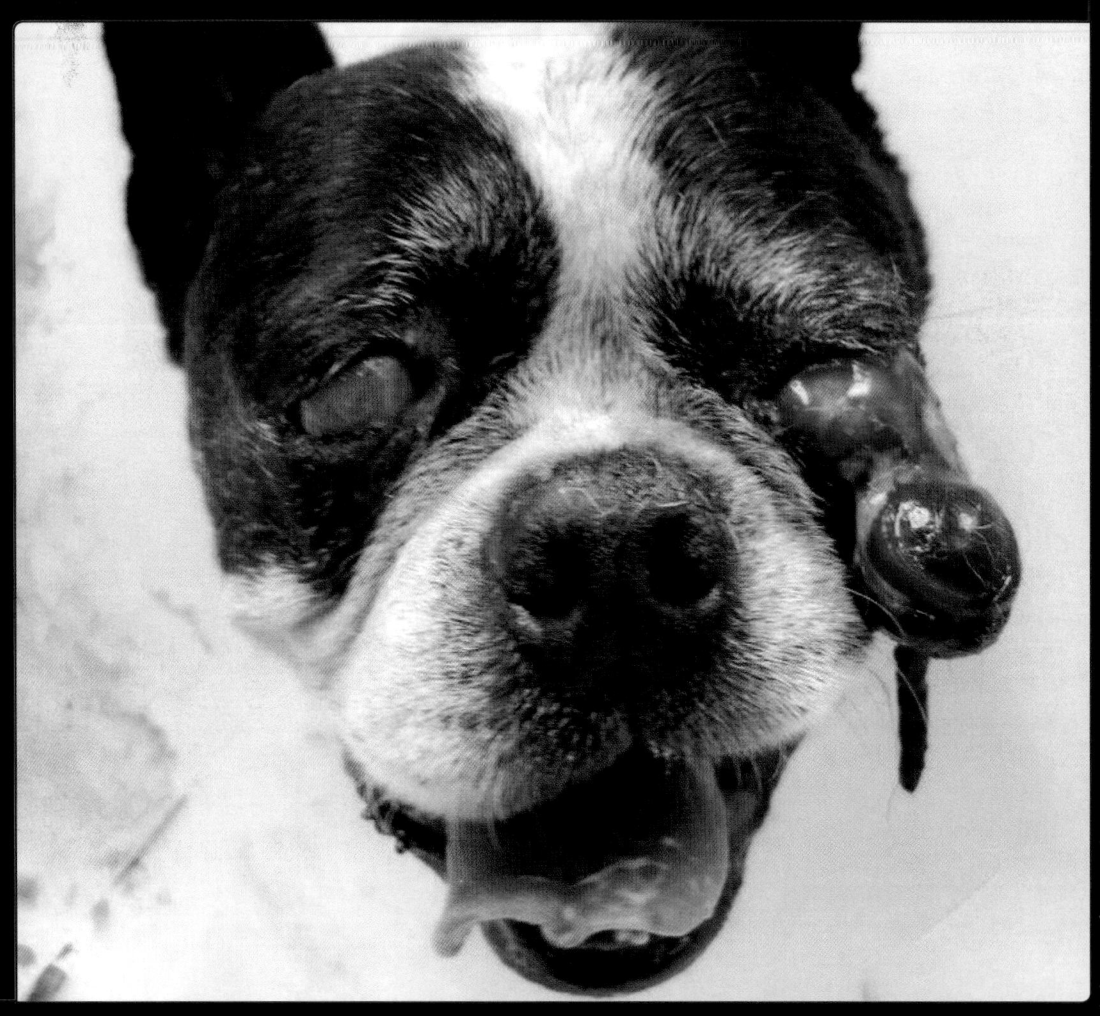

▲ This Boston Terrier has a severe traumatic proptosis of its left eye.

2

Ophthalmologic disorders

OPHTHALMOLOGY is derived from the Greek word *ophthalmos*, which refers to the eye. Disorders of the eye occur as primary entities or they can be manifestations of some other disease elsewhere in the body. The eye is sometimes referred to as the 'window to the body', because it allows a direct visualization of pathology that might not have originated in the eye. The clinician should have a basic understanding of diseases of the anterior and posterior segments of the eye and a basic knowledge of direct and indirect ophthalmoscopy. The lesions identified might very well be the first step to obtaining an expedient and accurate diagnosis. Some of the images found in this section would not have been possible without the gracious assistance of the ophthalmology section at the University of Florida, College of Veterinary Medicine.

2

Ophthalmologic disorders

- The eye is the window to the patient.
- A funduscopic examination should be done on every sick patient.
- Atropine eye drops are very irritating to the cat's oral cavity following drainage down the nasolacrimal duct. This can be avoided by using atropine ointment.
- Retinal hemorrhage is a common sign in hypertension.

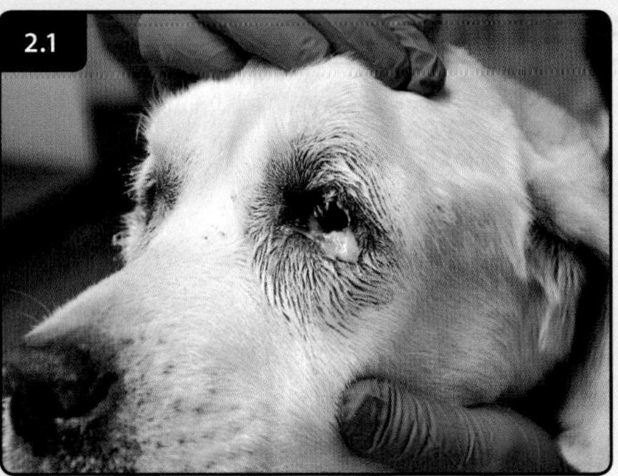

2.1. Keratitis sicca. This condition can be idiopathic but it can also occur in a dog with 7th cranial nerve palsy and with any disorder that can cause inflammation or destruction of the lacrimal apparatus. It can also occur from adverse drug reactions; for example, sulfa drugs. The Schirmer tear test is the diagnostic test of choice with abnormal levels being less than 15 mm/minute. Failure to treat with artificial tears will result in keratitis and ulcers. The temporal muscle atrophy in this dog reflects atrophy of the muscles of mastication.

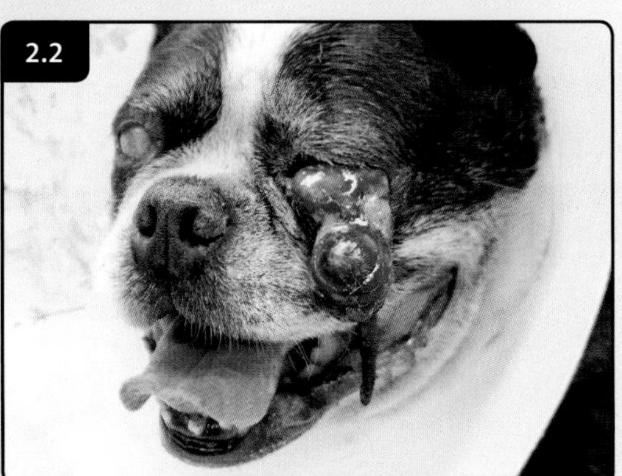

2.2. Proptosed eye in a dog. This Boston Terrier dog was attacked by another dog and quickly lost its eye. It was not amendable to being replaced in the globe because of the obvious tears in the extraocular muscles. The collar was being used to prevent any self-mutilation until enucleation was performed.

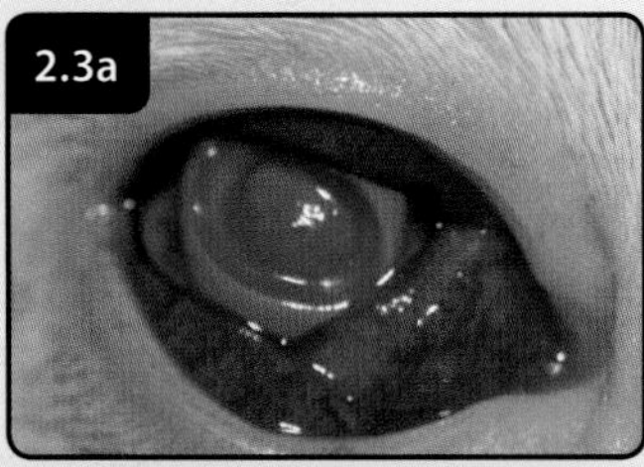

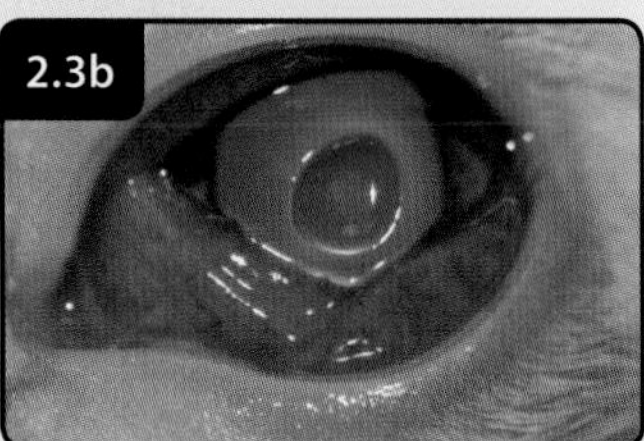

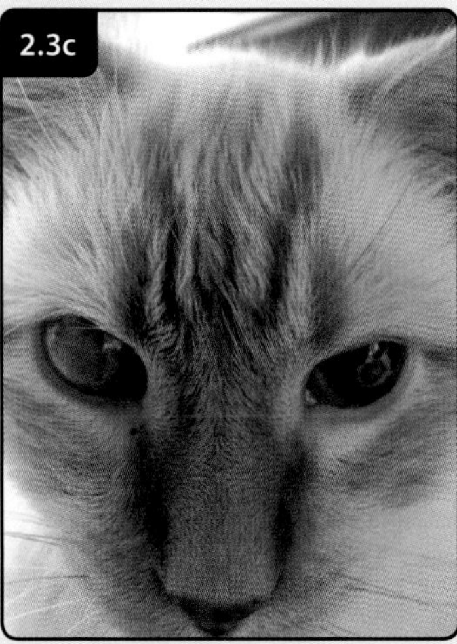

2.3a–c. Bilateral deep corneal ulcers. Despite being vaccinated for upper respiratory virus infection, this cat acquired conjunctivitis approximately 2 weeks after a new kitten was brought into the household. The corneal ulcers developed rapidly and extended deep to Descemet's membrane. Conjunctival flap surgery and topical horse serum saved both eyes. Figure 2.3c shows the cat 5 years later with corneal scars that did not impair vision.

2.4. Horner's syndrome in a cat. This image shows the classic signs of Horner's syndrome, namely ptosis, enophthalmos, and miosis. Lesion locations that can cause Horner's include the sympathetic nerve origin in the thalamic region extending through the cervical cord, the sympathetic branch that ascends the neck and chest, and the branch that passes through the tympanic bulla and ascends to the pupil dilator. Other clinical signs will help identify the exact lesion location.

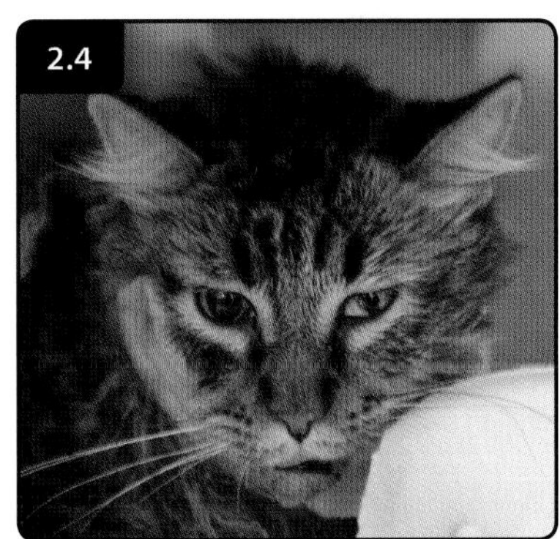

2.4

2.5. Thrombocytopenia-induced hyphema. This Boston Terrier has hyphema in its right eye. Hyphema has numerous causes including intraocular tumors, hypertension, infiltrative diseases, and coagulopathy. In this case the cause was immune-mediated thrombocytopenia. Treatment would entail treating the primary cause of the bleeding. Uveal inflammation can sometimes accompany the bleeding, thus calling for treatment for uveitis, which will include glucocorticoids and applying a mydriatic drug such as atropine topically.

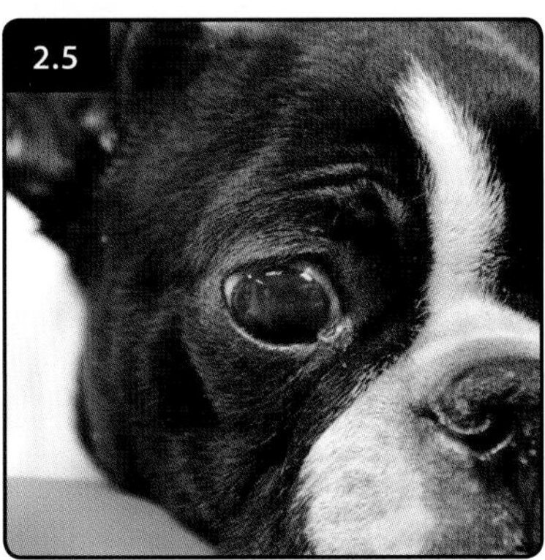

2.5

2.6a, b. Intraocular *Prototheca* infection. *Prototheca* spp. are algae type organisms for which there is no specific treatment. The systemic form can cause severe disease and often presents with clinical signs of diarrhea plus sudden onset of blindness from panophthalmitis and intraocular hemorrhage. Diagnosis is usually by fecal scrape with cytology, as shown in Figure 2.6b, or by tissue biopsy. The prognosis is usually poor.

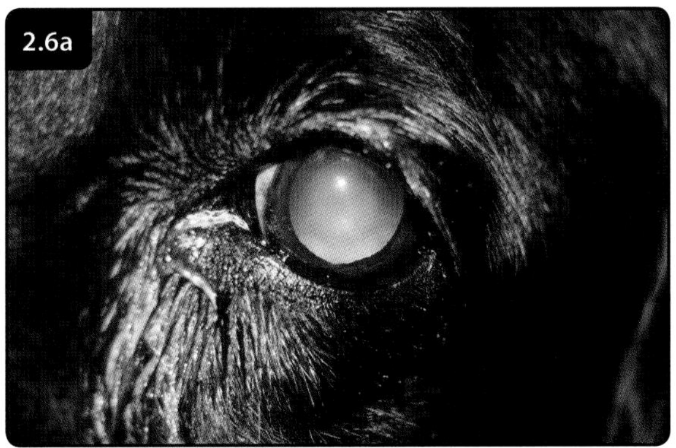

2.6a

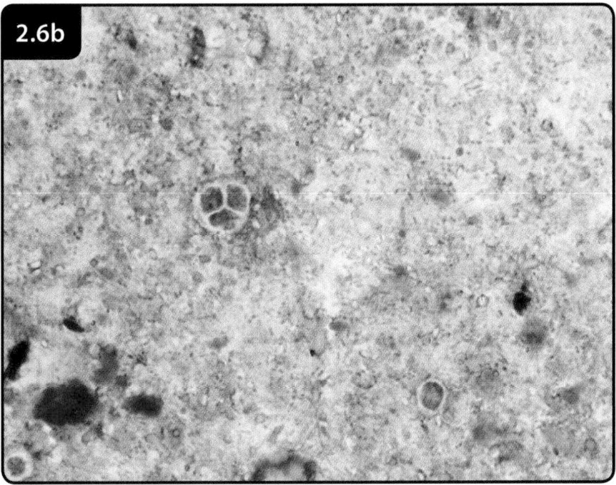

2.6b

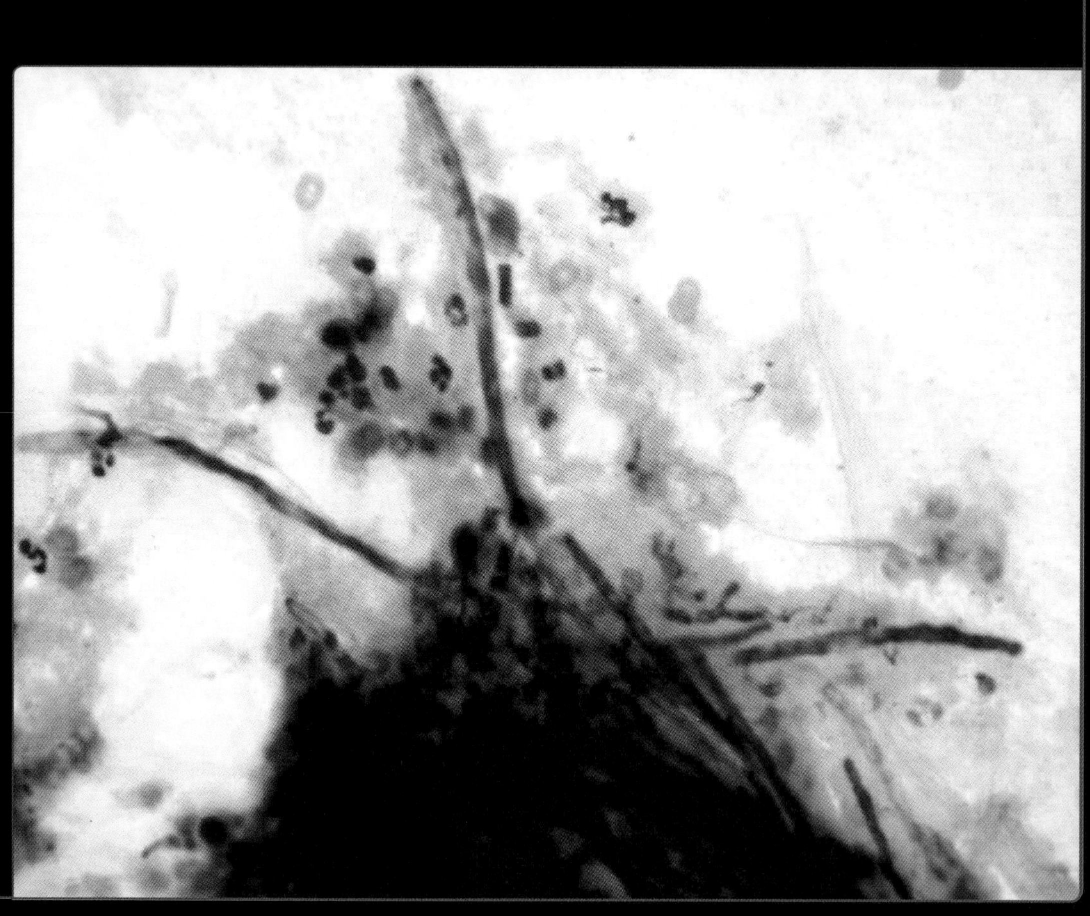

▲ This cytology specimen shows a septic exudate caused by fungi.

3

Infectious diseases

INFECTIOUS is derived from the Latin word *fectus*, meaning corrupt or infect. This group of disorders is a constant challenge to the clinician, because a timely diagnosis can often bring about a timely treatment, which can strongly influence the patient's prognosis. There are many infectious diseases of the dog and cat, but only a small selection of them will be illustrated in this chapter. Although the physical characteristics of certain infections are highly indicative of that particular disorder, it is strongly recommended that supportive diagnostic tests such a culture and sensitivity, biopsy, and serology are carried out to confirm any clinical suspicions. With the widespread availability of today's modern day transportation modalities, a thorough geographic and environmental history is an essential component in the accurate diagnosis of many of the disorders that follow.

3

Infectious diseases

- Use the strongest antibiotic for the most persistent and life-threatening bacterial infections.
- Patients in septic shock can be afebrile and have hypotension and thrombocytopenia.
- Fever has several different causes. Some of the more common causes include infection, hyperimmune reaction, autoimmune disease, cancer, necrosis, and drug reaction.
- Pneumonia with leukopenia can cause minimal radiographic signs.
- Immunocompromise can predispose to fungal infection.

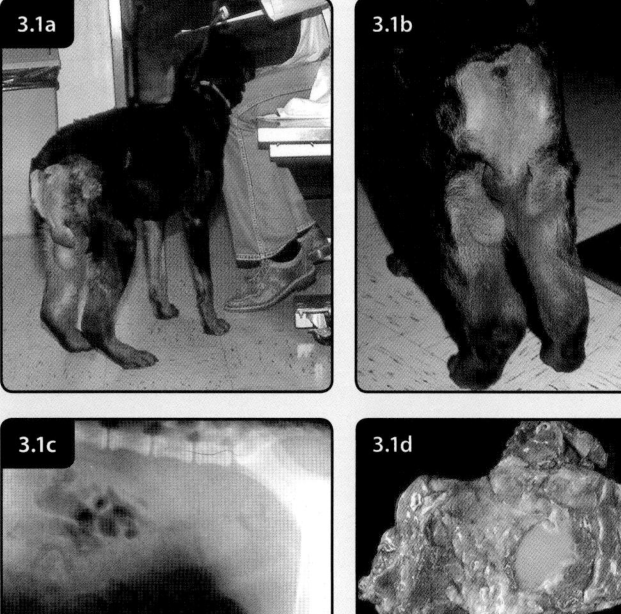

3.1a–d. Migrating foreign body infection and right hind leg lymphedema. This Rottweiler dog acquired a draining infected wound over its right hip that had not responded to 2 weeks of antibiotic treatment. Physical examination showed that the dog had right hind leg lymphedema, which extended the entire length of the leg, and a draining wound over the right ilium. Rectal examination revealed a mass effect originating from the dorsal caudal abdomen. The lateral abdominal radiograph showed ventral colonic displacement by an enlarged external iliac lymph node and an expanded retroperitoneal space. The lymphadenopathy was interfering with lymphatic fluid drainage from the right leg and was causing the lymphedema (clear fluid, noninflammatory). Antibiotics were administered pending culture and sensitivity results. The dog died while awaiting the owner's decision for surgery. Necropsy showed a large suppurative cavitation in the lumbar musculature that was probably caused by a migrating foreign body that had spread from a superficial draining wound over the right ilium.

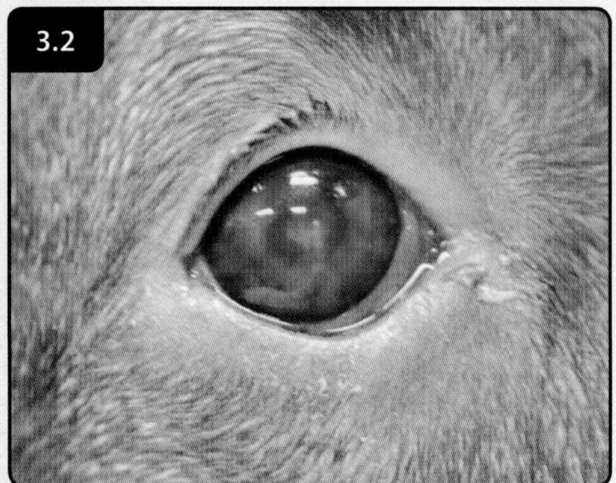

3.2. Fungal anterior uveitis. The uveitis in this dog was caused by a disseminated *Aspergillus terreus* infection that caused diskospondylitis, fungal pyelonephritis, and osteomyelitis involving the ribs. Diagnosis was made on culture after the fungal hyphae were identified on urinalysis. The prognosis was dismal and the dog was euthanized after not responding to attempted treatment with antifungal agents.

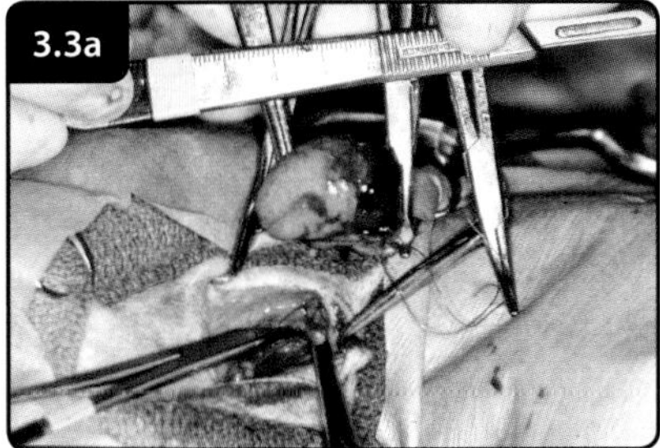
3.3a

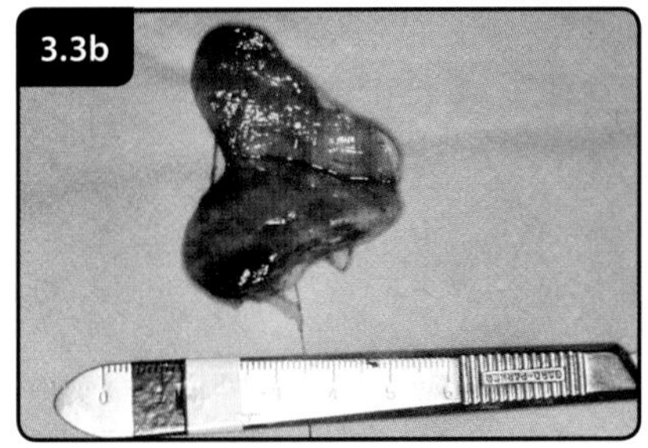
3.3b

3.3a, b. Fever and well-differentiated lymphadenopathy in cats. These surgical specimens of cervical lymph nodes were taken from a cat that had marked fever, anorexia, and depression. The clinical and histopathologic diagnosis was well-differentiated lymphadenopathy of unknown etiology (also known as distinctive lymph node hyperplasia in young cats), a syndrome that was recognized in cats in the 1980s and 90s. Many of these cats would eventually respond to time and various combinations of antibiotics. Today, this patient would be a strong suspect for having bartonellosis or perhaps feline immunodeficiency virus (FIV) infection, for which specific diagnostic tests are now available, using blood cultures and polymerase chain reaction for bartonellosis and serology for FIV.

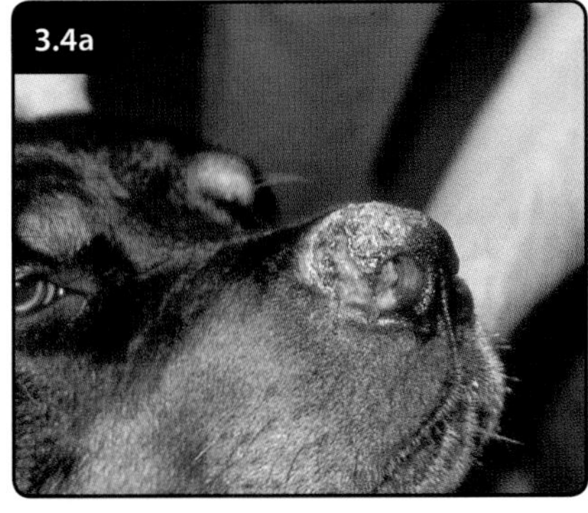
3.4a

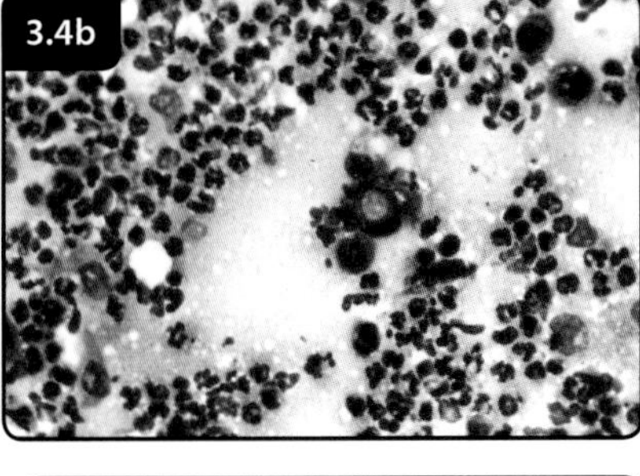
3.4b

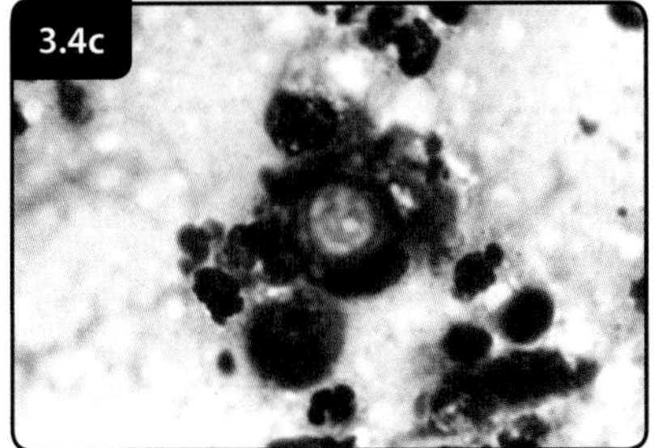
3.4c

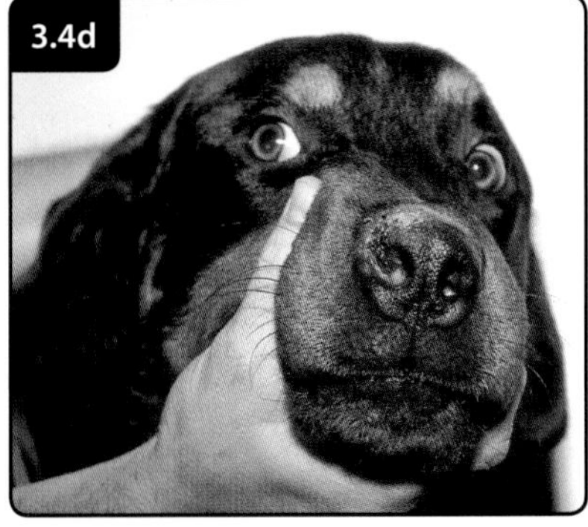
3.4d

3.4a–d. Blastomycosis in a dog. A young Rottweiler dog with a granulomatous lesion on its nose caused by *Blastomyces dermatitidis* is shown (Figure 3.4a). The dog also had cervical and prescapular lymphadenopathy from which cytology specimens were aspirated and diagnosed as *Blastomyces* (Figures 3.4b, c). The dog was treated with ketoconazole (before itraconazole became available) and it resolved well to extended treatment over 9 months. The dog is shown after it had improved after approximately 1 month of treatment (Figure 3.4d).

3.5. Blastomyces in a dog. This image shows lingual ulcers that were sampled with a touch prep impression for cytology evaluation. It showed organisms similar to those in Figures 3.4b, c. Blastomyces infections can cause lesions involving the lungs and other tissues of the body, particularly the skin. Diagnosis is easy to make on cytology, which shows the budding yeast cells amongst a neutrophilic infiltrate. Wright–Giemsa, PAS, and Diff-Quik® stains easily stain the organisms.

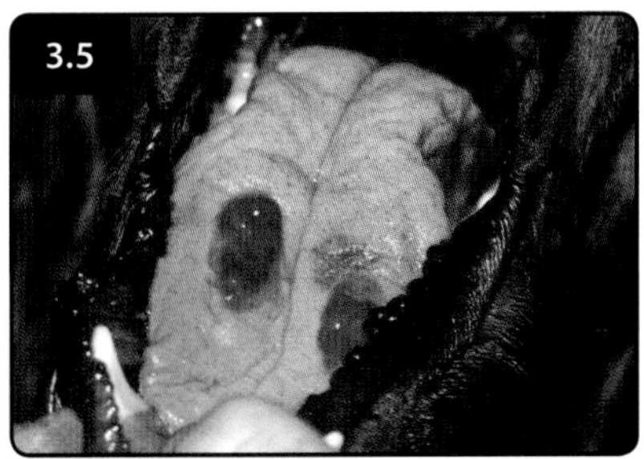
3.5

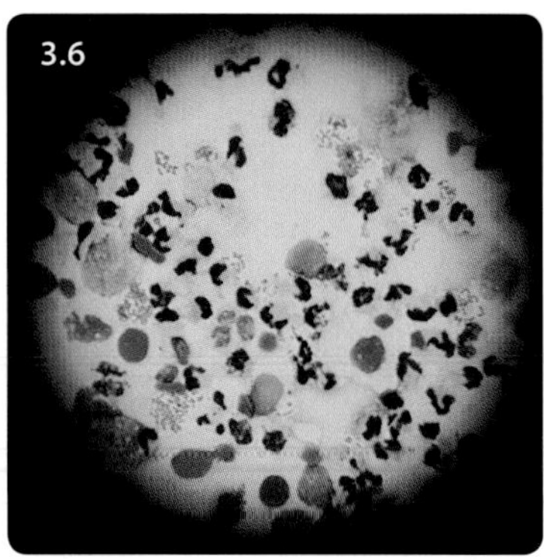

3.6. Spinal fluid cytology from a dog with bacterial meningitis. This cerebrospinal (CSF) fluid cytology sample came from an English Bulldog that had signs of neck pain, fever, and marked lethargy. The differential diagnosis included meningitis along with other conditions that can cause these signs. The cytology sample shows numerous free and phagocytosed bacteria and neutrophils. Such cases of sepsis are usually accompanied by primary infections of the inner ear, sinus, or penetrating head wound, but in this case there was no predisposing cause. More often, cases of meningitis in dogs are the sterile forms, but in this case the diagnosis was totally different to what was expected, calling for culture and sensitivity testing of the CSF and commencing parenteral antibiotics while providing the owner with a guarded prognosis until the dog clinically improves.

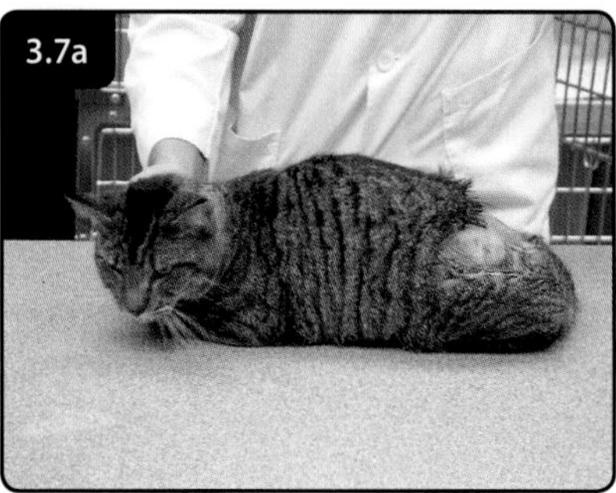

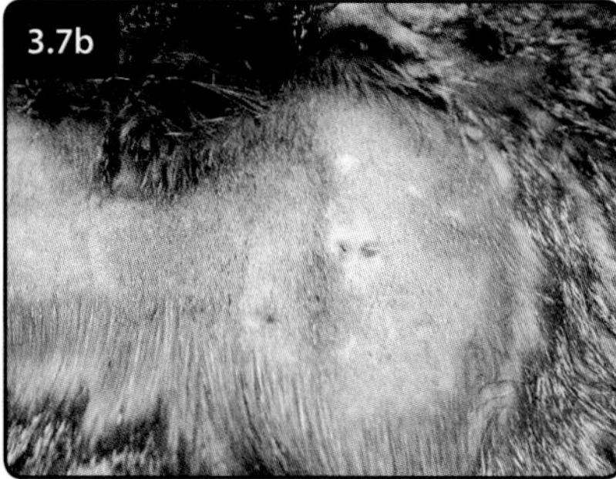

3.7a, b. Cat bite abscess. It is imperative to search for punctate bite wounds on a cat that presents for fever and lethargy and with a history of exposure to another cat. The wounds are often difficult to see, but a gathered tuft of fur might lead to the evidence shown in these images. Treatment calls for wound care, which might include hot packing and systemic antibiotics. The latter should cover for *Pasturella* amongst other species of bacteria. Any abscess that forms should be treated by lancing and drainage.

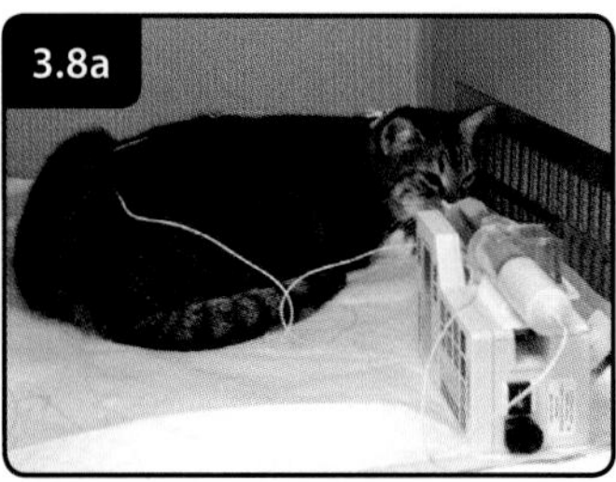

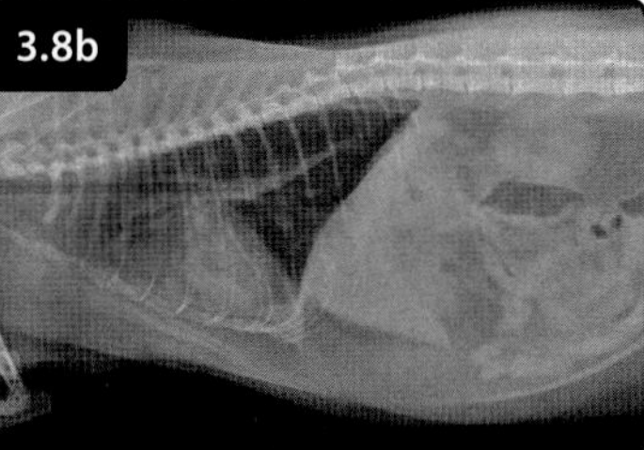

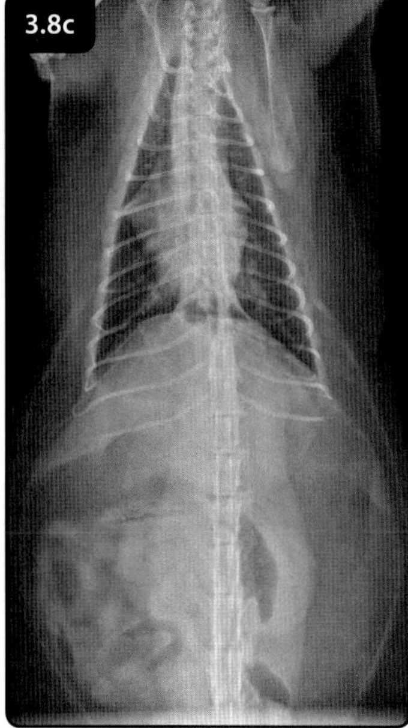

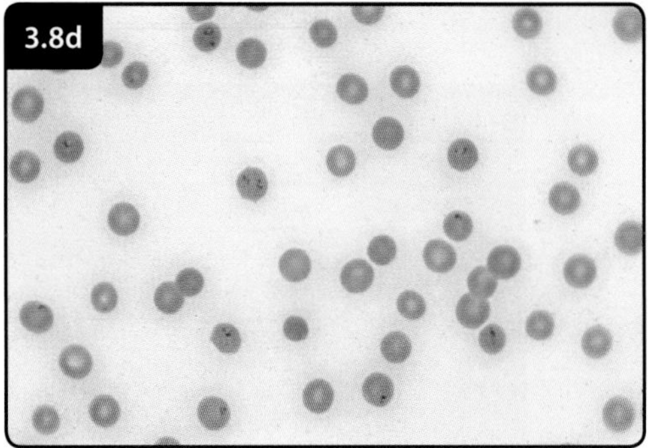

3.9. Canine distemper dentition. The young dog in this photograph has etched and discolored teeth due to enamel damage caused by prior canine distemper infection. The tooth damage was discovered on routine examination for another minor problem. The tooth damage is irreversible. This, along with 'hard pad', is an indicator of prior distemper virus infection.

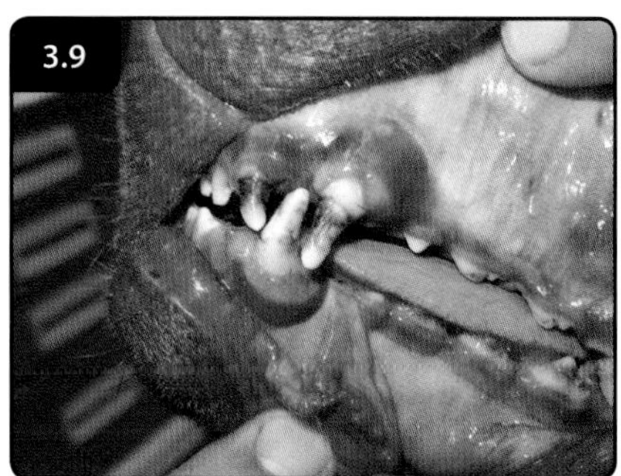

3.10a–c. Feline infectious peritonitis. Feline infectious peritonitis is a viral disease with a grave prognosis. The images show the typical gold-colored viscous sterile fluid exudate that can accumulate in the abdomen or thorax, a serum electrophoresis showing a polyclonal gammopathy, and a surgical view of the intestines showing the thickened bowel caused by microscopic pyogranuloma formation.

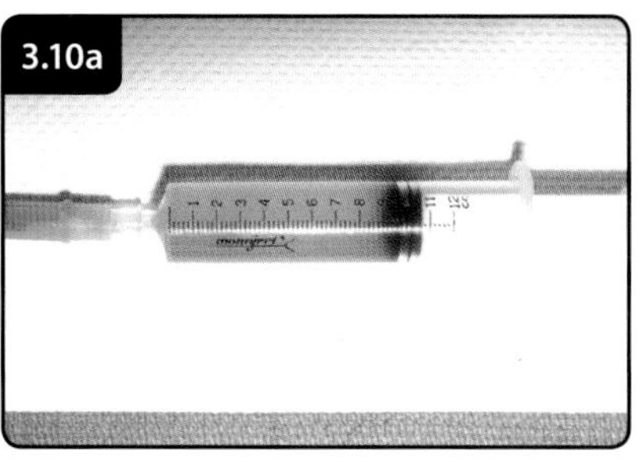

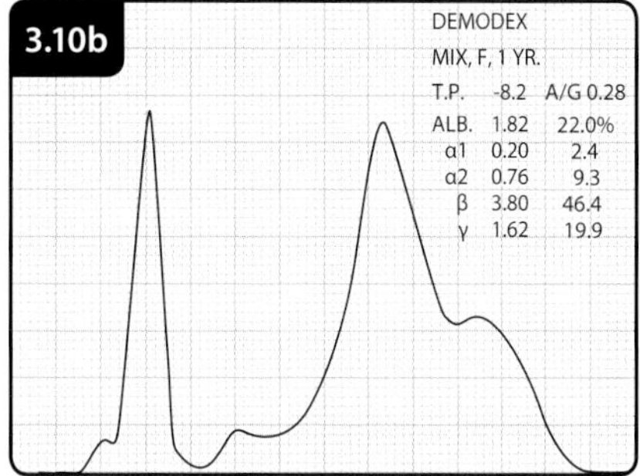

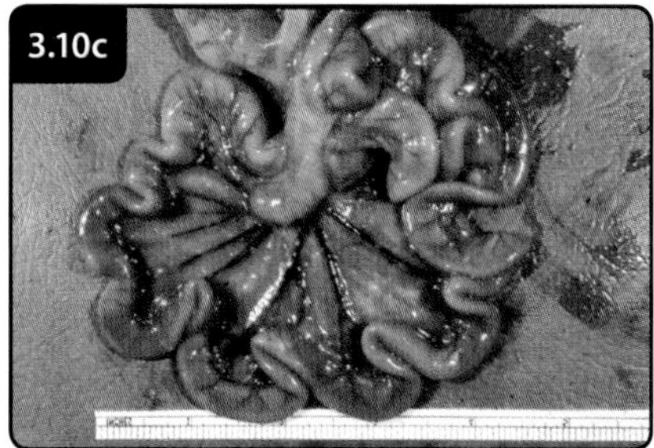

3.11. Oral thrush (*Candida* sp.) infection in a kitten. The whitish film on this kitten's tongue is due to *Candida* infection. Such fungal infections are usually caused by immune deficiency or some predisposing factor such as prior antibiotic treatment. It is important to discontinue all antibiotics and begin treatment with an azole drug such as ketoconazole.

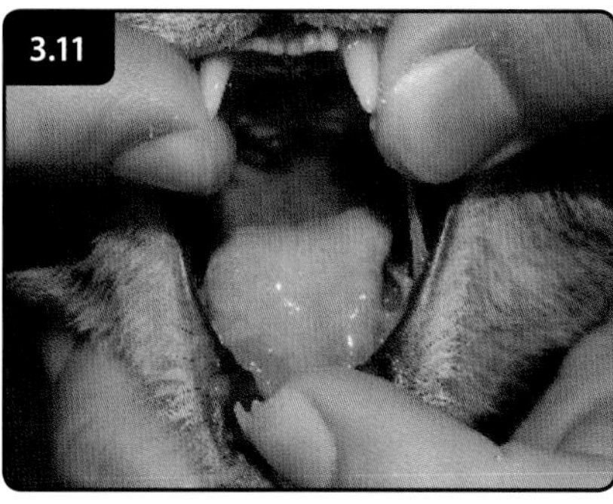

3.8a–d. Cytauxzoonosis in a cat. This cat was examined by its veterinarian for lethargy and anorexia of 2 days' duration. It was an indoor/outdoor cat. Clinical findings included fever, moderate labored breathing, and slight icterus. The radiographs show a marked interstitial pattern with focal areas of consolidation. The hemogram shows small piriform organisms on the red blood cells, which were identified as *Cytauxzooan felis*. The icterus was attributed to hepatic involvement by the organism. The prognosis is guarded but survival is possible with good patient support and administration of drugs such as imidocarb, atovaquone combined with azithromycin, or diminazene.

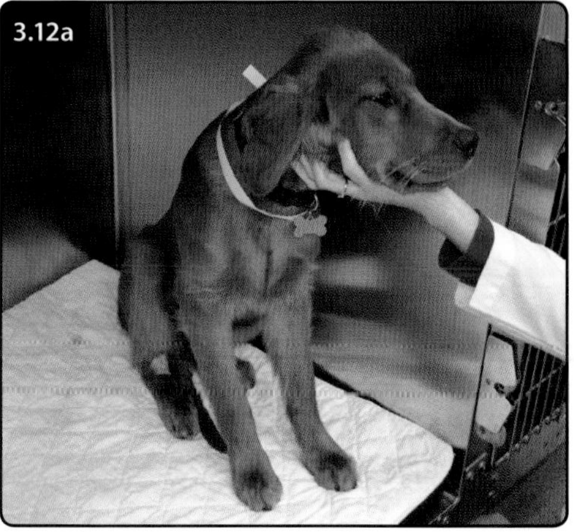

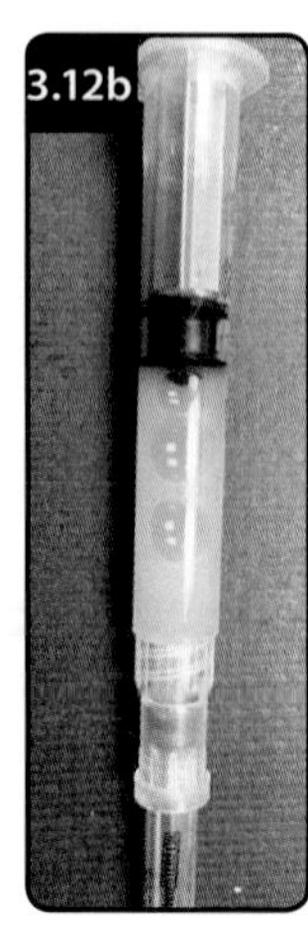

3.12a, b. Septic arthritis in a puppy. This puppy had signs of fever and right forelimb lameness. Physical examination showed a temperature of 104°F (40°C) and right carpal swelling. Sedation was induced and a joint tap performed for cytology and culture and sensitivity. The fluid was opaque and microscopically showed abundant numbers of neutrophils with karyolysis and the surprising absence of bacteria. Monoarticular disorders such as this are compatible with bacterial infection. The puppy responded to antibiotic treatment (amoxicillin and clavulanic acid). Joint irrigation with sterile saline can also help by eliminating the neutrophils and their destructive enzymes from the joint space.

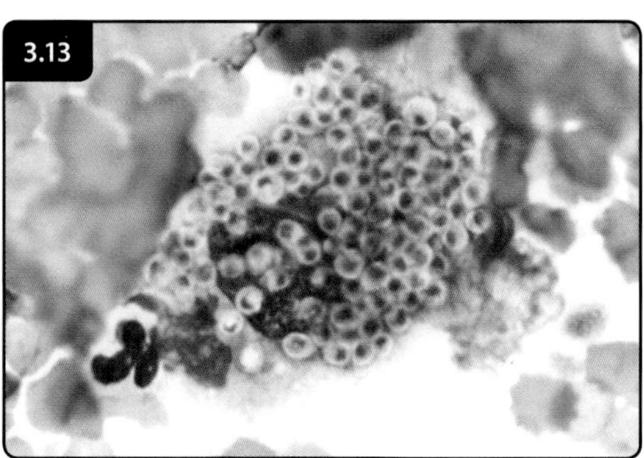

3.13. Histoplasmosis in a dog. This microscopic view of a fecal smear shows a macrophage fully packed with *Histoplasma* organisms. This patient had the gastrointestinal form and there was blood in the stool. In the USA this infection is usually confined to the midwestern states, but it can also occur in the southeast USA and in other parts of the world such as South America, Europe, and Africa. This dog would be screened for other organ system involvements such as the lungs. Treatment requires long-term azole-type drugs such as itraconazole.

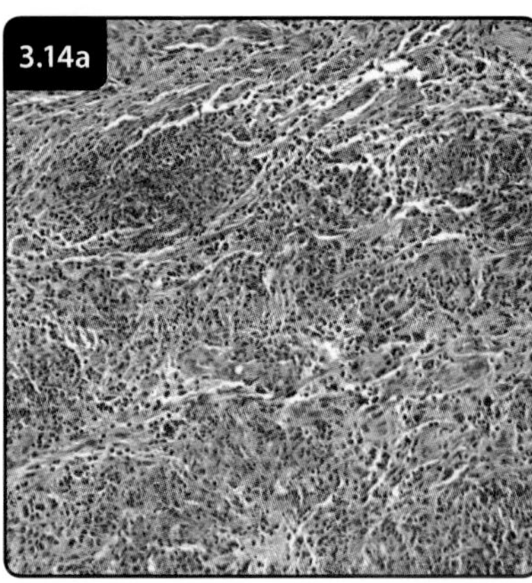

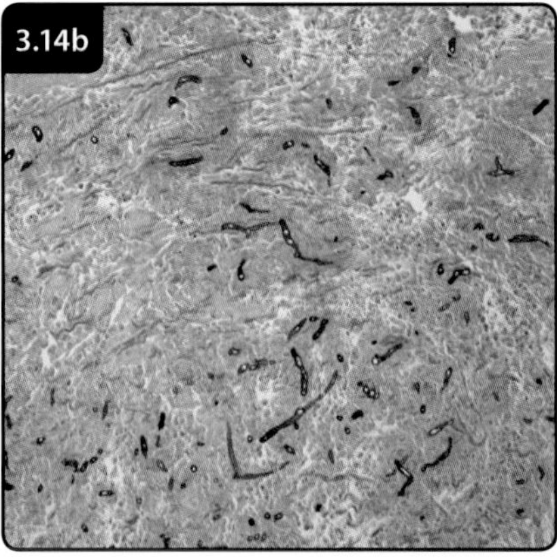

3.14a, b. *Lagenidium* sp. infection in a dog. This organism belongs to the class Oomycota and is often confused as being a pure fungal infection. The disease is similar to pythiosis and zygomycosis, which makes all of these disorders difficult to cure, thereby giving affected animals a very guarded prognosis. Radical surgical removal of the involved tissues, if possible, might be the best way to treat this disease. These microscopic views show the granulomatous inflammation using H&E stain (Figure 3.14a) and a more clear view of the organisms using Gomori methenamine silver stain (Figure 3.14b).

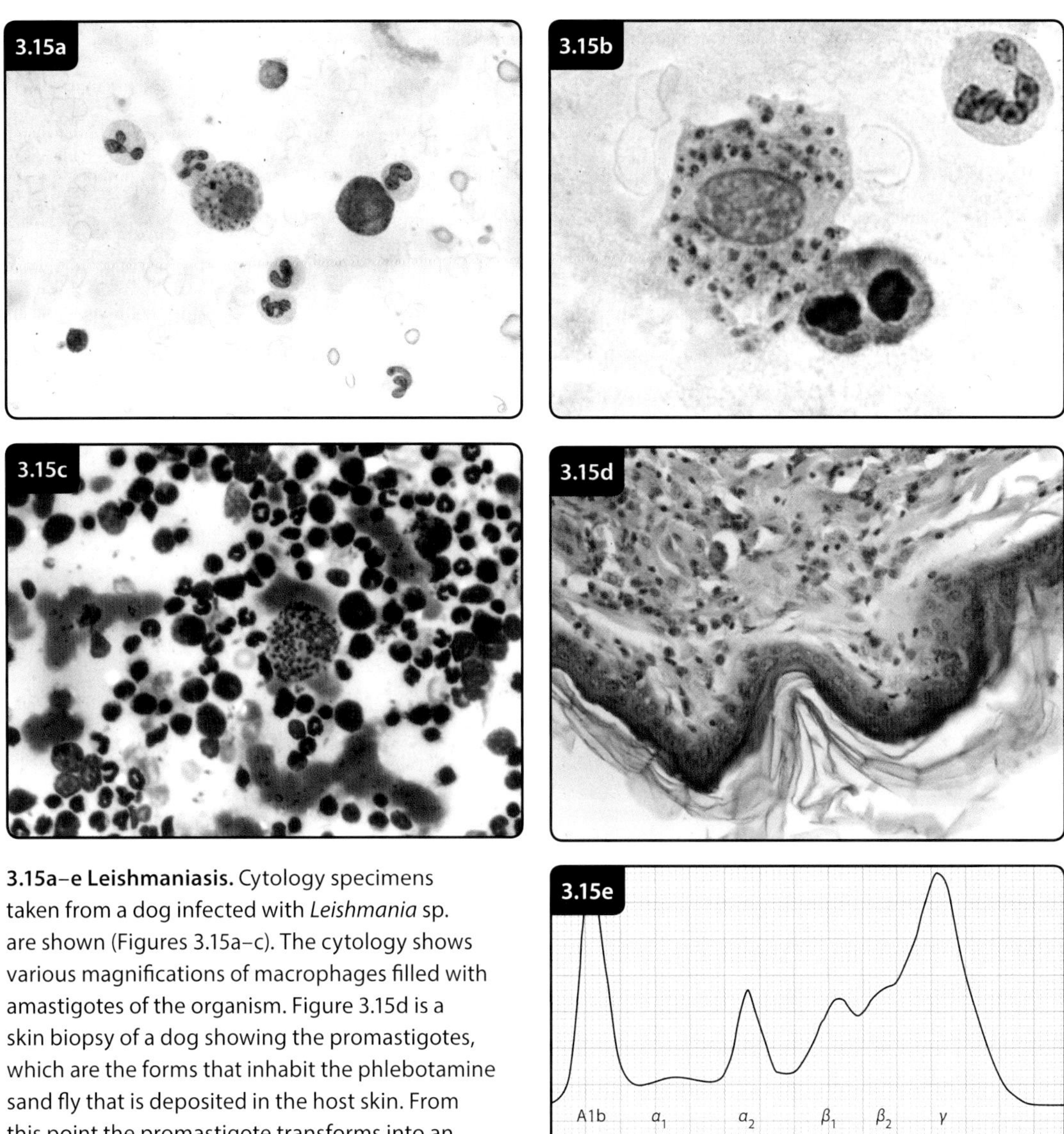

3.15a–e Leishmaniasis. Cytology specimens taken from a dog infected with *Leishmania* sp. are shown (Figures 3.15a–c). The cytology shows various magnifications of macrophages filled with amastigotes of the organism. Figure 3.15d is a skin biopsy of a dog showing the promastigotes, which are the forms that inhabit the phlebotamine sand fly that is deposited in the host skin. From this point the promastigote transforms into an amastigote, which parasitizes the host's tissues and cells such as the macrophage. The host will have an immunologic response that can be shown on the serum electrophoresis as a polyclonal gammopathy (Figure 3.15e). Organic antimonial drugs and allopurinol are used to treat this disease, with a variable response.

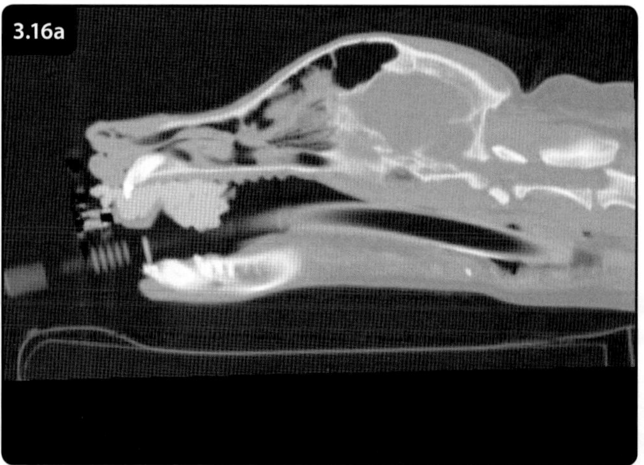

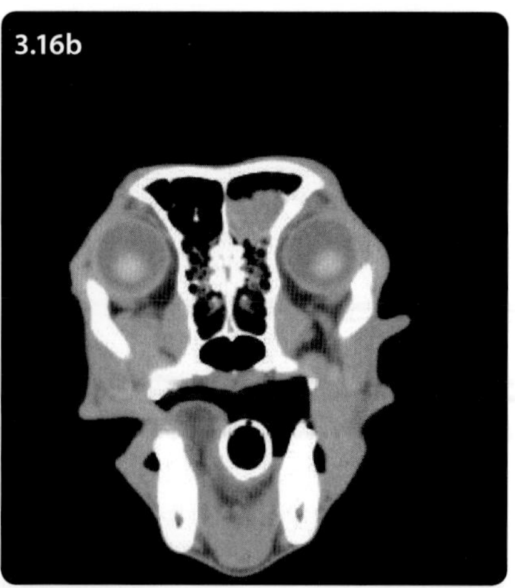

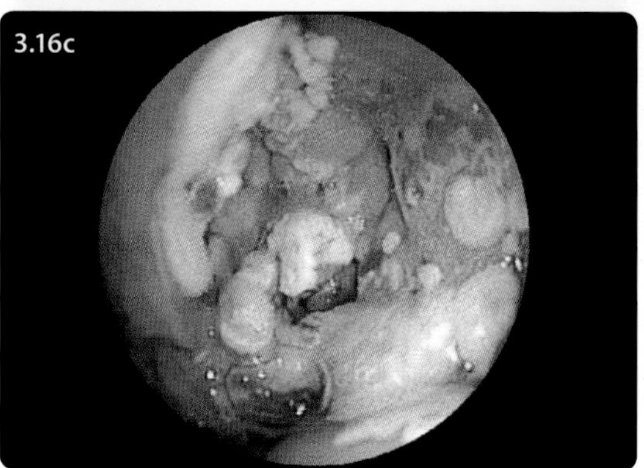

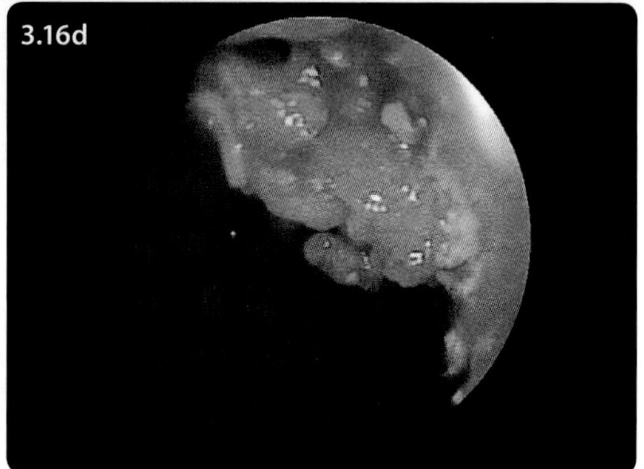

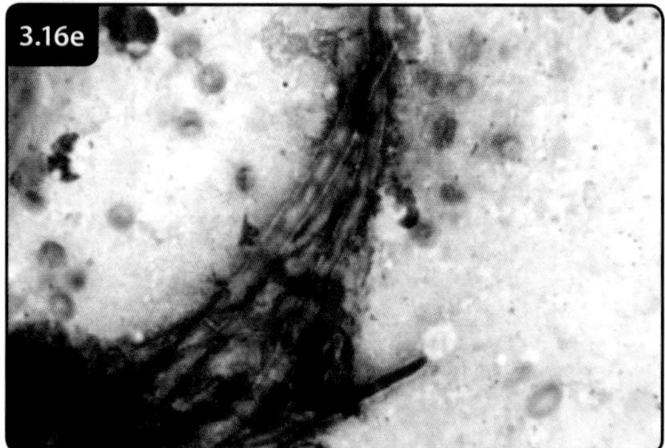

3.16a–e. Fungal rhinitis in a dog. Dogs with unilateral nasal discharge can have several different disorders including foreign body, tumors, and mycotic infection. The CT images of the skull show a lesion in the right frontal sinus and nasal cavity. The rhinoscopy images show fungal mats and the cytology preparation shows fungal hyphae. *Aspergillus* sp. is commonly isolated with these types of infections. (Rhinoscopy images courtesy Small Animal Internal Medicine Service, University of Florida)

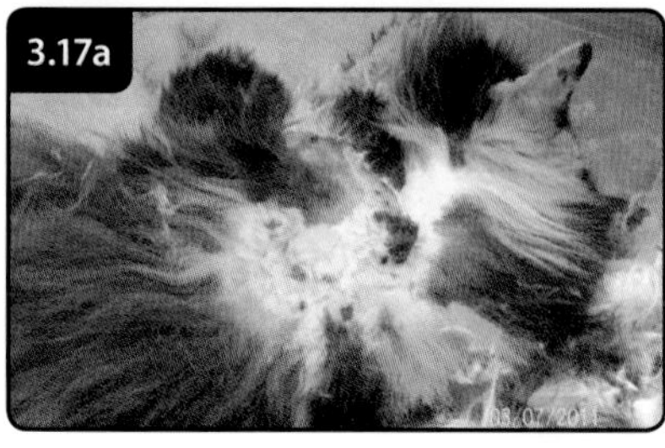

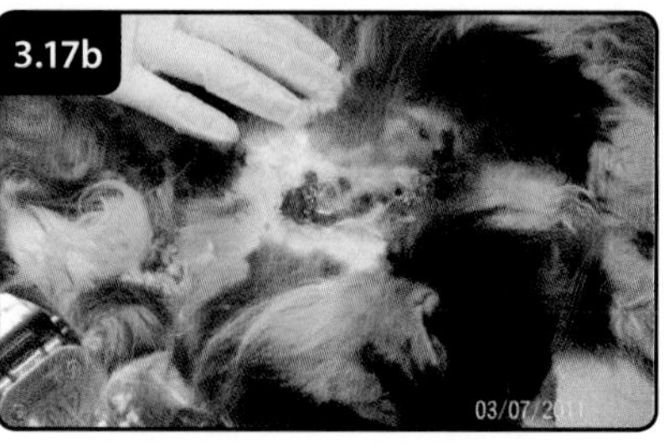

3.17a, b. *Nocardia* skin infection in a cat. Nocardiosis in the cat can involve several organ systems, especially the respiratory tract. This cat, however, has the cutaneous form, which causes chronic draining tracks and granulomas. *Nocardia* organisms are filamentous and will stain positive on acid-fast stains. Long-term sulfa drug therapy is the treatment of choice.

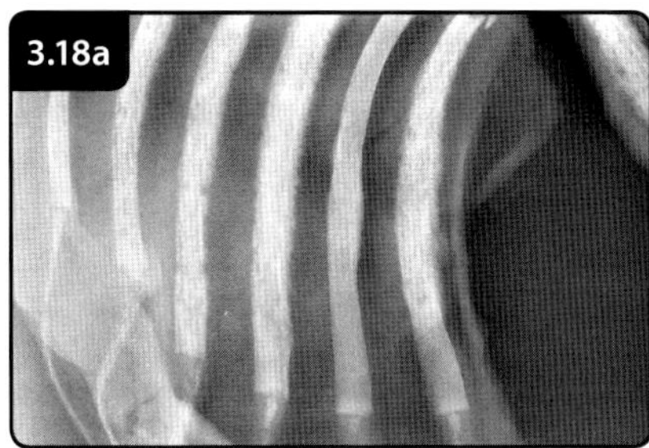

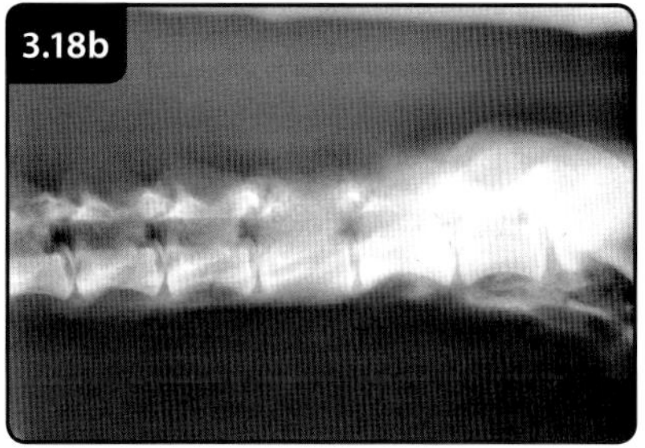

3.18a, b. Mycotic bone infection. These radiographs of the spine and ribs show marked periosteal proliferation. A bone biopsy would be indicated for a definitive diagnosis. Sometimes a fine needle aspirate for cytology can also be used diagnostically. Treatment requires long-term systemic antifungal drugs, but the prognosis is guarded.

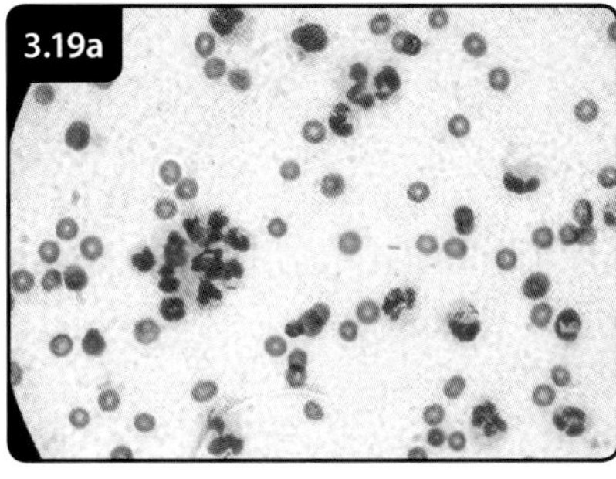

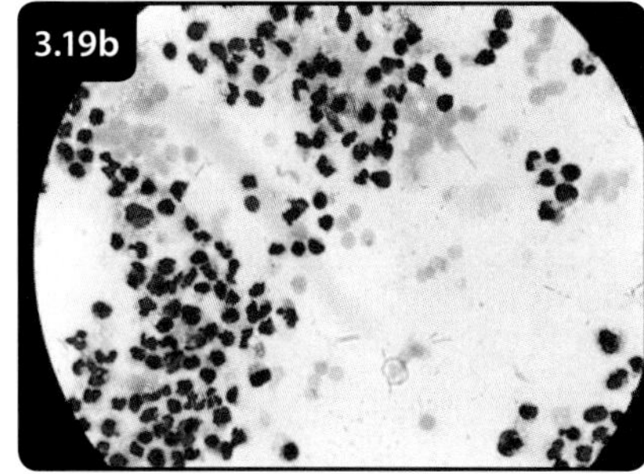

3.19a, b. Bacteria in neutrophils. These two cytology specimens show bacteria that have been ingested by neutrophils as well as free non-ingested bacteria. This is very characteristic of sepsis and calls for removal of the source of infection, good patient support, and antibiotic treatment. Bacterial culture and sensitivity would definitely be indicated.

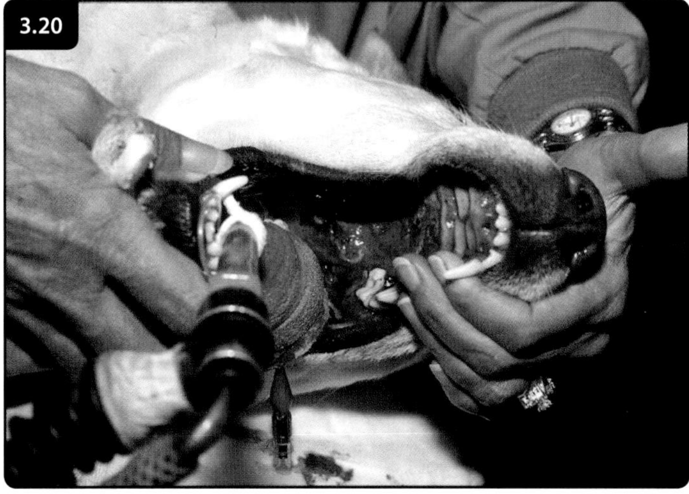

3.20. *Pythium insidiosum* in the oral cavity. Pythiosis is a serious disease because of its invasiveness, the delayed diagnosis, and its refractoriness to treatment. This image shows how the hard palate is diffusely infiltrated by this organism. Most cases are refractory to fungal treatment. Radical surgical resection is usually best if the lesion is amenable to treatment.

3.21. Critical care. Animals with septic shock are critically ill if they require a multitude of drugs to maintain adequate life support. This image leaves one with the impression that the medical situation for this patient is indeed critical. Animals with septic shock often receive an oxygen-rich environment in addition to intravenous crystalloids, antibiotics, antacids, analgesics, and vasopressors that are slowly infused by individual syringe pumps. One can postulate that the severity of the disease is directly proportional to the number of different syringe pumps attached outside of the cage. Such polypharmacy should invoke frequent assessments to avoid drug interactions and adverse drug reactions.

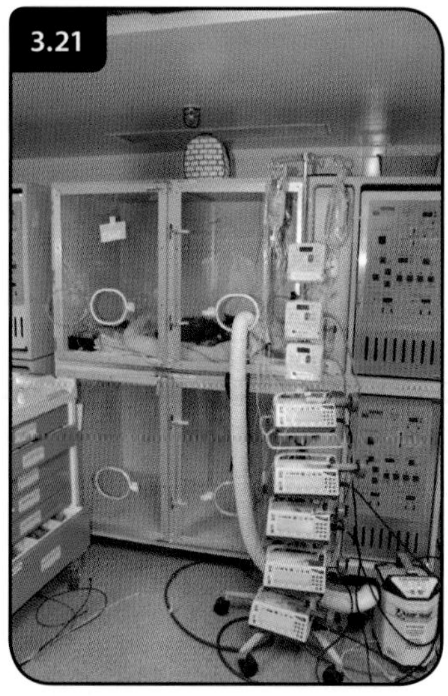
3.21

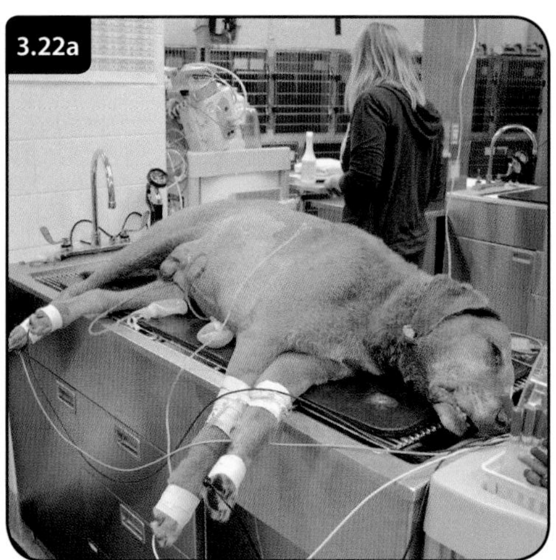
3.22a

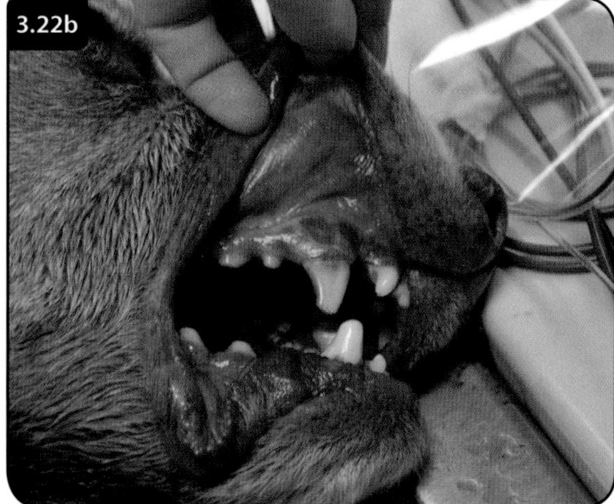
3.22b

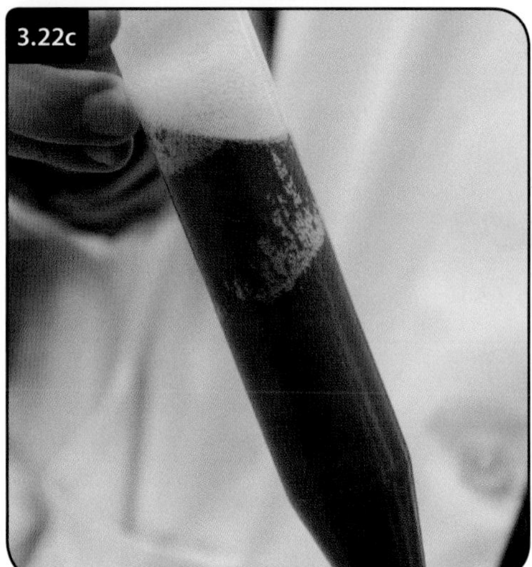
3.22c

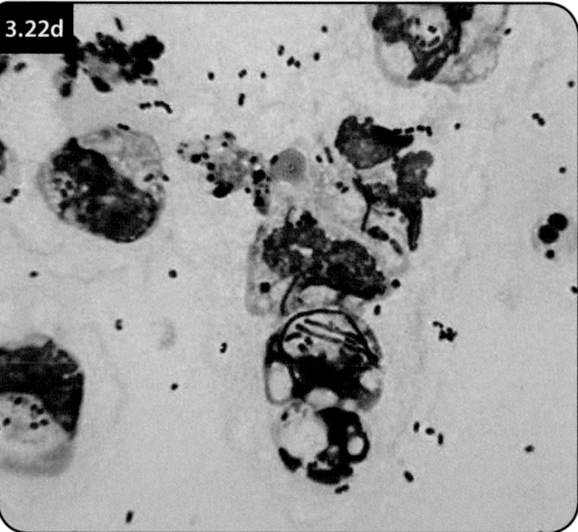
3.22d

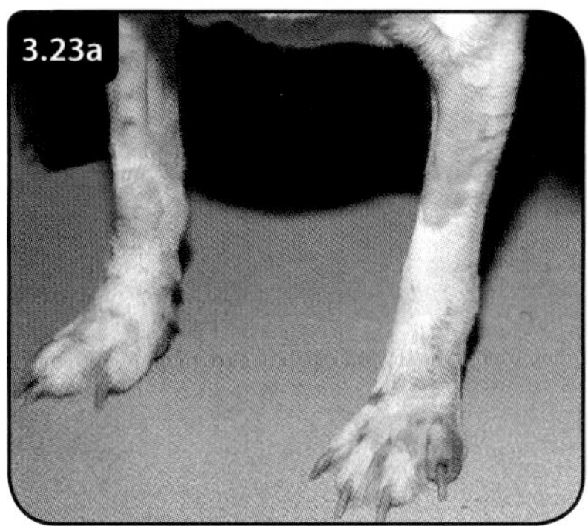

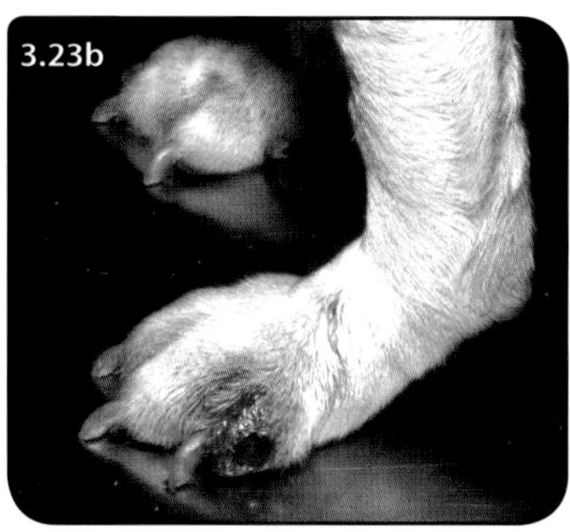

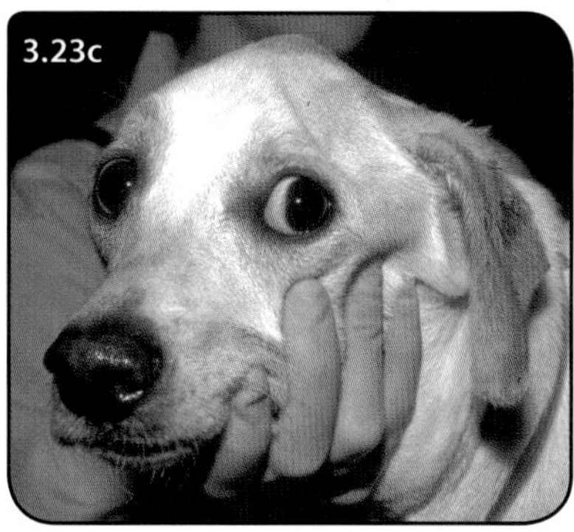

3.23a–c. Fungal infection secondary to prednisone-induced immunosuppression. This dog had immune-mediated hemolytic anemia that responded well to prednisone treatment. After several weeks treatment at a dosage of 1–2 mg/kg, the dog acquired a fungal infection involving her digits that spread to become lymphangitis. Amphotericin B treatment was necessary while the prednisone dose was reduced and then discontinued and replaced with another drug. The 'dropped carpus' from ligamentous laxity and the facial muscle atrophy are additional adverse effects of glucocorticoid.

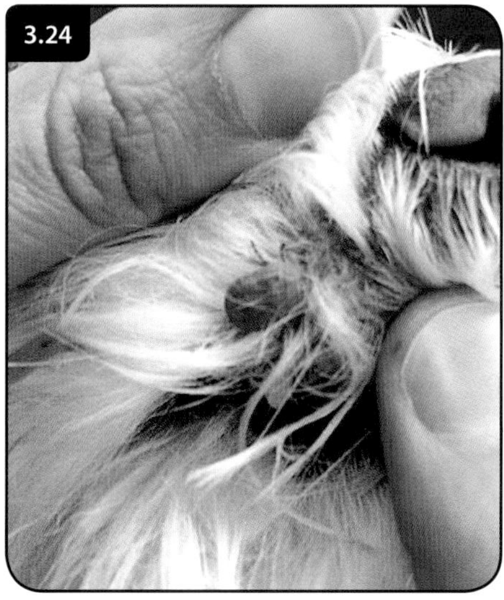

3.24. Tick bite. Many diseases are tick borne. Therefore, a thorough examination for ticks is an important part of the evaluation in all dogs that are suspect for having a tick-transmitted illness such as ehrlichiosis or anaplasmosis.

3.22a–d. Septic peritonitis. This dog is in the hyperdynamic phase of septic shock where the oral mucous membranes are characteristically very hyperemic. This will eventually progress to the hypodynamic stage, which is associated with cardiovascular collapse and the refractoriness of hypotension to intravenous crystalloids. Figure 3.22c shows a brownish colored free abdominal fluid sample that was described as feculent (fecal-like) and septic, as shown on the microscopic evaluation of the fluid (Figure 3.22d). Note the presence of bacteria both inside and outside of the neutrophils. This dog would require immediate medical stabilization and surgery.

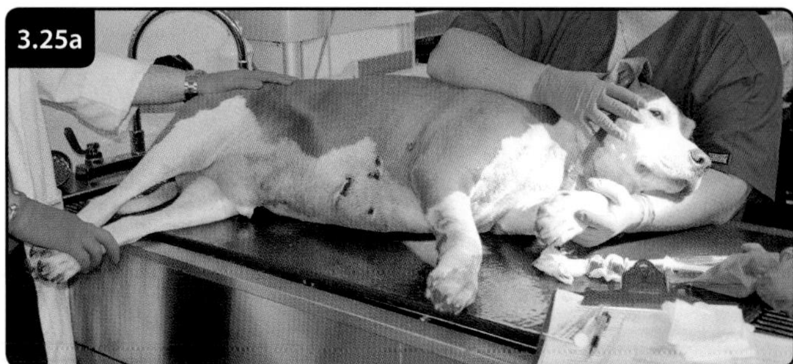
3.25a

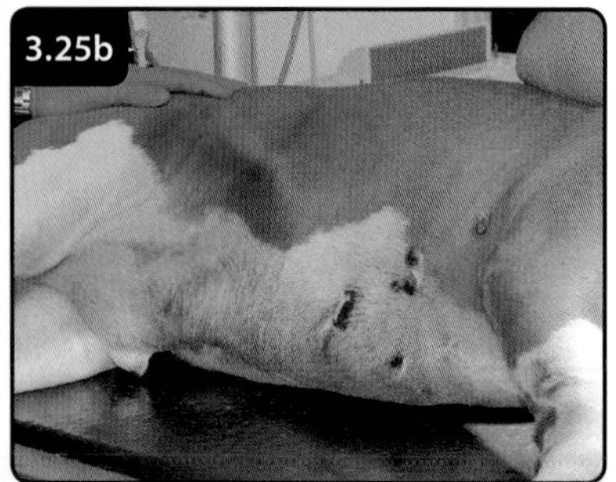
3.25b

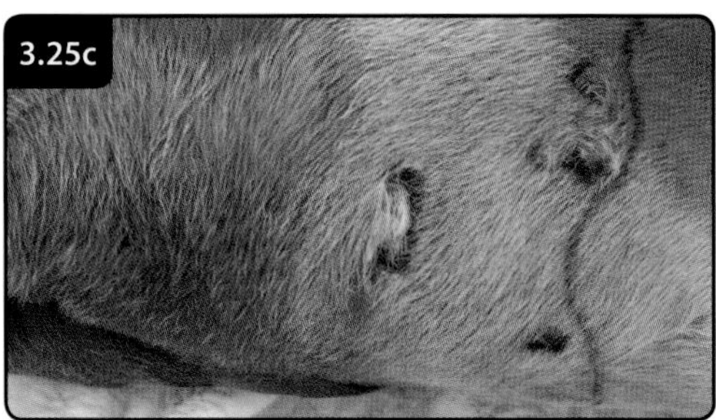
3.25c

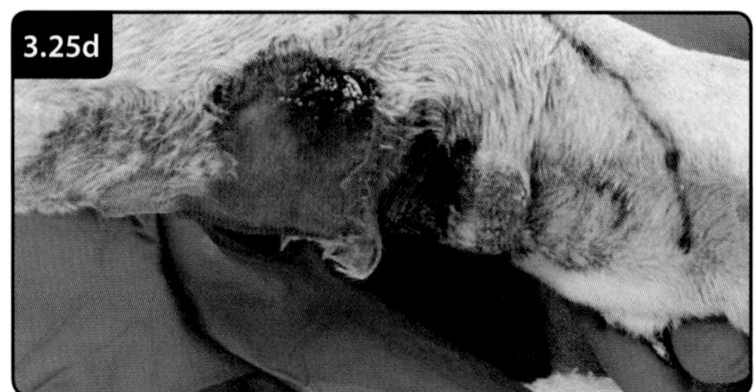
3.25d

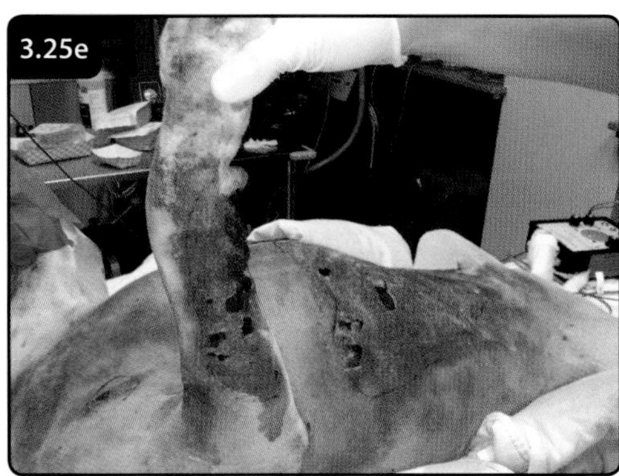
3.25e

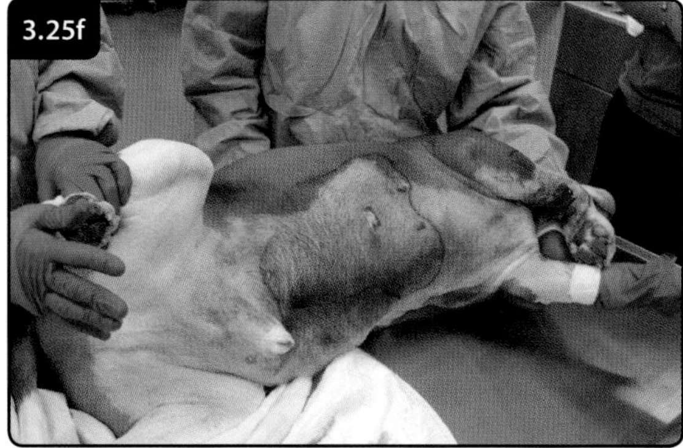
3.25f

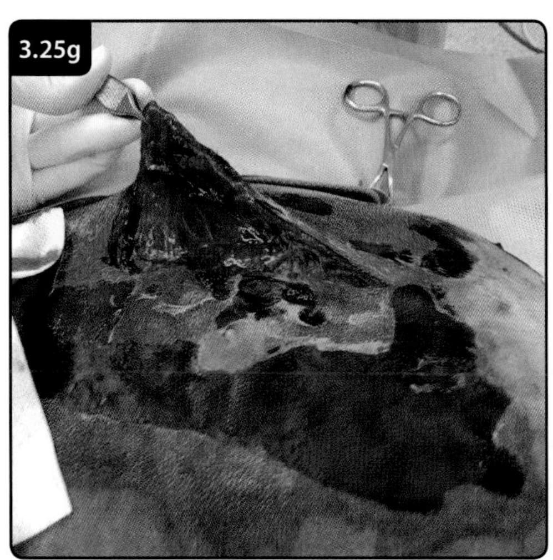
3.25g

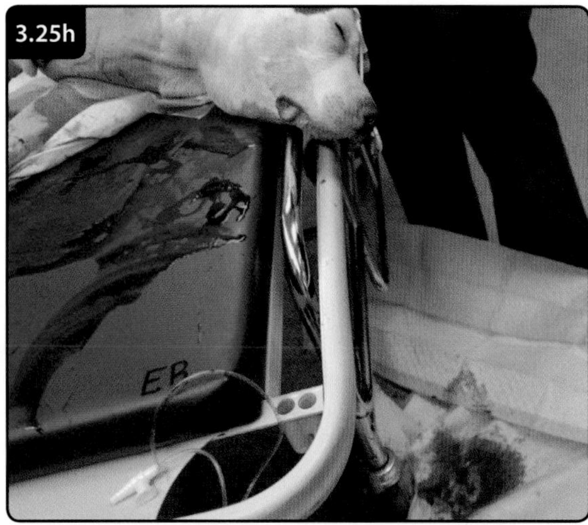
3.25h

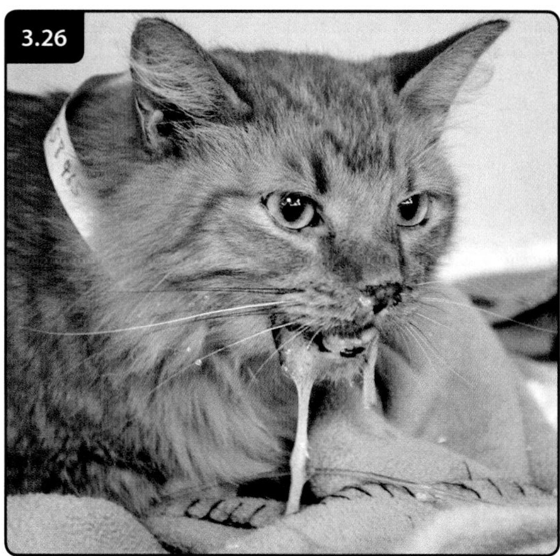

3.26. Viral upper respiratory infection in a cat. Both rhinotracheitis virus and calicivirus in the cat cause debilitating infection involving both the upper and lower respiratory tracts. Pharyngitis is a common sign and might be the only clinical feature when the patient is initially examined. Failure to detect this as an early sign of contagious disease will result in exposure of all cats housed in the same ward, resulting in widespread disease. The main signals for this involvement are the ptyalism, open-mouth breathing, and inflamed oral mucous membranes.

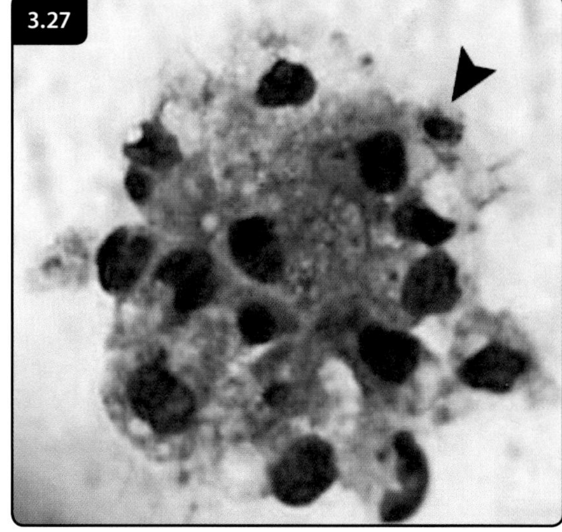

3.27. *Candida* sp. sepsis in a dog. This abdominal cytology image is from a dog that had a bowel perforation and septic shock. The cause of sepsis in most of these patients is bacterial, but occasionally *Candida* can be the culprit, especially if the animal had been on antibiotics for several days during the preceding days or weeks. Such infections are always life-threatening and offer a very guarded to grave prognosis. The arrowhead points to the yeast organism. (Courtesy Dr. Jen Owen)

3.25a–h. Streptococcal toxic shock-like syndrome in a dog. This Terrier dog was admitted as an emergency after it had an animal encounter in the woods and subsequently became critically ill over the next 24 hours. Figures 3.25b–g are a sequence of images taken over 2 days showing how rapidly the tissue necrosis advanced despite immediate surgical débridement and parenteral antibiotics to cover *Streptococcus* sp. shortly after admission. Figure 3.25h shows the dog in the terminal stages of septic shock, when acute respiratory distress syndrome occurred and killed the dog.

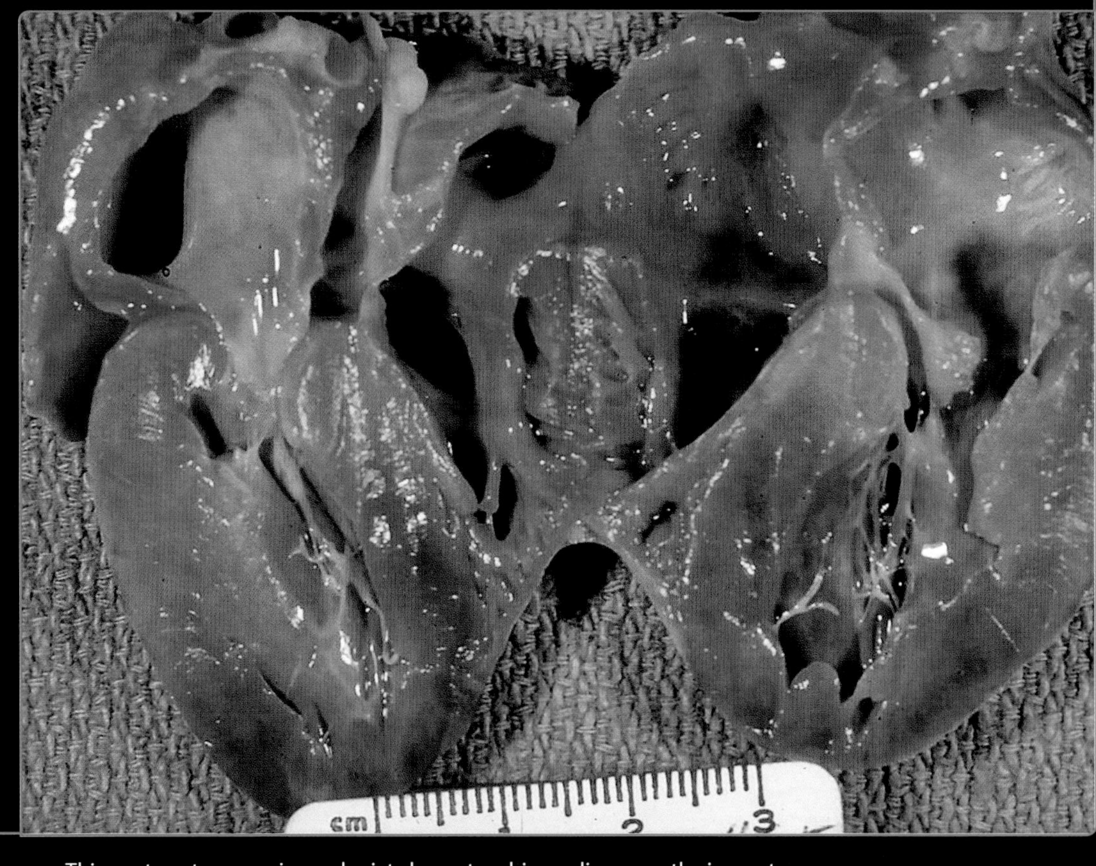

▲ This postmortem specimen depicts hypertrophic cardiomyopathy in a cat.

4

Cardiovascular disorders

CARDIO comes from the Greek word *kardia*, meaning heart. Cardiac disease presents with clinical signs that vary from the subtle to very dramatic. The physical signs can likewise vary, but when they reach a high degree of severity the patient can have severe respiratory distress from pulmonary edema, impaired circulating blood volume as can occur with pericardial effusion, abdominal distension from ascites, or perhaps acute arterial occlusion as occurs with a saddle thrombus. Most of the time the experienced clinician can identify the significance of these lesions, but the first encounter might be accompanied by some self-doubt. The potential lethal consequences of untreated heart disease demands early diagnosis, and most of these diseases can be diagnosed with a thorough history and physical examination, chest radiographs, and an electrocardiogram. With the discovery and application of echocardiography to clinical practice, the clinician can now appreciate the actual pathologic anatomy and abnormal function associated with cardiovascular disease during the early phase of the medical evaluation.

4 Cardiovascular disorders

- Cardiomegaly does not always cause tall ECG complexes.
- With proper placement of leads, a standing ECG can be performed, which will give good information regarding rate, rhythm, and interval measurements.
- Do not use beta-blockers until pulmonary edema resolves.
- Cats with heart disease rarely cough.
- Echocardiogram for diagnosing vegetative endocarditis.
- Heartworm treated dog at discharge: dispense prednisone and furosemide for the earliest signs of pulmonary thromboembolism.
- Many animals die without ever showing open-mouth breathing.

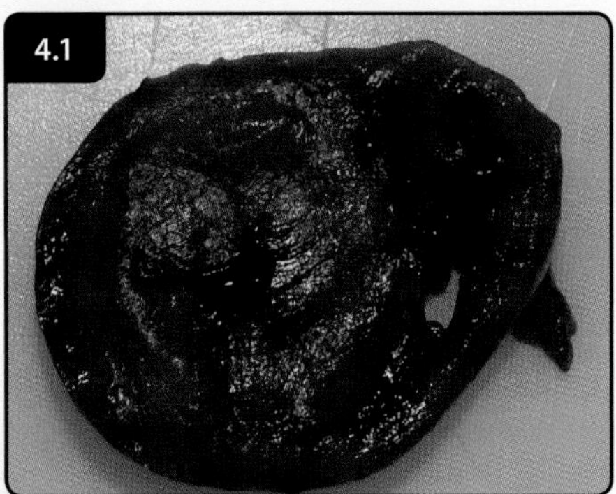

4.1. Endomyocarditis. This postmortem heart specimen is from a cat that presented in congestive heart failure. Note the hypertrophied left ventricle and the markedly compromised left ventricular lumen diameter because of the very thickened left ventricle. Histopathology described the lesion as endomyocarditis.

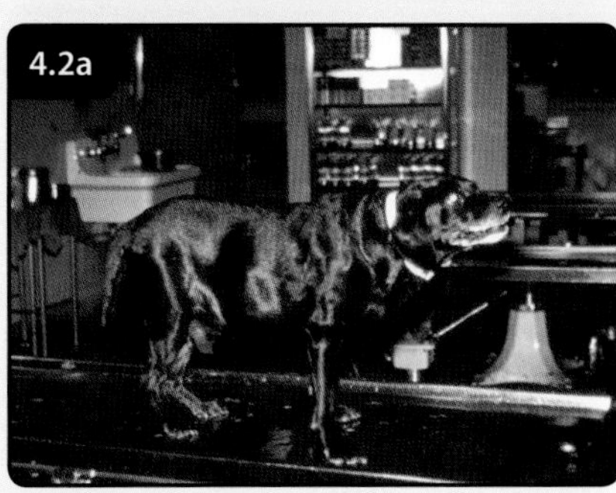

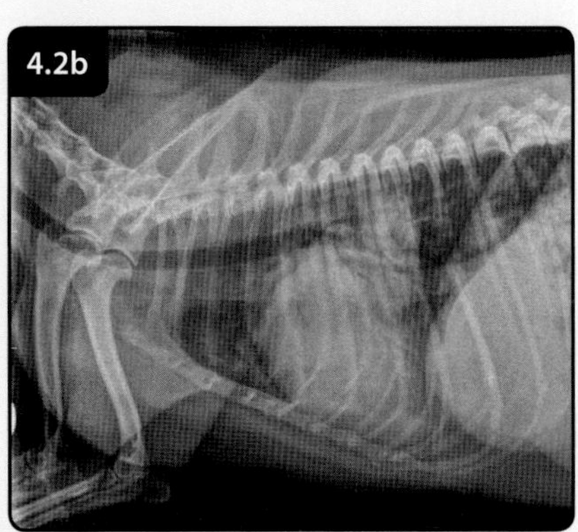

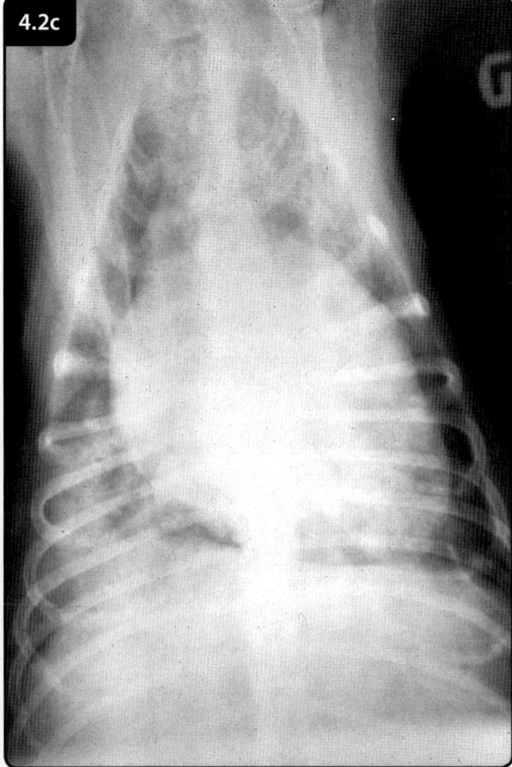

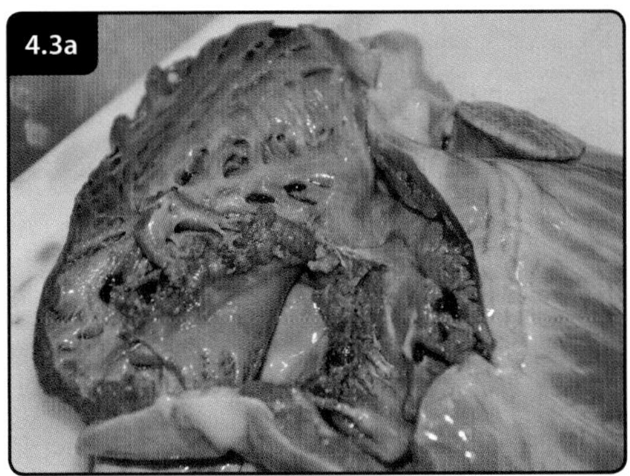

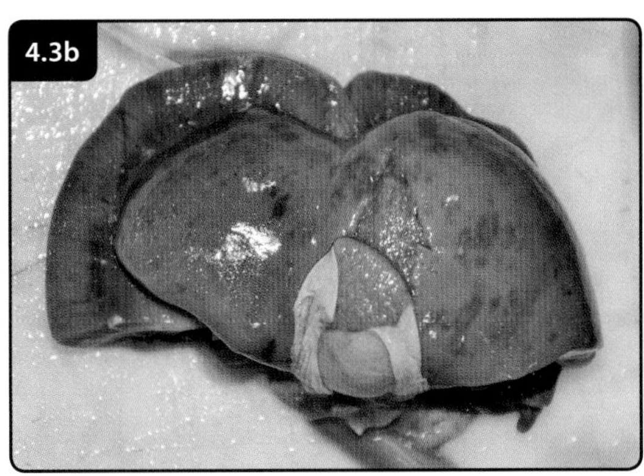

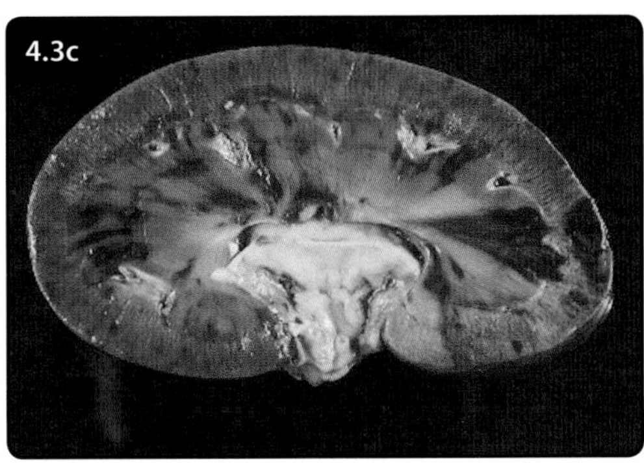

4.3a–c. Vegetative endocarditis. Animals affected with vegetative endocarditis can die from four main causes, namely sepsis, fatal emboli, cardiac arrhythmias, or congestive heart failure. This dog's mitral valve is totally destroyed and this probably led to its demise. The kidneys show the infarcts that were caused by emboli originating in the heart. Some patients can incur acute kidney injury from this insult.

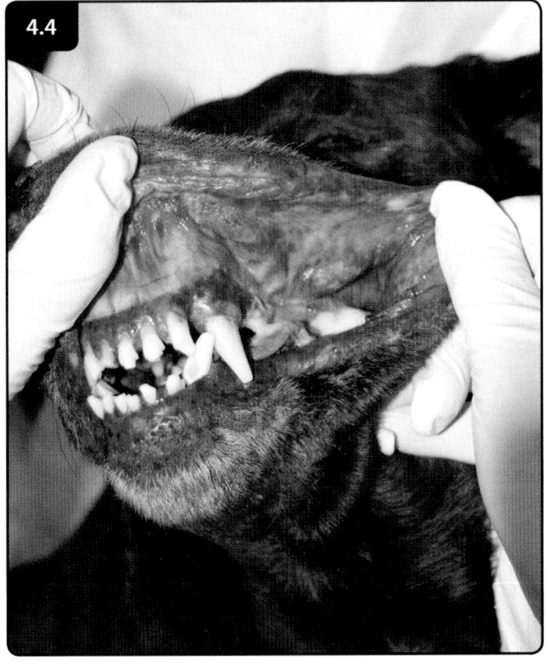

4.4. Hyperemia. The hyperemic oral mucous membranes in this dog represent the hyperdynamic phase of cardiac function as a result of sepsis. The pulses in this dog would be bounding and full. These signs characterize the first phase of septic shock, which is subsequently followed by the hypodynamic phase, which is characterized as a hypofunctioning heart and poorly perfused peripheral tissues and weak thready pulses.

4.2a–c. Congestive heart failure. This geriatric male Labrador Retriever shows posture typical of respiratory distress. He had a loud systolic murmur and a sinus tachycardia that was accompanied by diffusely moist lung sounds heard on auscultation. The thoracic radiographs show left heart enlargement and diffuse alveolar infiltrates typical of left-sided congestive heart failure. The elevated and split mainstem bronchi are a result of left atrial enlargement.

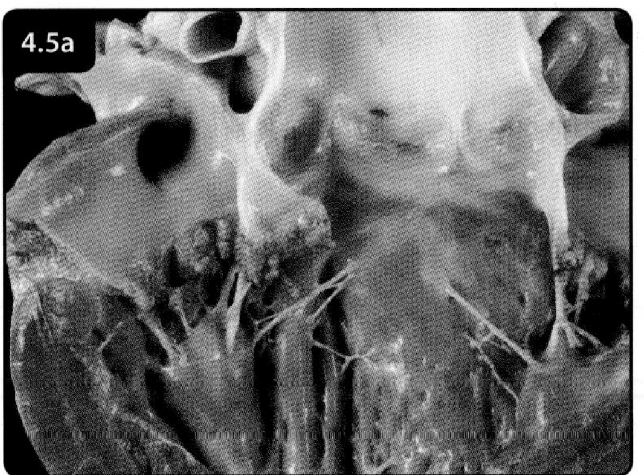

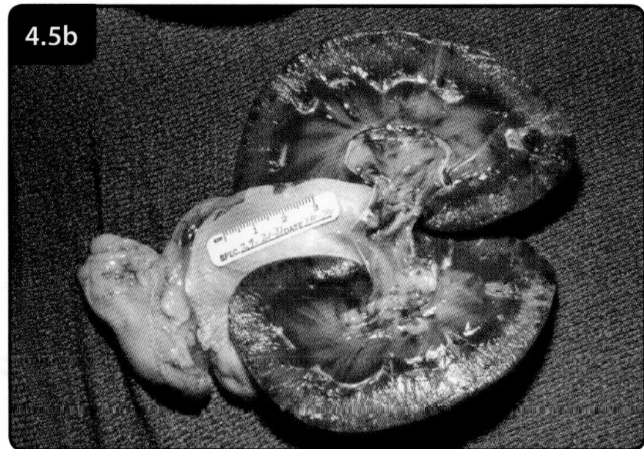

4.5a, b. Vegetative endocarditis and emboli. The vegetations on the atrioventricular valve can eventually cause tearing of the valve, thus causing fulminating left-sided congestive heart failure. The same can happen with an affected aortic valve. This kidney specimen shows evidence of an embolic shower caused by the release of vegetative fragments into the circulation. The bright red lesions represent more acute injury, and the result can be acute kidney injury.

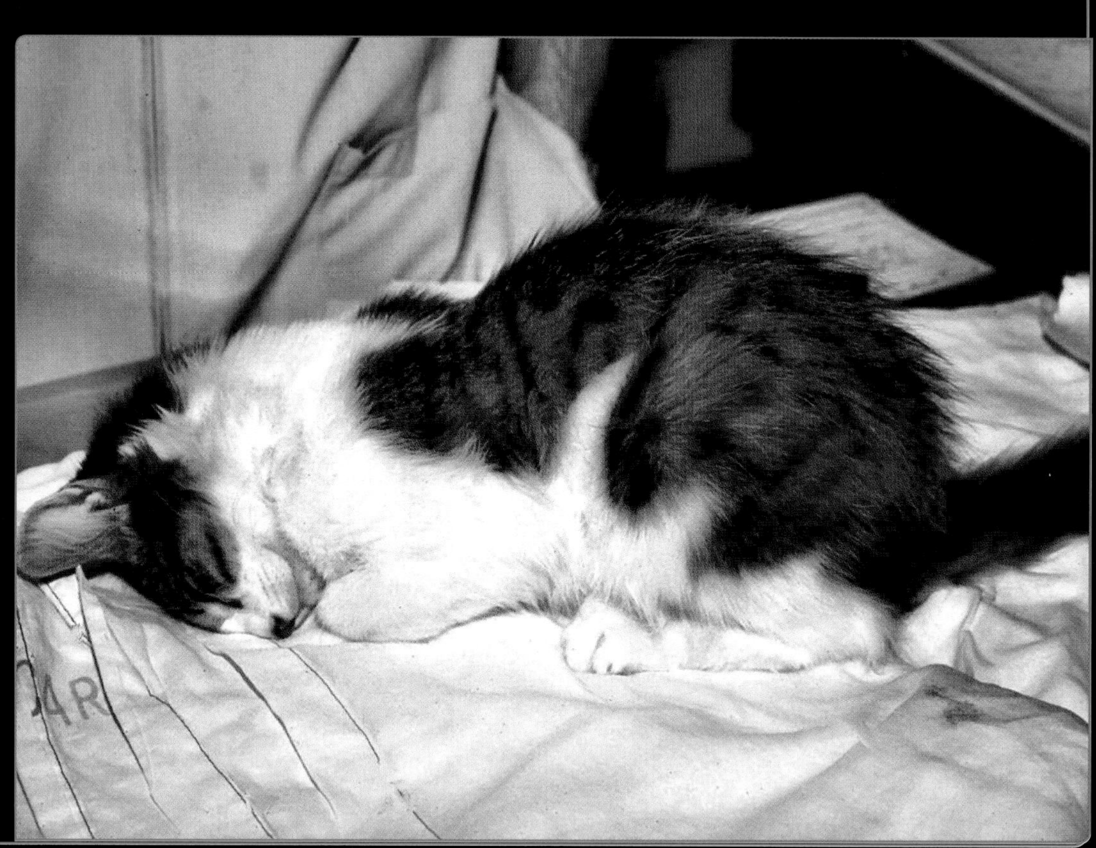

▲ This kitten is markedly weak because of hypokalemic myopathy.

5

Serum electrolyte disorders

The suffix 'lyte' is derived from the Greek word *lutos*, meaning soluble. In medicine, the term refers to a substance that can be decomposed by a specific process. In clinical medicine this would apply to a salt that dissolves in a fluid medium. The electrolytes are found in all body fluids, and they are the vital constituents of all cellular and tissue functions. The main electrolytes in the extracellular fluid (ECF) compartment are sodium, potassium (only 2% of total body potassium in ECF), chloride, magnesium, calcium, phosphorus, and bicarbonate, while the most important electrolytes in the intracellular fluid compartment include potassium (98% of total body potassium), magnesium, sodium (much less than the sodium in the ECF), phosphorus, and bicarbonate. Normally, the body maintains strict control of fluid and electrolyte homeostasis, and when disease disrupts this balance, severe consequences can occur to various organ systems.

The most important disruptions involve disorders in sodium, potassium, and calcium metabolism because hypo- and hypernatremia cause marked adverse effects on the brain, while hypo- and hyperkalemia cause adverse effects on the heart and skeletal muscle. Hypo- and hypercalcemia adversely affect membrane transport and neuromuscular integrity. The clinical examples found in this section illustrate the adverse effects of some of these clinical disorders. Luckily most of the disorders are amendable to treatment if caught early enough. Grave consequences await marked delays in diagnosis.

5 Serum electrolyte disorders

- Metabolic alkalosis plus hypokalemia common with upper GI obstructions.
- 0.9% NaCl plus KCl – best for treating upper GI obstructions.
- TCO_2 >40 mEq/l is always metabolic alkalosis (usually with hypokalemia).
- TCO_2 <10 mEq/l – usually means severe metabolic acidosis.
- When giving SC fluids avoid hypokalemia – add 3.5 mEq KCl/150 ml lactated Ringer's solution (LRS) and give SC (for adult sized cat).
- All intravenous maintenance fluids should contain 7–10 mEq KCl/250 ml; exceptions are oliguria and untreated addisonian crisis.
- Avoid tissue edema by restricting excess fluids with severe pulmonary, brain, and general trauma.
- To make up 2.5% dextrose solution increments, add 12.5 ml D-50-W to 250 ml of fluids or add 50 ml of D-50-W to a liter of isotonic crystalloid (LRS, NaCl).

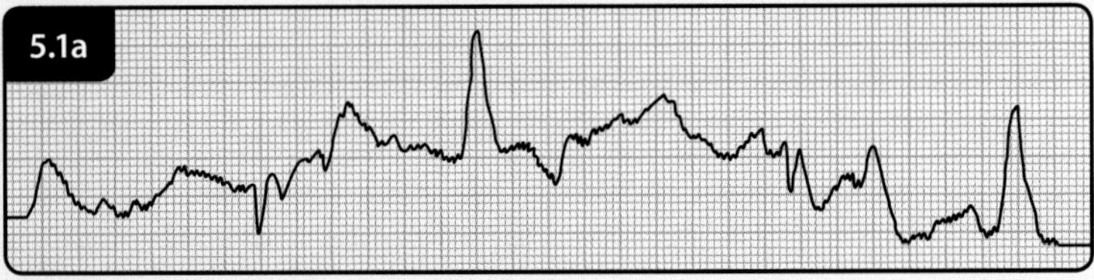

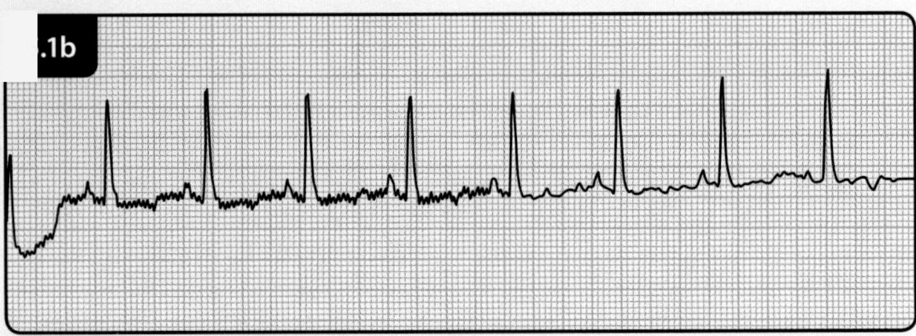

5.1a, b. Hyperkalemic cardiotoxicity. Figure 5.1a depicts a lead II ECG rhythm strip showing abnormal ventricular conduction (accelerated idioventricular conduction) associated with marked hyperkalemia (normal 3.5–5.5 mEq/l [3.5–5.5 mmol/l]). The cat associated with this life-threatening situation had urethral obstruction with hyperkalemia. Serum potassium levels over 7.0 mEq/l (7.0 mmol/l) typically show this cardiac abnormality before progressing to ventricular fibrillation and cardiac arrest. This cardiac abnormality is associated with the heart muscle being in a sustained depolarized state. Treatment for the hyperkalemia alone involves administration of intravenous isotonic crystalloid solutions, along with calcium gluconate, +/- insulin and dextrose, +/- sodium bicarbonate. Beta-adrenergic drugs can also counteract the cardiotoxicity. Figure 5.1b shows the return of normal cardiac conduction several hours after treatment. Sixty cycle interference due to background electrical activity from the ECG machine is also present. This is causing artifactual waves in the early complexes.

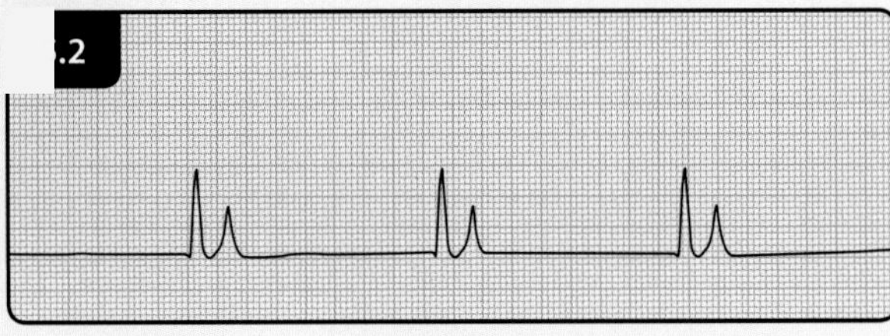

5.2. Hyperkalemic cardiotoxicity. This lead II rhythm strip from a 9-month-old male Dalmation experiencing an addisonian crisis shows atrial standstill defined as bradycardia and absent p waves. The same treatment as described in Case 5.1 above, in addition to glucocorticoid and mineralocorticoid drugs, would be indicated for this dog.

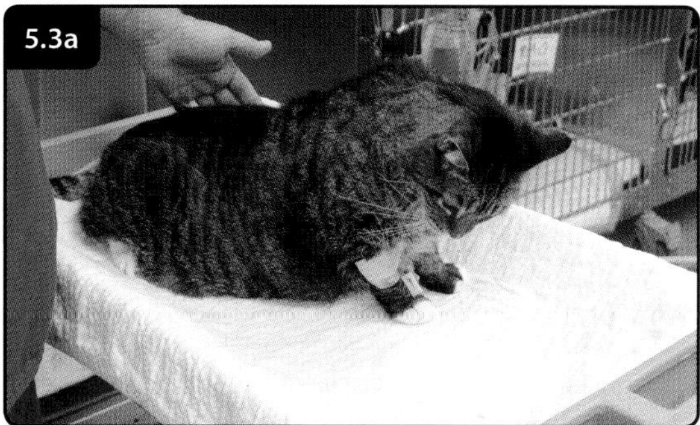

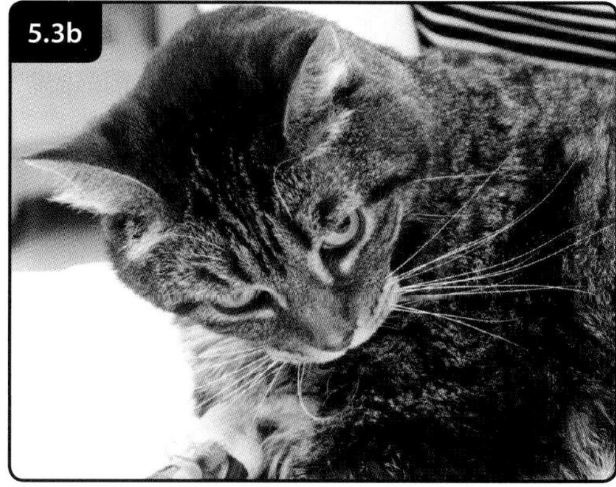

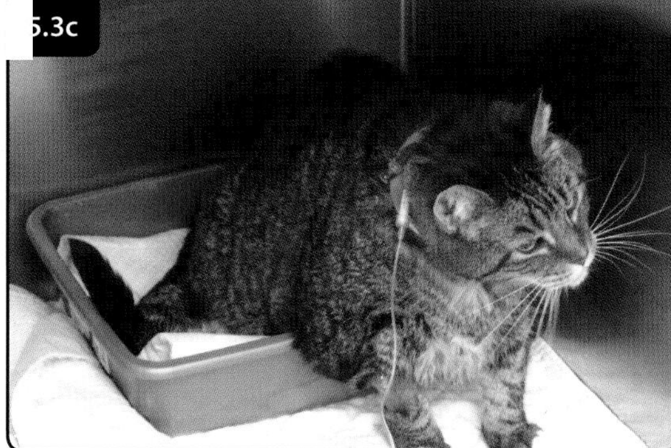

5.3a–c. Hypokalemic myopathy in a cat. This cat postures with flaccid ventral cervical flexion and generalized muscular weakness (Figures 5.3a, b) associated with hypokalemia (serum potassium = 2.8 mEq/l [2.8 mmol/l]; normal = 3.5–5.5 mEq/l [3.5–5.5 mmol/l]). The cat showed significant improvement in neuromuscular function after it received approximately 8 mEq of KCl/kg body weight intravenously over a 24-hour period (Figure 5.3c).

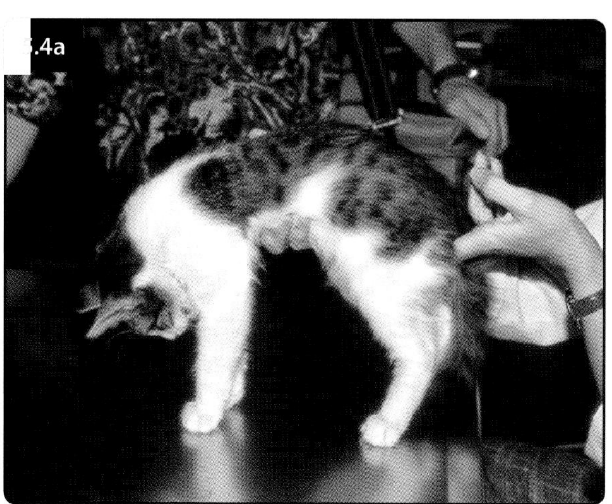

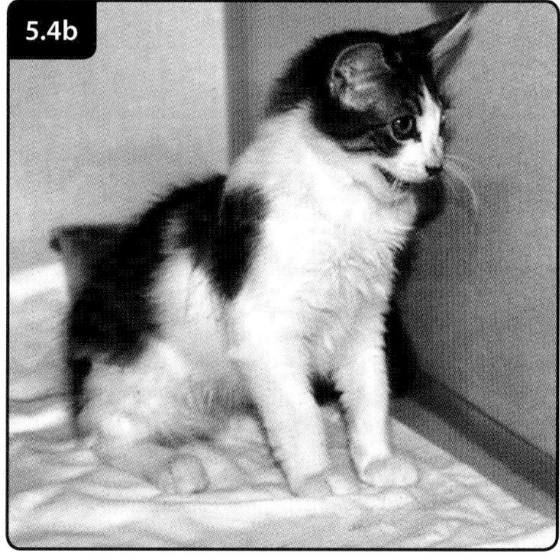

5.4a, b. Hypokalemic myopathy in a cat. This kitten also has hypokalemic myopathy that was associated with a potassium deficient diet. The weakness is due to a hyperpolarized myoneural junction, which can go on to a depolarized state. Overnight potassium chloride administration produced a return to normal function by the next day.

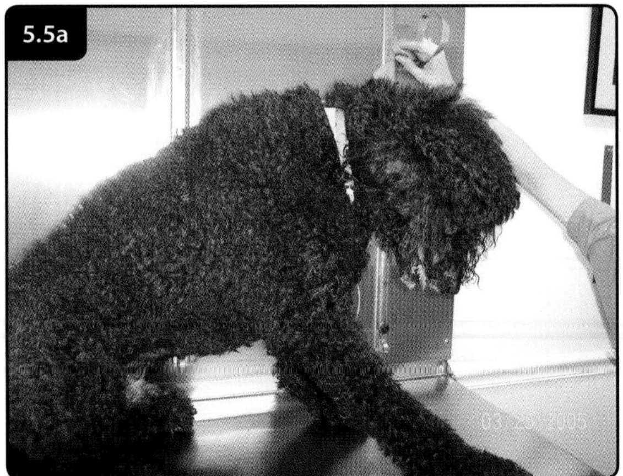

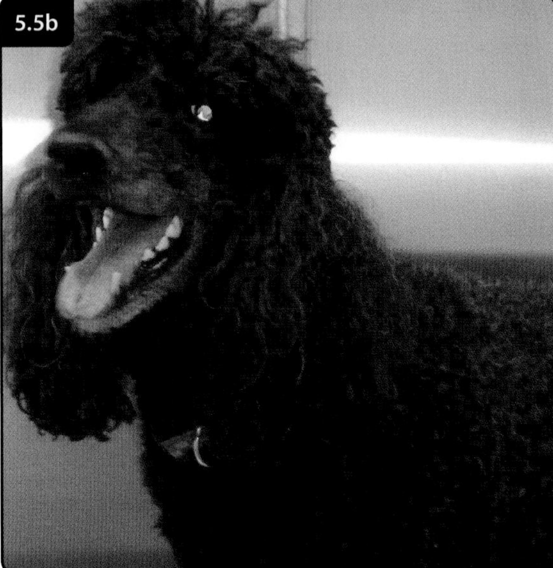

5.5a, b. Hypokalemic myopathy in a dog. These before and after images show a Standard Poodle with hypokalemic myopathy that resolved after it received potassium chloride supplementation in its intravenous fluids. It was caused by too large a dose of deoxycorticosterone pivalate (DOCP). Treatment was continued with oral potassium chloride until the effects of the DOCP lessened over the following 2 weeks.

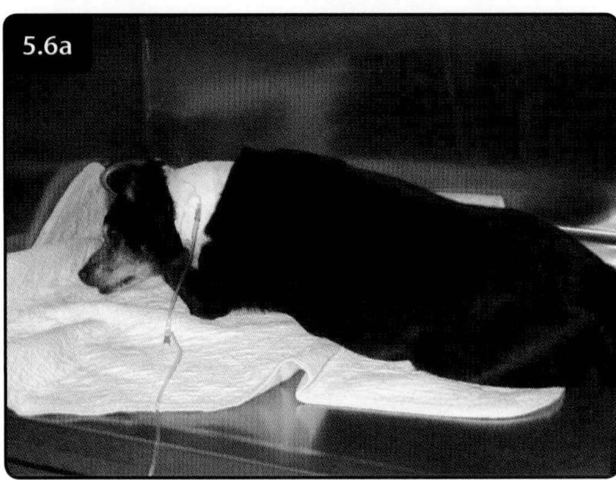

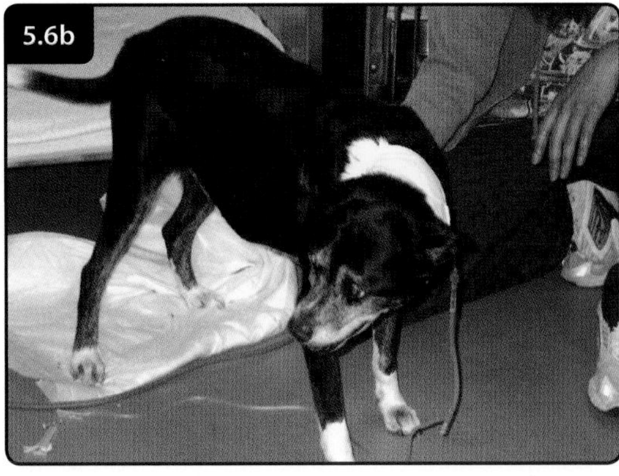

5.6a, b. Hypokalemic myopathy in a diabetic dog. The kaliuresis that can occur with untreated diabetes mellitus can cause myasthenia in dogs and cats. This dog was probably weak from several factors associated with its ketoacidosis, but a potassium level of <3.0 mEq/l (<3.0 mmol/l) was highly contributory. Figure 5.6b shows a dramatically improved patient after normokalemia was restored.

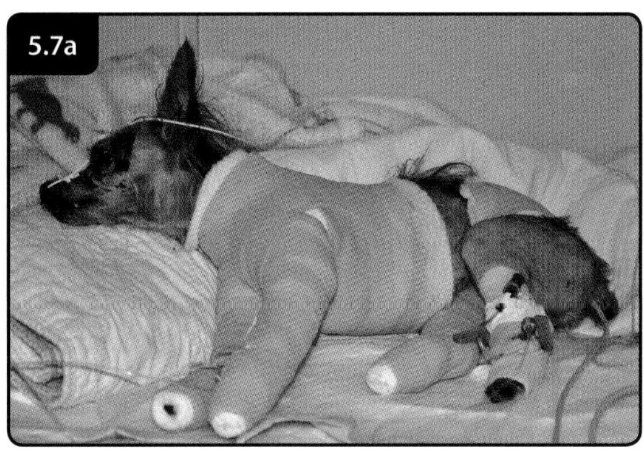

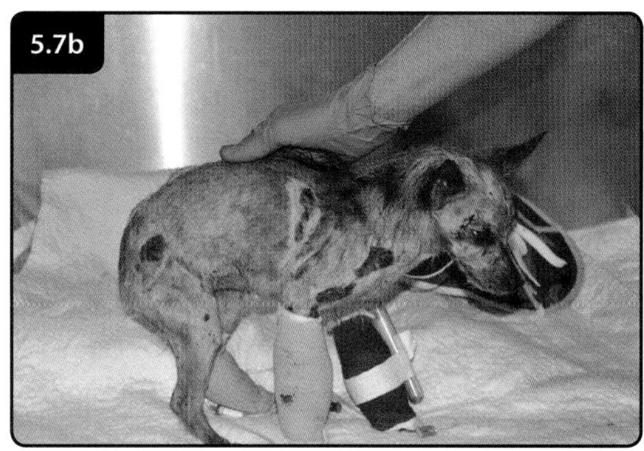

5.7a, b. Hypernatremic encephalopathy. This dog acquired diabetes insipidus after head trauma disrupted the production or secretory pathway of antidiuretic hormone (ADH; vasopressin). The water diuresis in the absence of adequate compensatory drinking caused hypernatremia (serum sodium 171 mEq/l [171 mmol/l]) and hypertonic encephalopathy, which produced a comatose state. Slow-onset hypernatremia requires the administration of hypotonic intravenous solutions slowly over a 72-hour period. Administering desmopressin acetate (DDAVP®) as a replacement for ADH will assist with water conservation at the distal renal tubule and collecting duct. The dog responded well to this treatment over a 3-day period (serum sodium 144 mEq/l [144 mmol/l]).

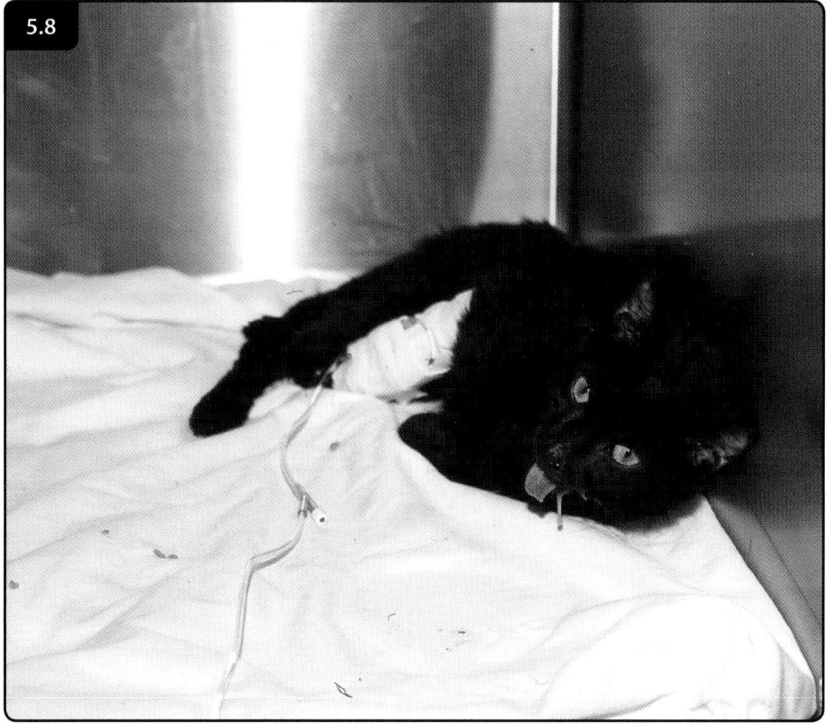

5.8. Hypernatremia in a cat. This cat had severe sublingual muscular hypertrophy from Duchenne's muscular dystrophy that interfered with its ability to drink. The desiccation caused the serum sodium to increase to >180 mEq/l (>180 mmol/l), which required a slow return to normonatremia over the next 72 hours using hypotonic intravenous fluids. Slow-onset hypernatremia must not be corrected any more rapidly than 8–12 mEq/l (mmol/l) per 24 hours in order to avoid fatal cerebral edema.

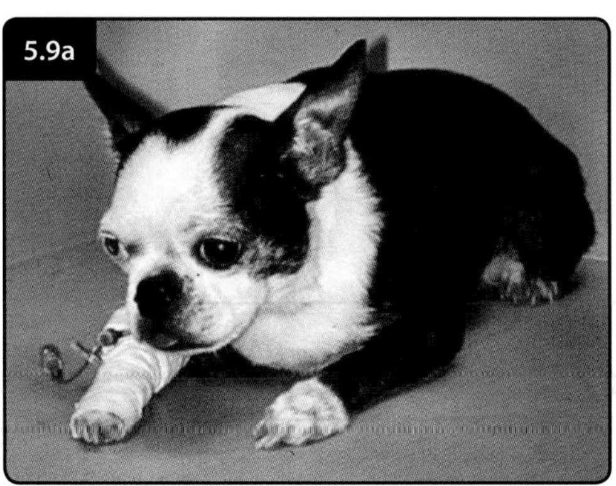

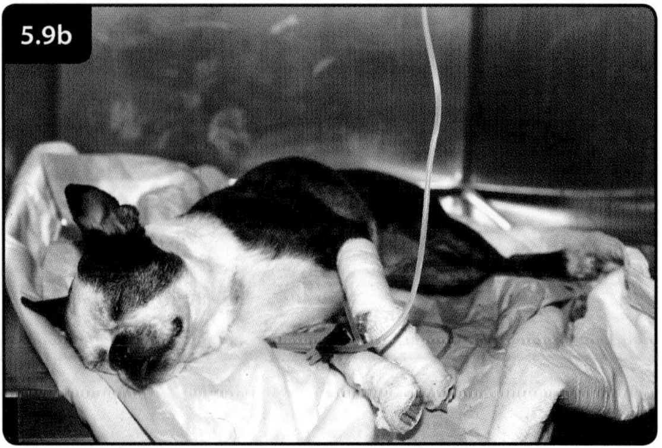

5.9a, b. Hyponatremic encephalopathy in a dog. This Boston Terrier had Addison's disease and a serum sodium concentration of 110 mEq/l (110 mmol/l). The sodium level was inadvertently increased to 134 mEq/l (134 mmol/l) over the next 24 hours, which caused the dog to lapse into a coma from central pontine myelinosis (osmotic disequilibrium syndrome). Brain function remained abnormal after 2 weeks and the owner had the dog euthanized. More time might have brought about more improvement. Slow-onset hyponatremia (i.e. that occurs over 48 or more hours) should be corrected slowly over a 48–72-hour period at a rate not exceeding 8–12 mEq/l (8–12 mmol/l) per 24 hours.

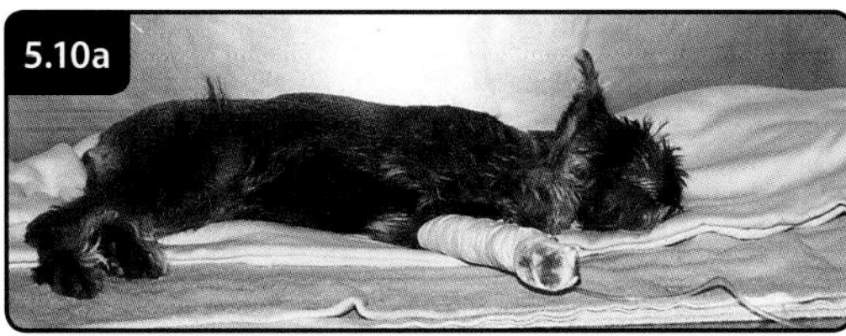

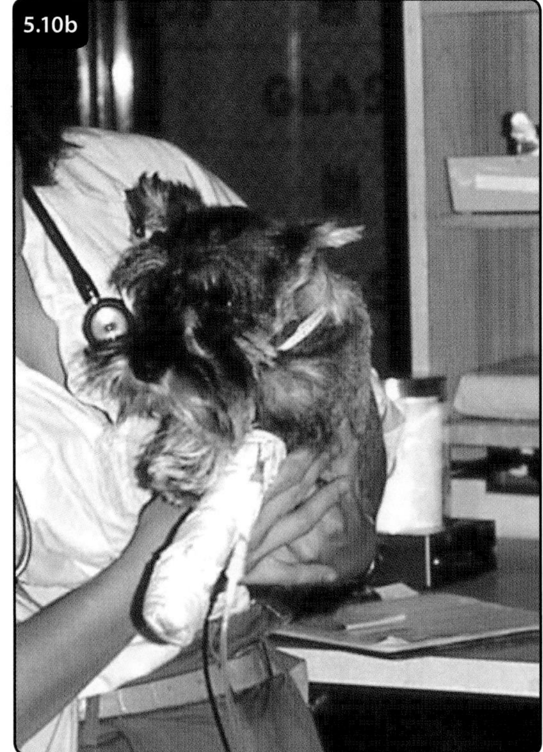

5.10a, b. Essential hypernatremia in a young Schnauzer. This dog presented in a coma because of its serum sodium measuring 190 mEq/l (190 mmol/l) owing to essential hypernatremia. This condition occurs when the thalamic supraoptic and paraventricular nuclei do not respond to increases in serum osmolality with increased antidiuretic hormone (ADH) secretion. There is also an accompanying hypodipsia. Normally, ADH secretion responds to as little as a 3% increase in serum osmolality. As a result, the serum sodium increases and the patient lapses into a life-threatening hypertonic encephalopathy. The slow onset of disease requires a slow correction in the serum sodium level over a 72-hour period of time. The daily decrease should not exceed 10–12 mEq/l (10–12 mmol/l) per 24 hours through the administration of hypotonic saline or dextrose in water solution. This dog improved by day 3. Its long-term water requirements were met by adding its calculated daily water needs to its moist dog food diet.

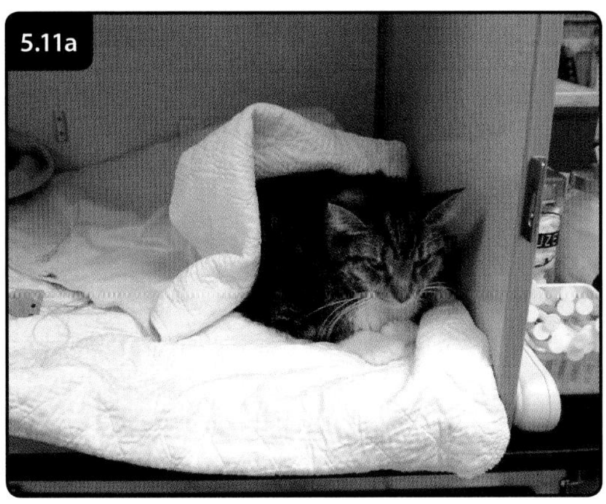

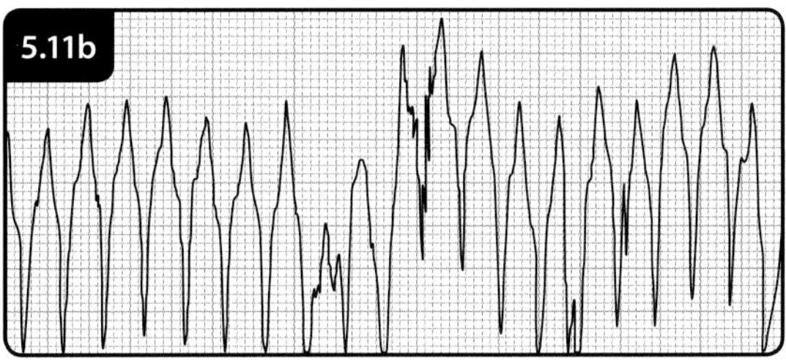

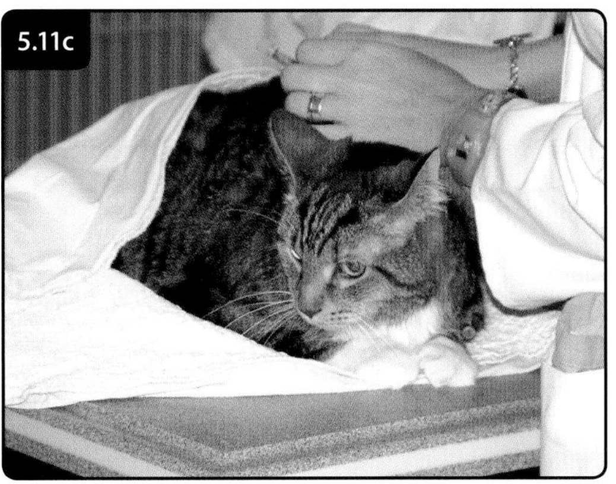

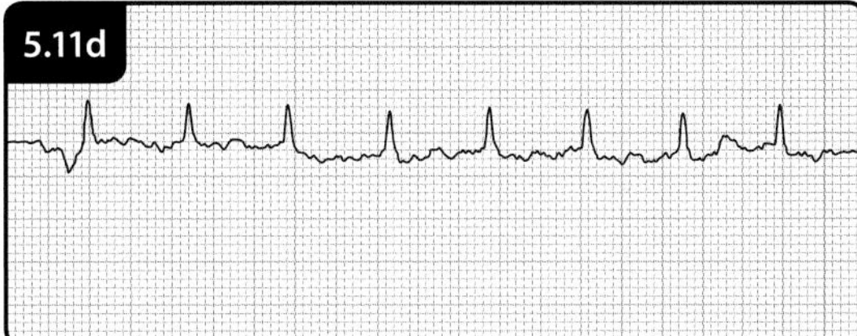

5.11a–d. Hypokalemia in a diabetic cat. On admission (Figure 5.11a) this diabetic cat had marked hypokalemic-induced ventricular tachycardia (Figure 5.11b). Treatment with intravenous lactated Ringer's solution with added potassium chloride at 60 mEq/l (60 mmol/l) brought about a marked improvement in the cat and its ECG pattern. Insulin therapy should be delayed for 12–18 hours under these circumstances because it will further drive extracellular potassium into the cells, which will cause further lowering of the serum potassium concentration.

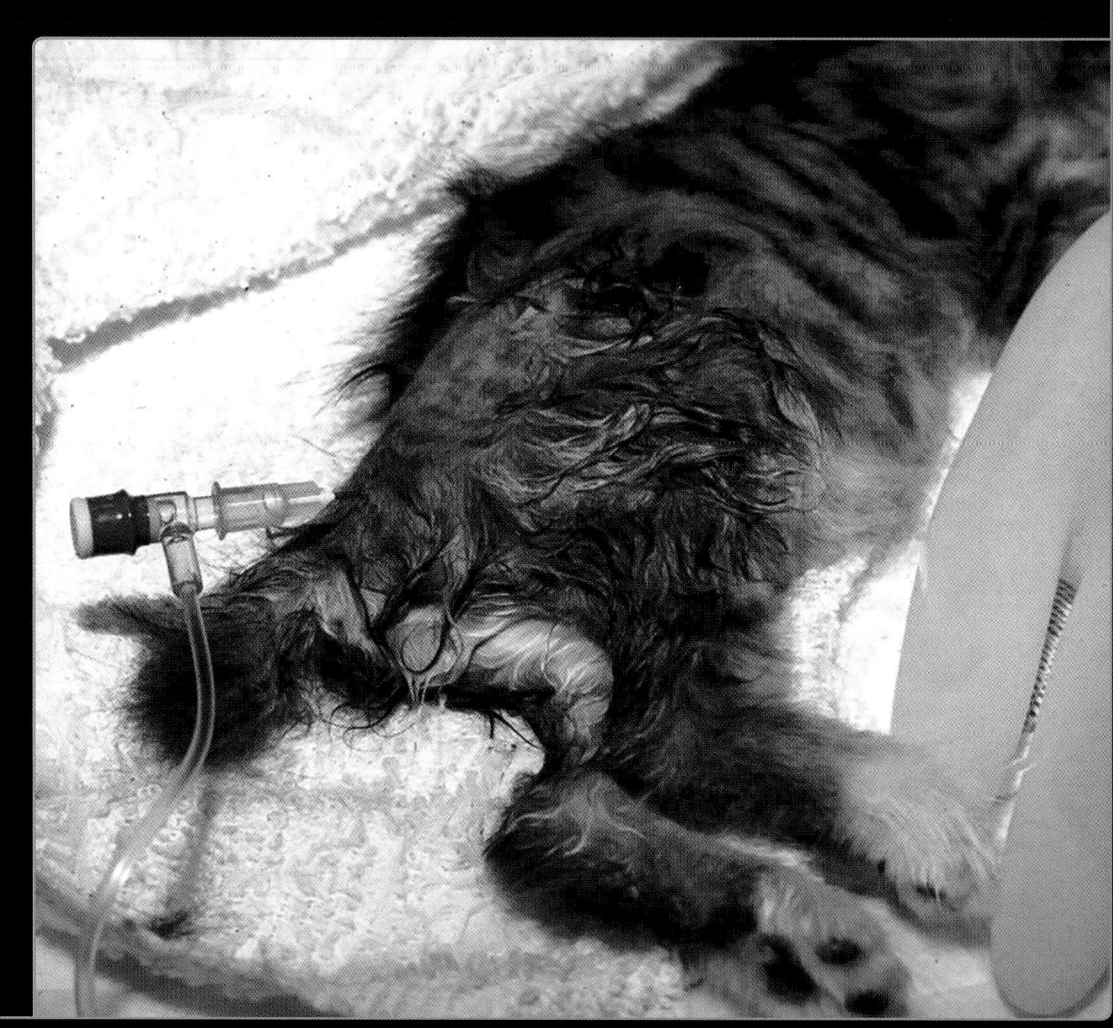

▲ This kitten is being administered parenteral fluids intraosseously using a 20 gauge needle.

6

Fluid therapy complications

There are several definitions of the word 'fluid'. Merriam-Webster describes fluid as: 'having particles that move and easily change their relative position without a separation of the mass and that easily yield to pressure: capable of flowing.' Because the total body water of most land mammals ranges between 50% and 70% of the body weight, depending on age and body fat content, it is no surprise that disturbances in fluid physiology can have a major impact on the host. There are two major fluid compartments in the body: intracellular, comprising 65% of the total body water; and extracellular, comprising 35% with three-quarters comprising the interstitial space and one-quarter the intravascular space. In clinical medicine, we are usually more focused on disorders of the extracellular space because of our frequent encounters with dehydration and hypovolemia, but disorders involving intracellular water can have devastating consequences in an organ such as the brain.

To accomplish most of our therapeutic objectives in critically-ill patients, intravenous catheters are often used to deliver the fluid and electrolyte deficits and to provide for maintenance fluid needs. Unfortunately, there are inherent complications associated with catheters and the medications they might deliver. The main complications include catheter-related infections, thromboses, and cannula dislodgement in the blood vessel becoming an embolus. This section will illustrate some of these conditions.

6 Fluid therapy complications

- Subcutaneous fluid administration – isotonic, 18 gauge needle for animal >5.0 kg, gravity flow.
- Intraosseous cannulas can be life-saving.
- A heparinized syringe might contain as much as 200 units heparin – too much for puppies and kittens.
- Subcutaneous fluid administration – stay behind the scapula and in front of the wing of the ilium. Use 18 gauge needle and 50 ml/site (adult cat).

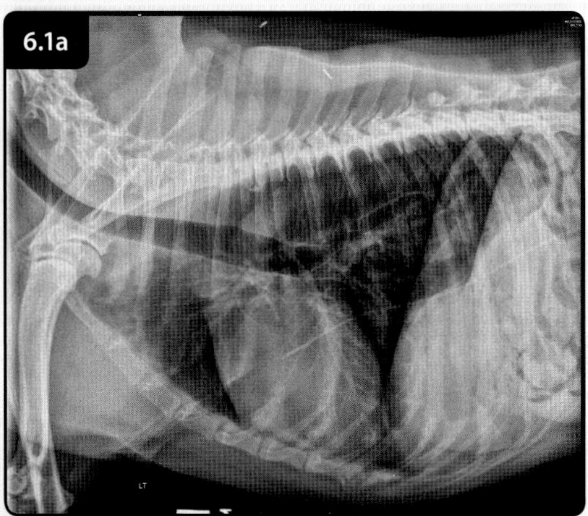

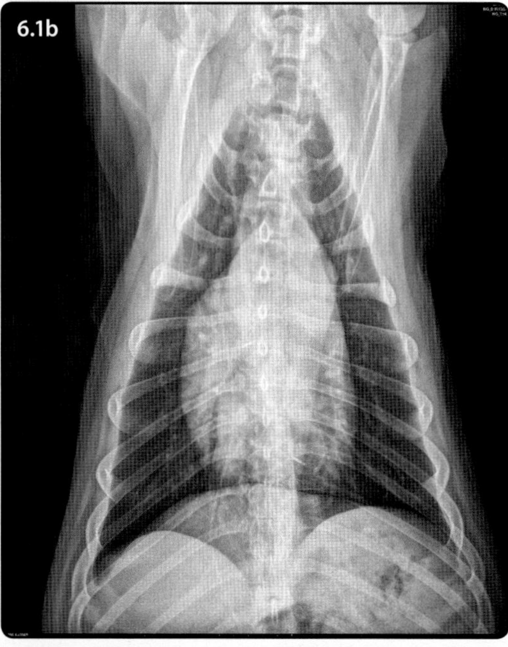

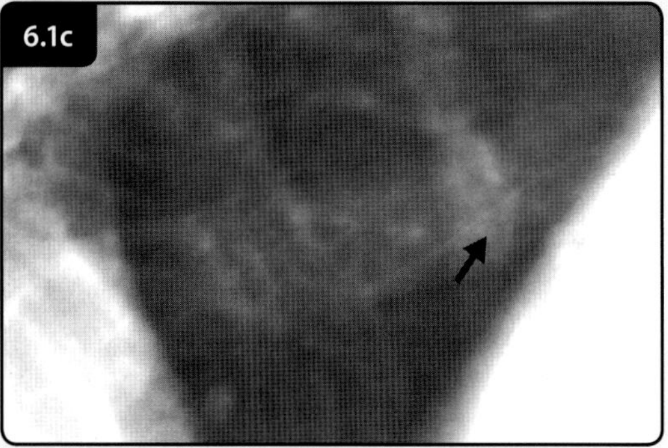

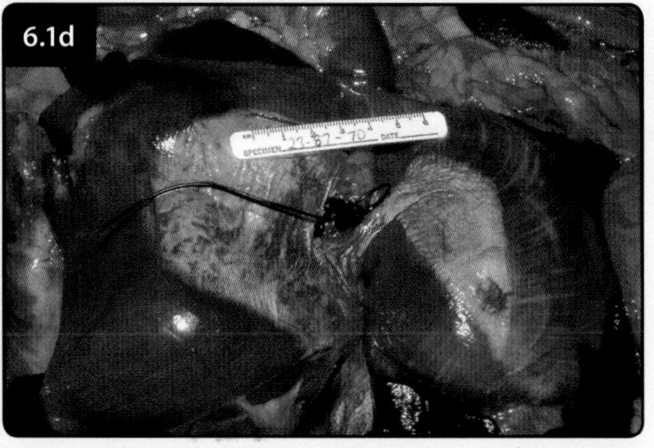

6.1a–d. Intravenous catheter embolus. This iatrogenic condition creates the obvious nightmare for all parties concerned. The embolus can occur in any major vessel that contains the catheter. Figures 6.1a, b show a dislodged peripherally inserted central catheter that fragmented off the main line and migrated into a pulmonary artery. Intra-arterial thrombus formation is a likely sequela. Associated clinical signs will vary, but all clinicians feel obligated to attempt its removal, if feasible. Figure 6.1c show a jugular catheter embolus in the caudal vena cava (arrow). There will often be a thrombus formed around the catheter, as occurred in this necropsy specimen (Figure 6.1d).

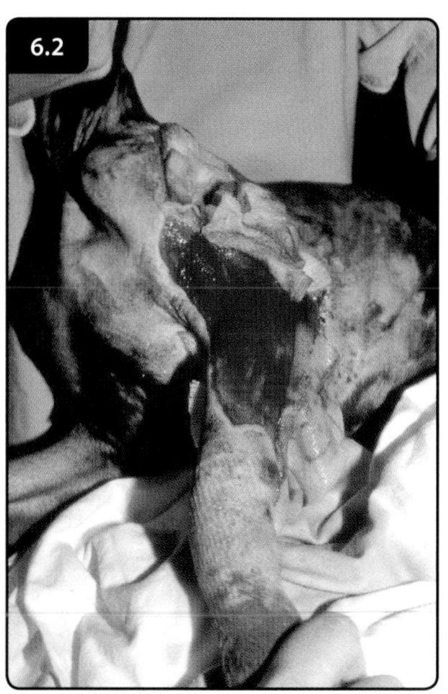

6.2. Subcutaneous fluid-induced tissue slough. The sloughed shoulder skin of this Dobermann puppy occurred because an excessive deposit of subcutaneous fluids was given at this site. Such large deposits can disrupt the hypodermal blood vessels and compromise tissue perfusion. In general, subcutaneous fluids should not be deposited over the region of the scapula or the pelvis because the fluid will gravitate down the appendage, where it is poorly accommodated.

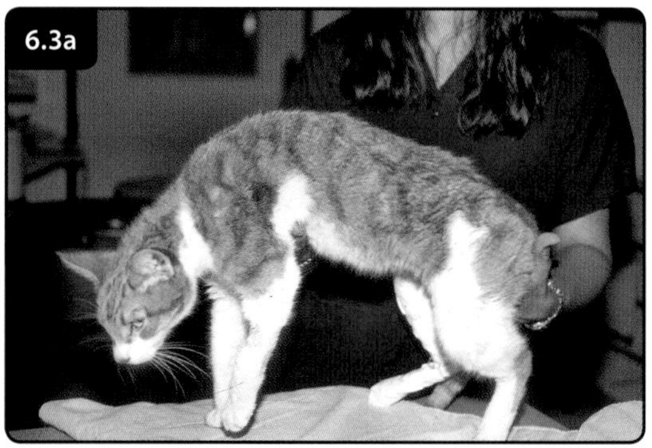

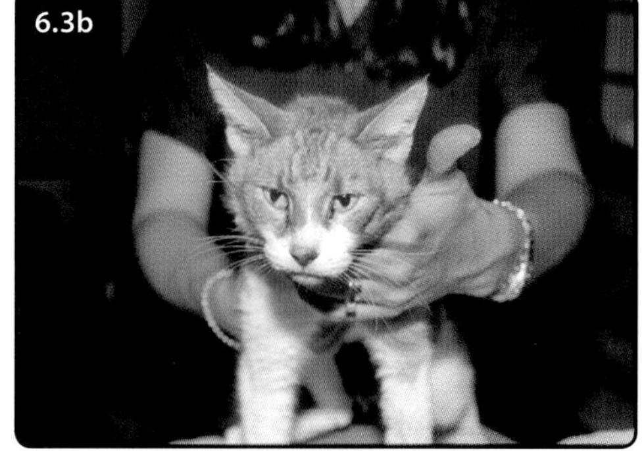

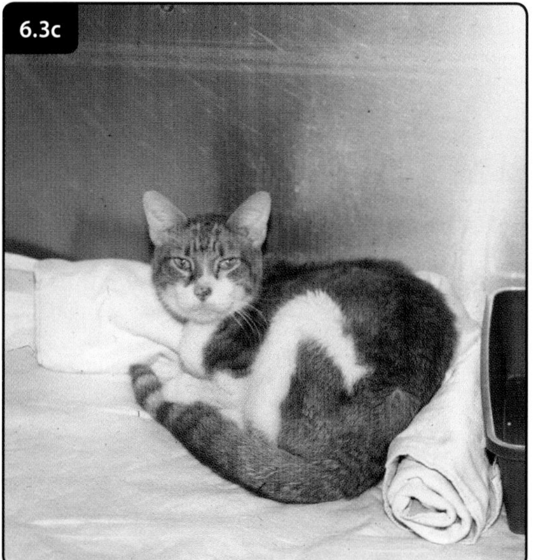

6.3a–c. Dehydrated cat. Cats show minimal tolerance for dehydration. This patient was dehydrated from decompensated chronic kidney disease and showed typical signs of moderate dehydration with skin tenting, third eyelid protrusion, and retracted eyes in sockets (Figures 6.3a, b). Clinical signs of improvement were readily apparent after rehydration with intravenous isotonic fluid administration (Figure 6.3c).

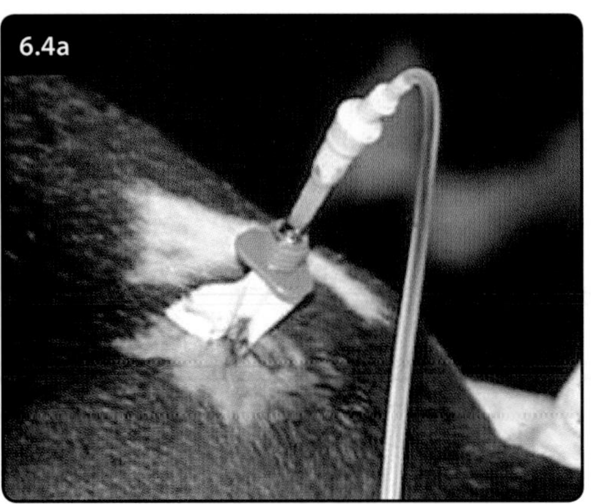

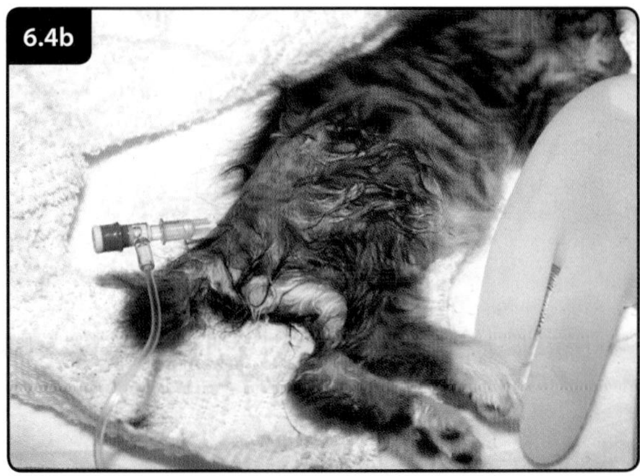

6.4a, b. Intraosseous (IO) fluid administration. The Basset Hound in Figure 6.4a is being volume resuscitated using a Jamshidi bone marrow needle. After being hit by a car, there were repeated failed attempts to place an intravenous catheter, which was remedied by using an IO needle. Administering fluids into the bone marrow is just like depositing them in a large vein. Figure 6.4b shows a modification of the technique for a 0.5 kg kitten where a simple 20 gauge needle functioned perfectly as an IO needle. It is important to make a small skin nick incision to prevent a skin plug from blocking the needle orifice. The IO needle can be replaced with the usual intravenous catheter and insertion site once the patient is stable. Most medications that are administered intravenously can also be given IO.

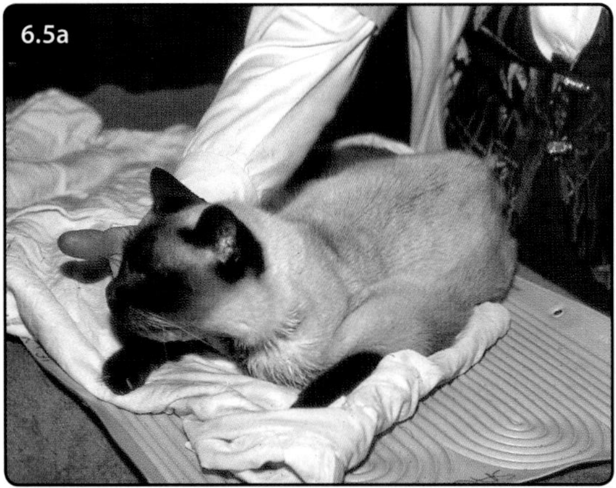

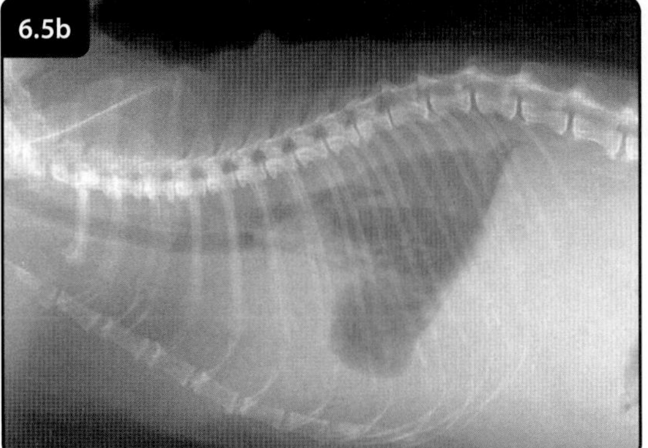

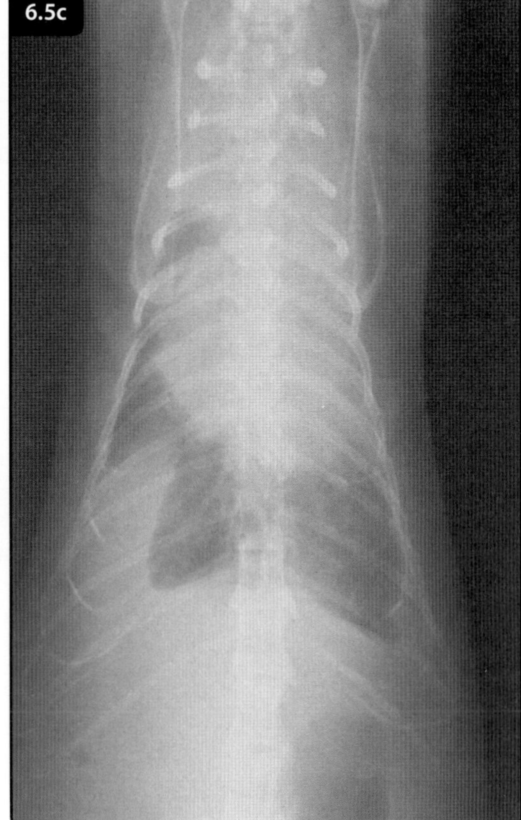

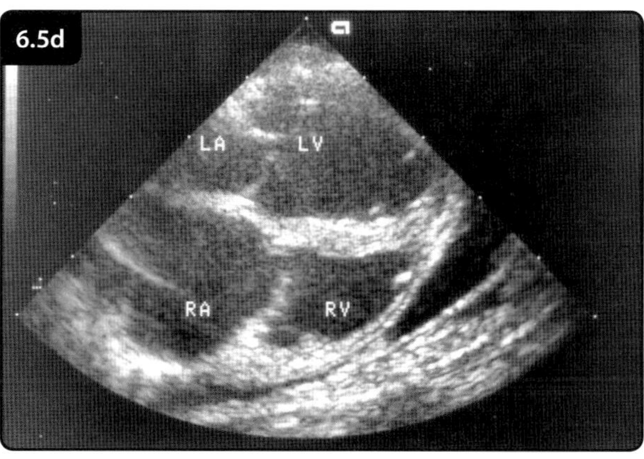

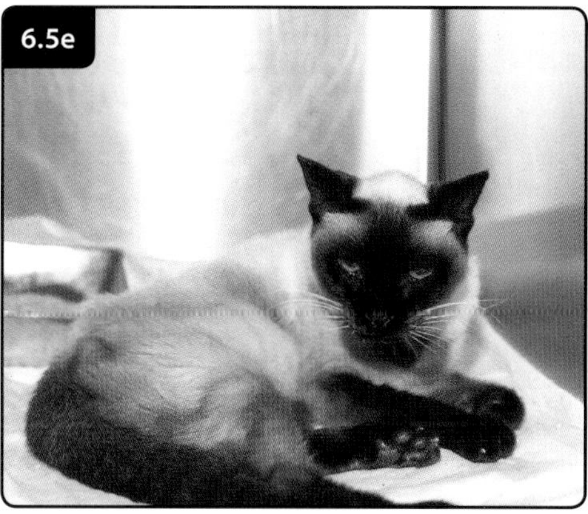

6.5a–e. Intravenous fluid overload. This Siamese cat (Figure 6.5a) was treated with "lots of fluids" for her severe flea bite anemia. As a result of the excess fluid accumulation, she showed overt signs of overload including 'spongy skin' along with intrathoracic effusion, which was pure transudate. Fresh whole blood or packed red blood cells in saline is what she really needed. This was administered slowly over several hours because of her overload condition, while all other fluids were restricted. Thoracic radiographs (Figures 6.5b, c) showed cardiac enlargement from the fluid overload, but the wall structure was normal on echocardiogram (Figure 6.5d). Figure 6.5e shows a clinically improved cat that no longer shows signs of fluid overload.

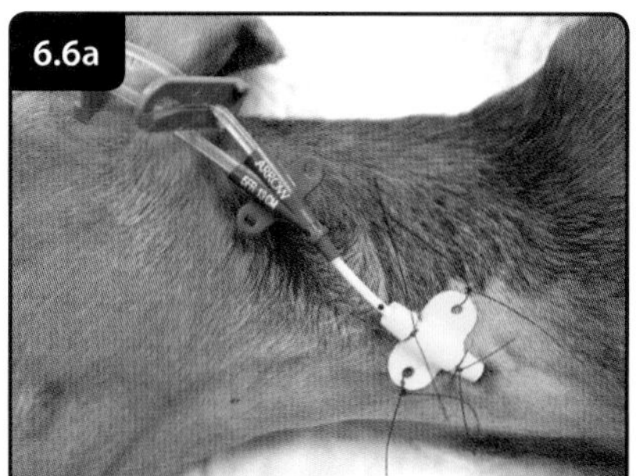

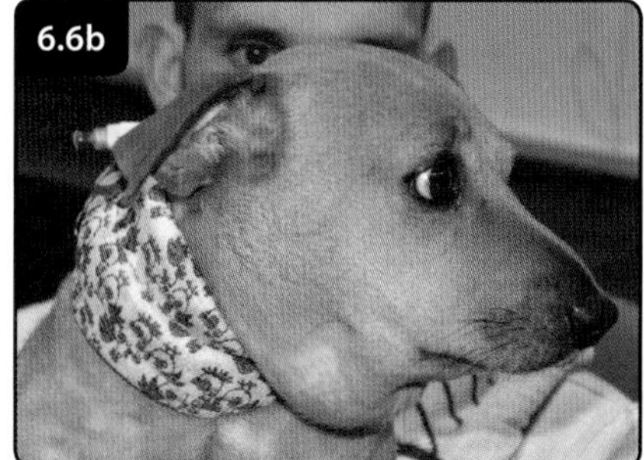

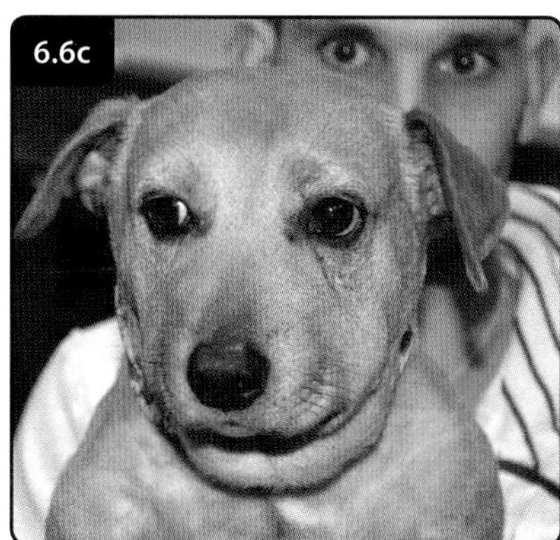

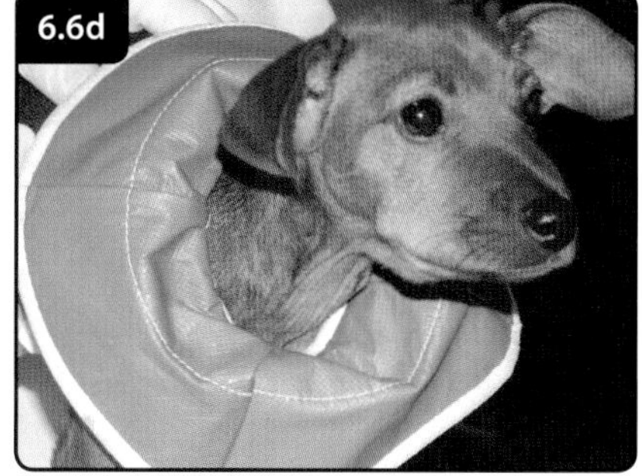

6.6a–d. Cranial vena cava syndrome. This dog had acute kidney injury and was treated with dialysis through a jugular vein hemodialysis catheter (Figure 6.6a). After 1 week of treatment, the dog's head developed pitting edema as a result of a cranial vena cava thrombus that developed from the intravenous dialysis catheter (Figures 6.6b, c). There was no sign of phlebitis, but catheter removal was essential. Over the next few days the fluid slowly resorbed (Figure 6.6d) and the venous drainage became re-established.

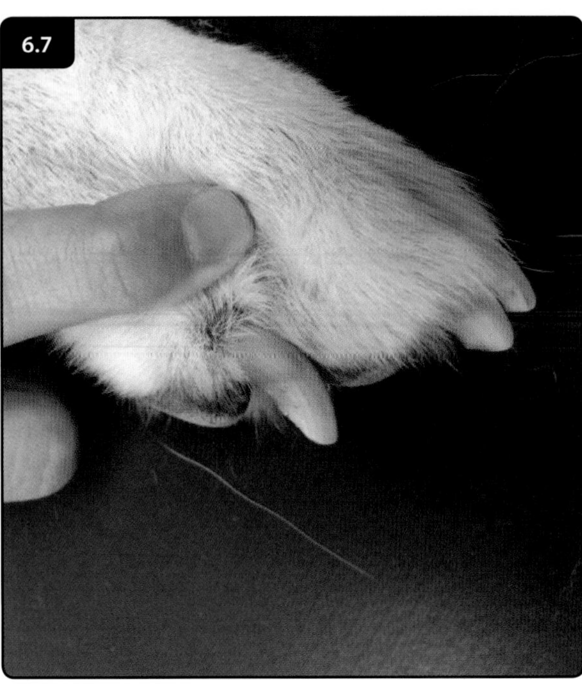

6.7. Poor perfusion. The digits on this paw have a mildly cyanotic hue because of poor peripheral perfusion that was due to hypovolemia from hemorrhagic gastroenteritis. The dog's packed cell volume was approximately 60% (0.6 l/l). Bolus intravenous crystalloid treatment, giving 20 ml/kg every 15 minutes for 4 boluses, restored the normal vital signs and the nail beds returned to their normal pink color.

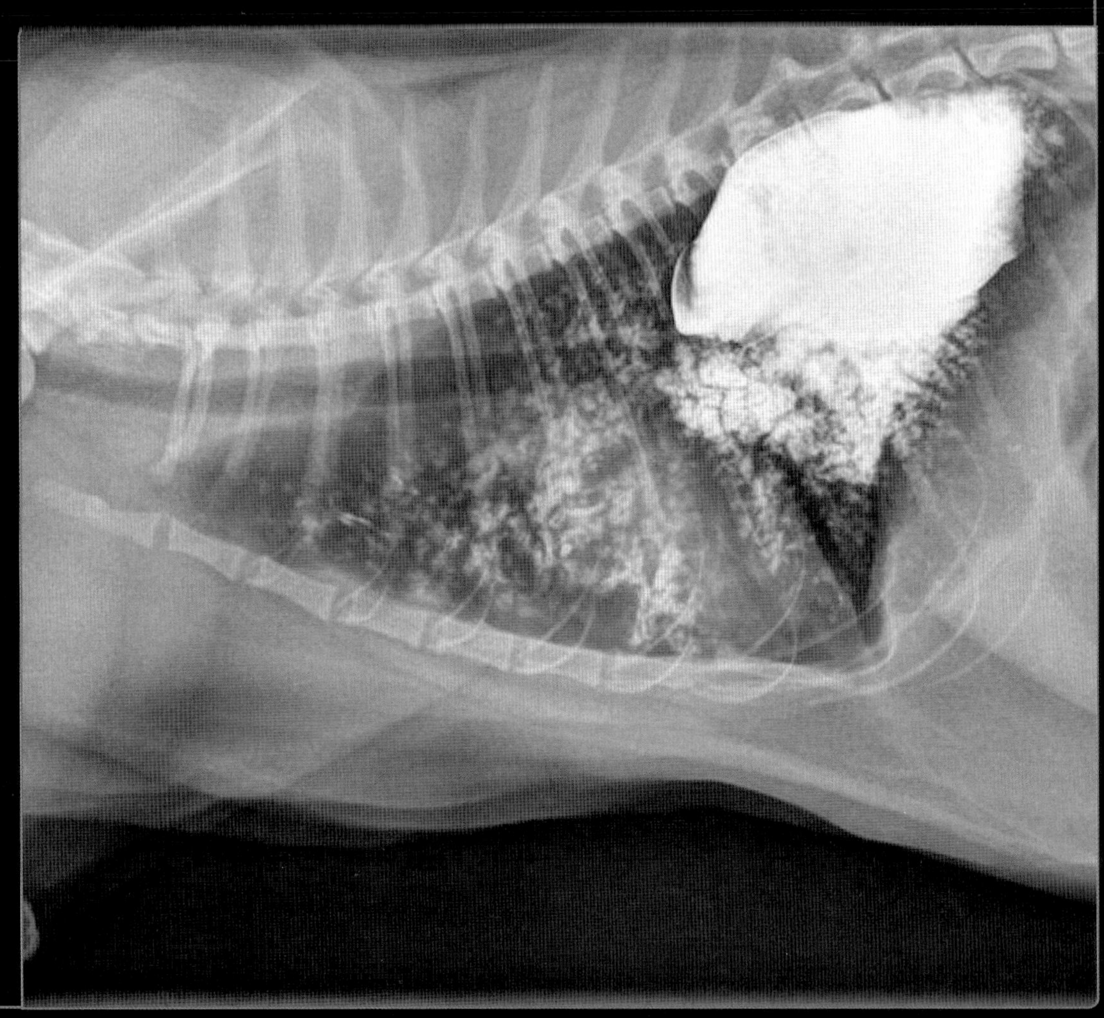

▲ This radiograph shows severe aspiration pneumonia associated with a barium swallow procedure.

7

Respiratory disorders

RESPIRATION is derived from the Latin word *respirare*, meaning breathe again. The various clinical disorders of respiration can vary from those that are relatively minor to those that are life-threatening. It behoves the clinician to have a sound understanding of the pathophysiology of these disorders, because life-saving treatment might depend on it. Above all, the clinician should remember that the airway must be patent and that oxygen must be available at all times. It is also essential to remember that the two main functional disorders are defects in ventilation and defects in perfusion. The ability to recognize this in the patient will dictate the diagnostic and therapeutic plan. This is one group of diseases where a tissue diagnosis can be difficult to obtain, thus making it much more important for the clinician to use all available diagnostic information as accurately as possible.

7 Respiratory disorders

- Watch for the exaggerated abdominal component.
- Muffled chest sounds: fluid, mass, air, obesity, deep chested, 'plugged ears'.
- Coughing cats: allergic bronchitis, flukes, lungworms, heartworms, hair or foreign body in trachea, tumor or granuloma in trachea or bronchus.
- Cats with heart disease rarely cough.
- Sudden-onset diffuse pulmonary infiltrates – think acute respiratory distress syndrome.
- Bacterial pneumonia plus leukopenia (bone marrow associated) – causes minimal radiographic infiltrates.
- Only pulmonary edema can clear from the lungs after 36–48 hours.

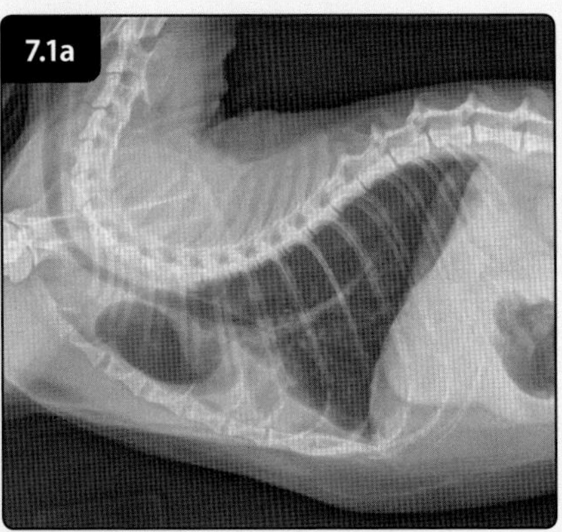

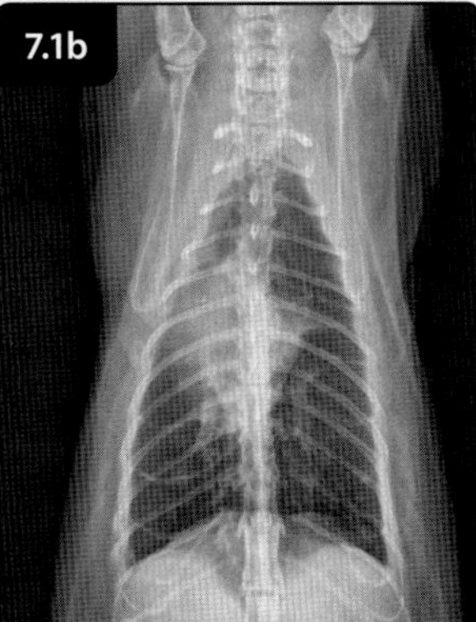

7.1a, b. Feline allergic bronchitis. These thoracic radiographs depict classic signs of this syndrome. There is diffuse bronchial thickening with 'doughnut-shaped' bronchioles. There is also atelectasis of the right cranial lung lobe as a result of mucous plugs obstructing the bronchus. The lung collapse will reinflate with treatment and time. (See 7.5c for higher magnification.)

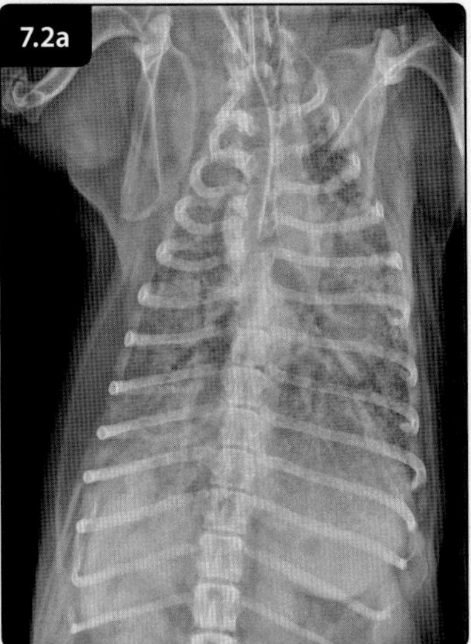

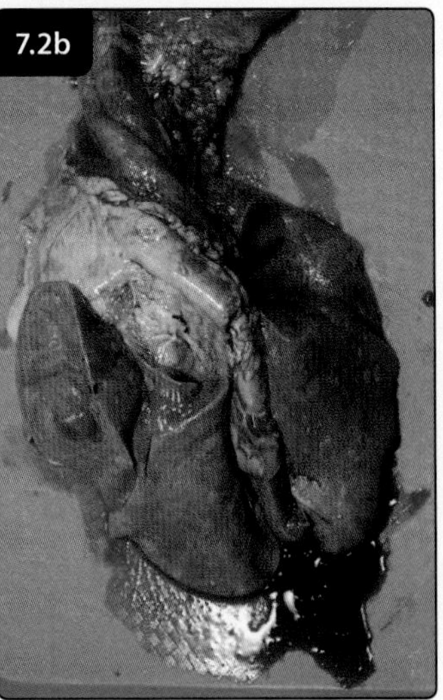

7.2a, b. Acute respiratory distress syndrome (ARDS) accompanying coral snake envenomation in a dog. The dog associated with these images had been bitten by a coral snake and had to be put on a ventilator because of the effects of the neurotoxin, which was causing respiratory paralysis. It became very hypoxemic and the radiograph shows the diffuse 'white out' alveolar pattern that suggested ARDS. The postmortem specimen has diffuse pulmonary infiltrate and edema typical of this syndrome, which has a very grim prognosis. Barotrauma from the ventilator could have contributed to the problem if the pressures had been set too high. This complication was unusual for a dog with this toxidrome.

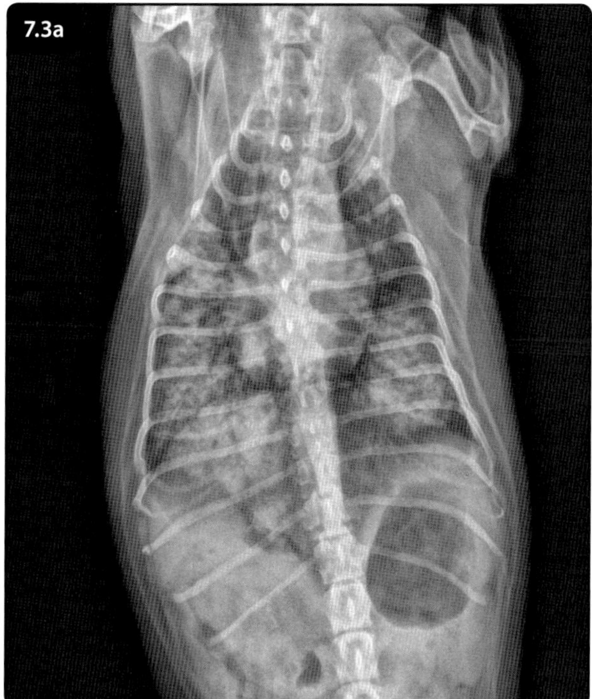

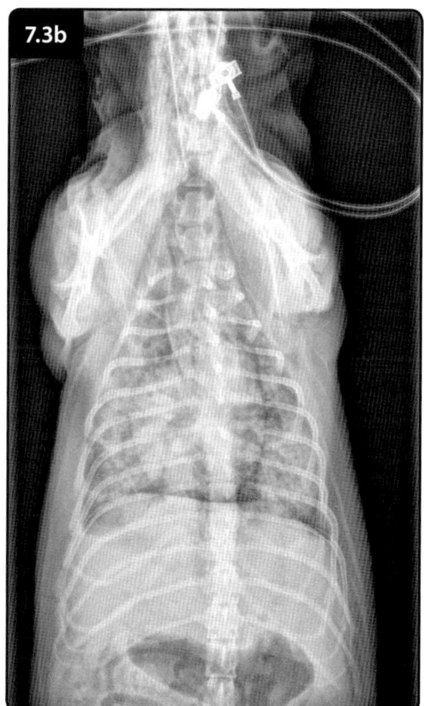

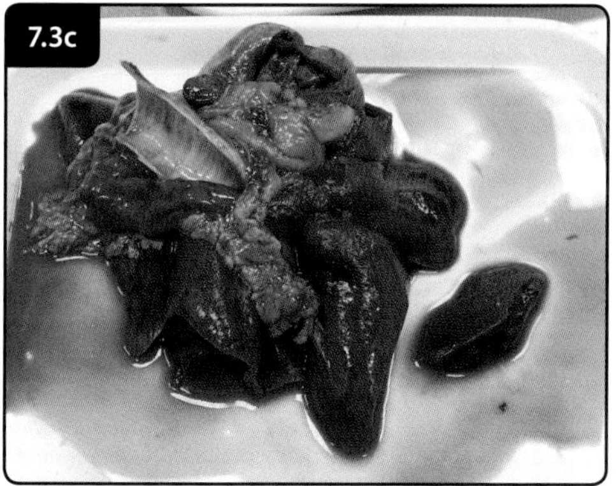

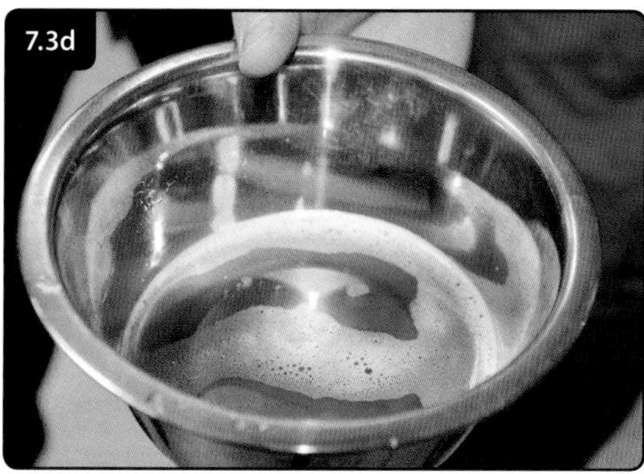

7.3a–d. Acute respiratory distress syndrome (ARDS). The general description of ARDS is a representation of a systemic inflammatory response syndrome involving the lungs. It can occur from a multitude of causes including diffuse pulmonary hemorrhage and infection, trauma, sepsis, etc. It progresses rapidly and appears as a diffuse alveolar infiltrate ('white out') on the radiograph. Figure 7.3a shows ARDS evolving, while Figure 7.3b shows severe involvement of both lungs. Figure 7.3c shows the characteristic congested appearance of lungs with ARDS. Histopathology will reveal inflammatory cells and protein-containing fluid in the alveoli (the author likens it to 'inflammatory soup'). Figure 7.3d shows the large amount of fluid that came from the lungs of a dog during its agonal termination from ARDS.

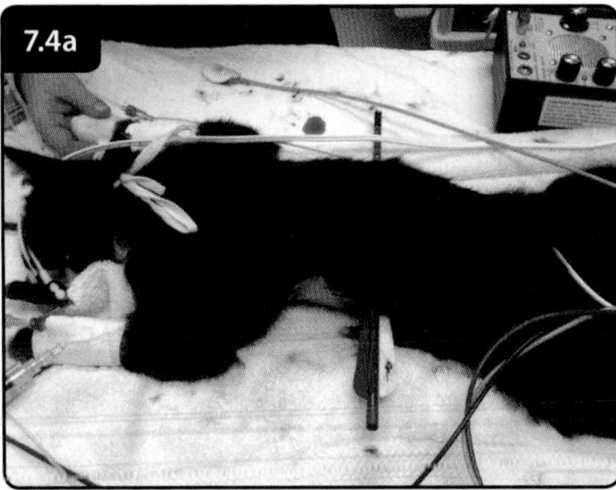

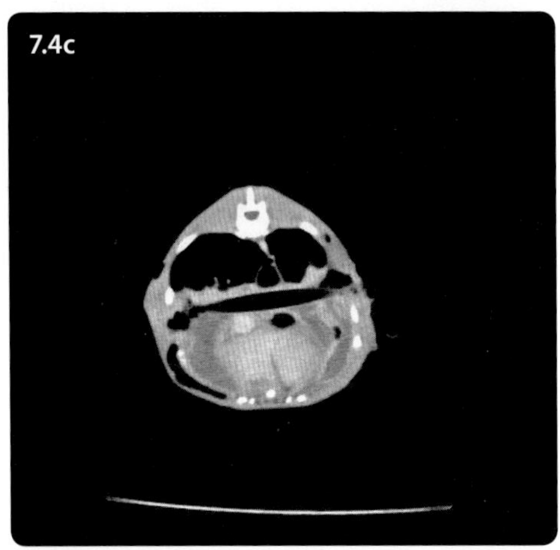

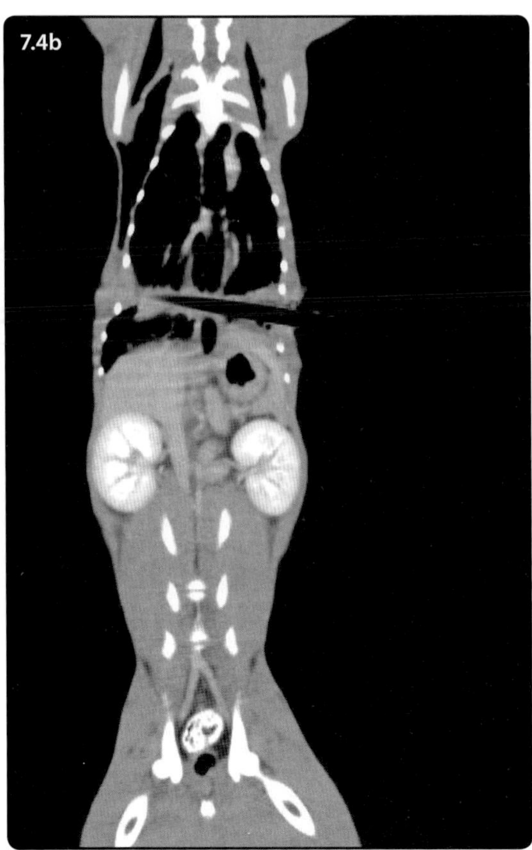

7.4a–c. Cat with an arrow in its chest. This cat was shot with an arrow and miraculously survived. The CT images clearly show the arrow and its relationship with surrounding structures.

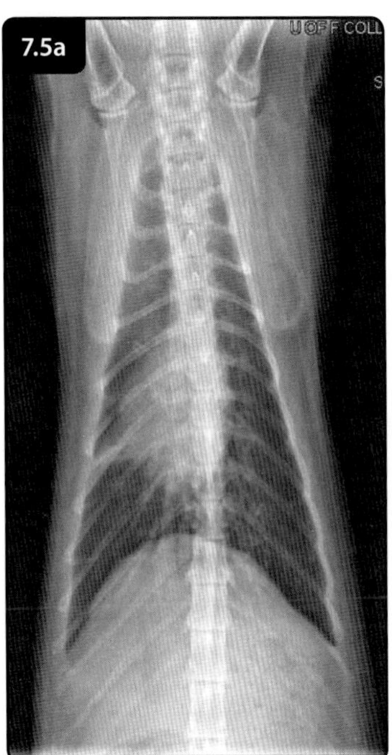

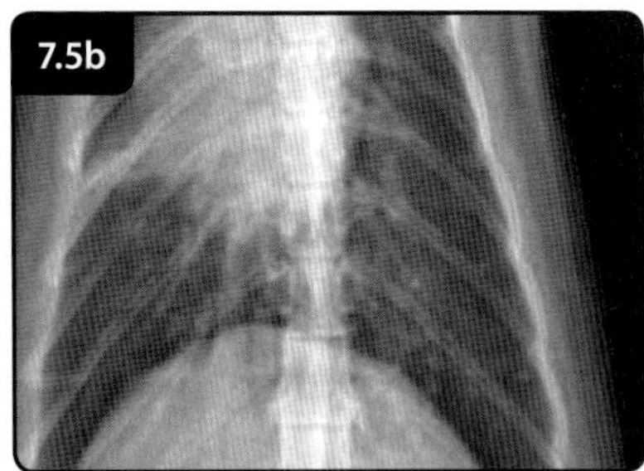

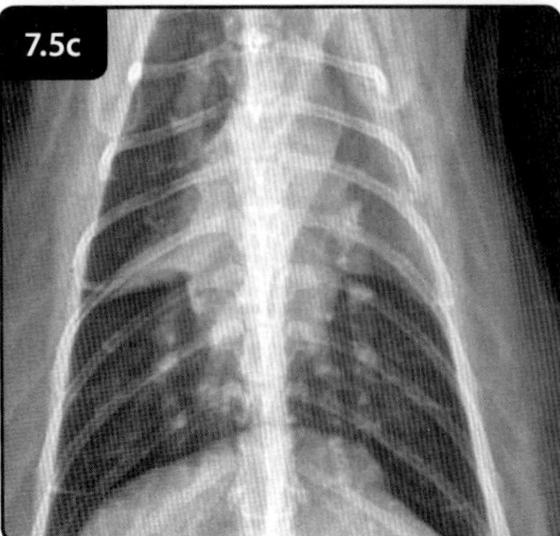

7.5a–c. Feline allergic bronchitis. Figures 7.5a, b depict feline allergic bronchitis, again showing atelectasis, as in Case 7.1, but here involving the right caudal lung lobe. Bronchial thickening is subtle. Figure 7.5c is taken from another bronchitic cat showing thickened bronchi that are easily seen in addition to collapse of the right middle and left cranial lung lobes.

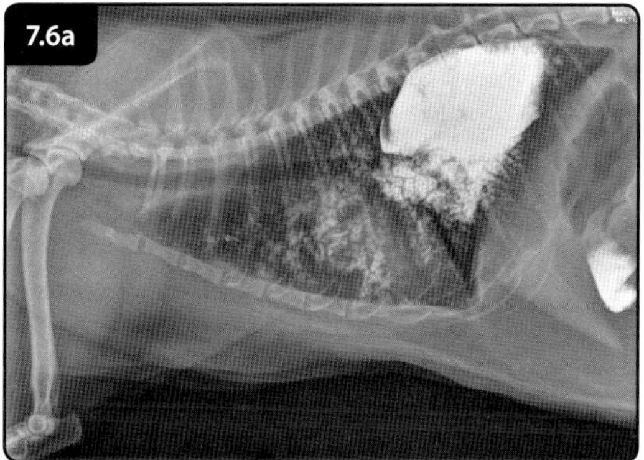
7.6a

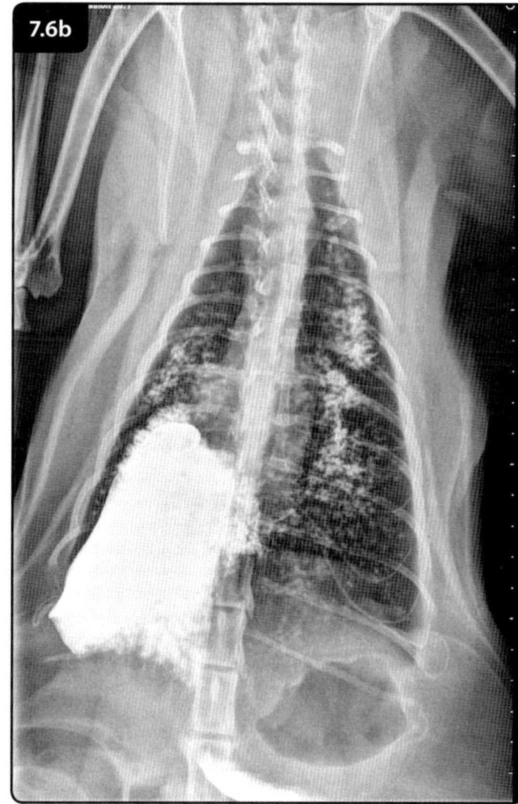
7.6b

7.6a, b. Barium aspiration. This cat was given a barium swallow and it aspirated. Although barium is thought to be rather inert, it can cause a severe granulomatous inflammatory reaction in the lungs, which can sometimes be fatal. There is no treatment for this other than general patient support. The radiographs show barium diffusely distributed in many lung lobes, with the right caudal lobe being the most affected.

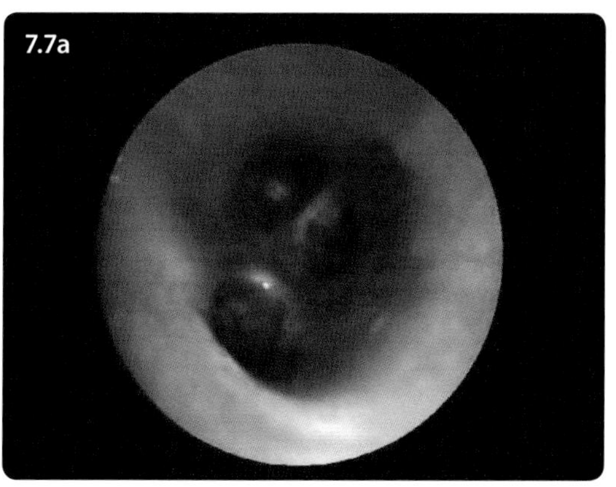
7.7a

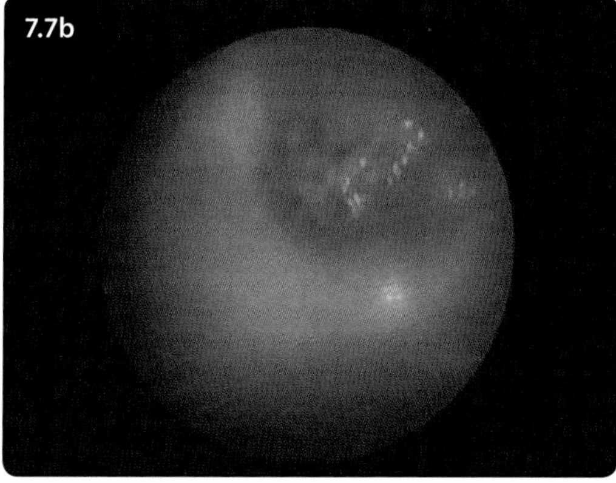
7.7b

7.7a, b. Bronchoscopic view of bacterial pneumonia in a dog. Figure 7.7a shows a normal bronchial appearance while Figure 7.7b shows exudate surrounding the bronchial openings. Samples of the exudate are accessible for culture and sensitivity and cytology.

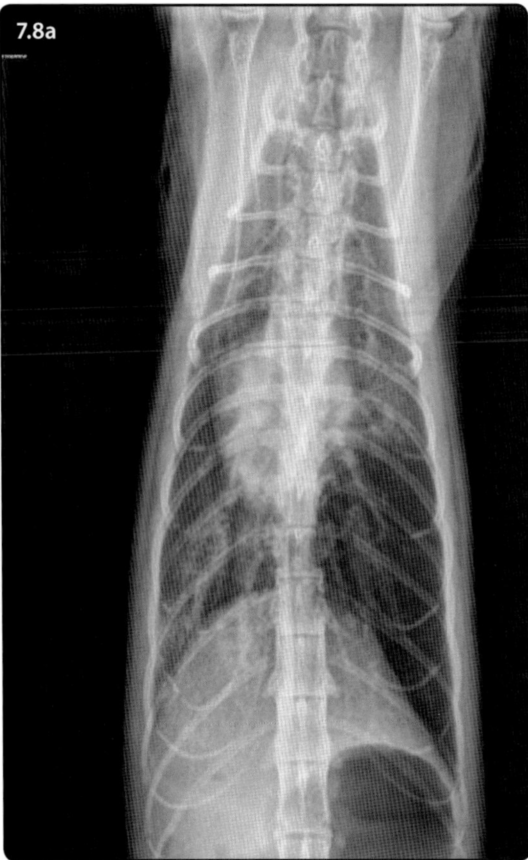

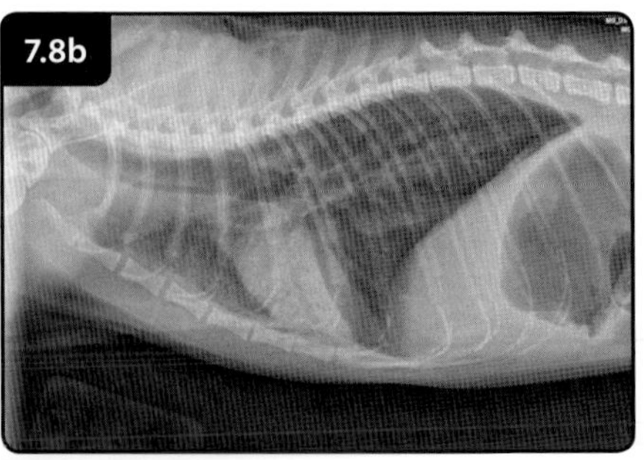

7.8a, b. Aspiration pneumonia in a cat. Figure 7.8a shows infiltrates in the left apical and right caudal lung lobes. Consolidation of the right middle lung lobe is demonstrated by the appearance of air bronchograms and alveolograms on the lateral projection (Figure 7.8b). Aspiration pneumonia is a complication that many sick animals acquire while in the hospital, especially when they have an alteration in consciousness from their illness or from administered sedatives. The bacteria involved are usually gram negative, but anaerobic bacteria can also be involved. Initially, a chemical pneumonitis occurs if the gastric aspirate is acidic (pH <2), while bacterial pneumonia usually does not occur until the second to third day after the aspiration event.

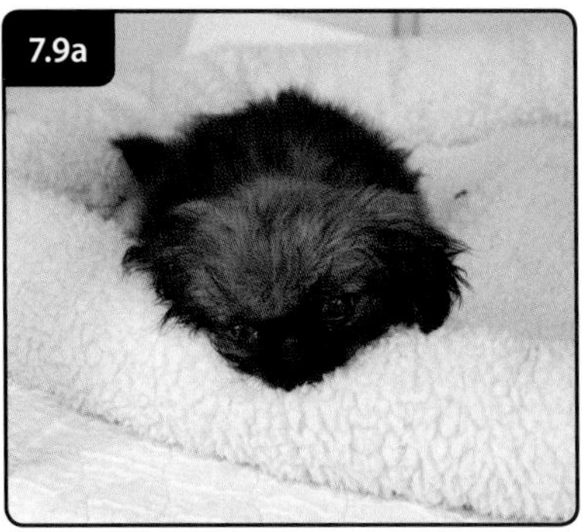

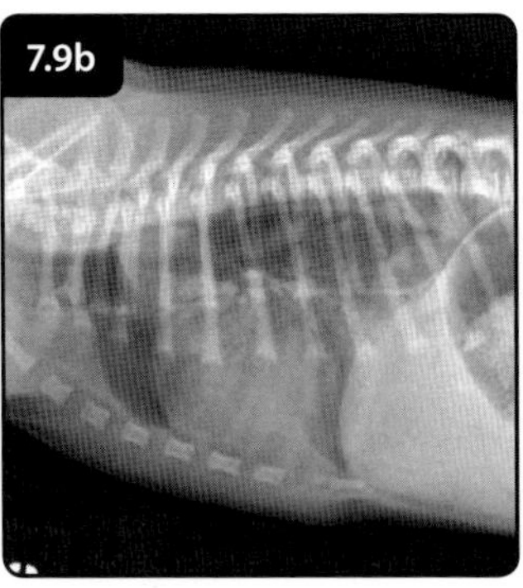

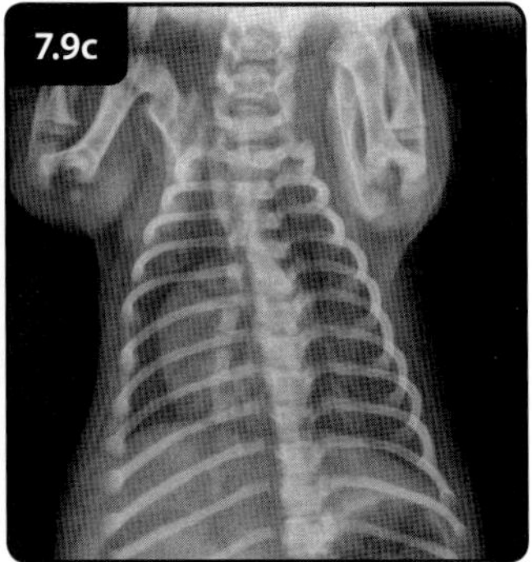

7.9a–c. Choke-induced neurogenic pulmonary edema. This puppy presented in severe respiratory distress after it had pulled on its leash. The sudden onset of labored respiration and the prominent caudal dorsal lung infiltrate are compatible with neurogenic pulmonary edema. The distended esophagus was transient and attributed to aerophagia. Treatment calls for oxygen administration. Some clinicians give furosemide for one or two treatments because there is an increased hydrostatic pressure component in the underlying pathophysiology. There is always a guarded prognosis for the first 24 hours.

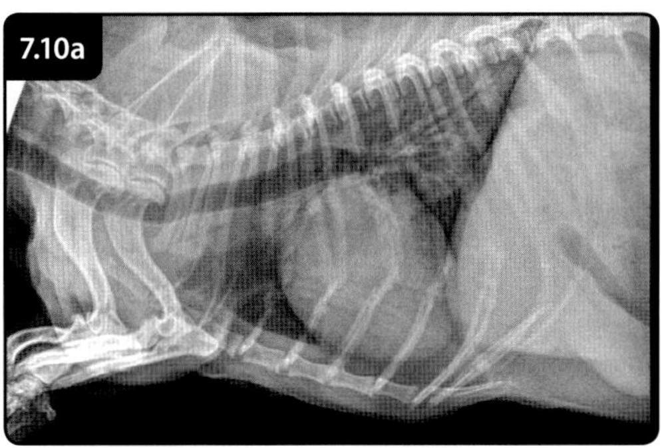

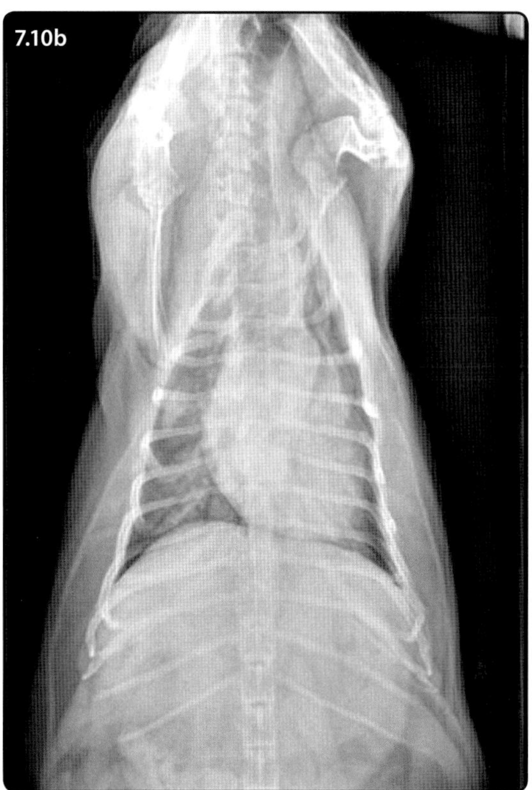

7.10a, b. Neurogenic pulmonary edema caused by choking in a dog. These radiographs show the typical caudal dorsal alveolar infiltrates caused by choking. Strangulation, choking, seizures, and electric cord bite are known causes of neurogenic (noncardiogenic) pulmonary edema. This results from central sympathetic nervous system stimulation that causes vaso- and venoconstriction of the large blood vessels in the cardiopulmonary circulation, causing plasma and red blood cells to penetrate the pulmonary alveolar–capillary network, resulting in pulmonary edema.

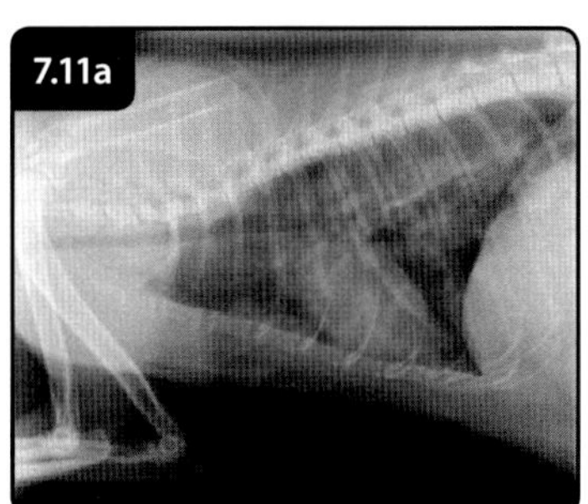

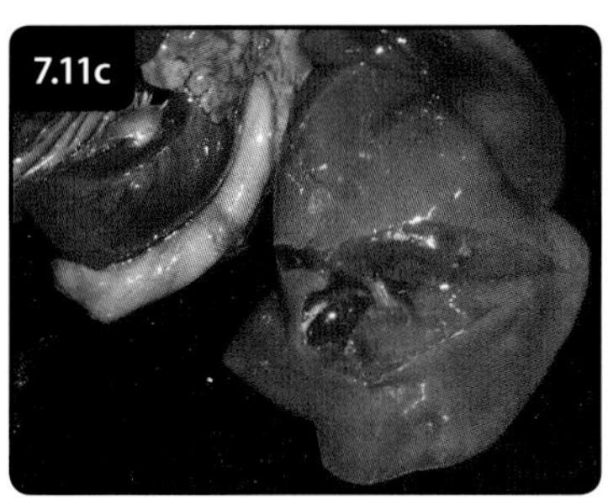

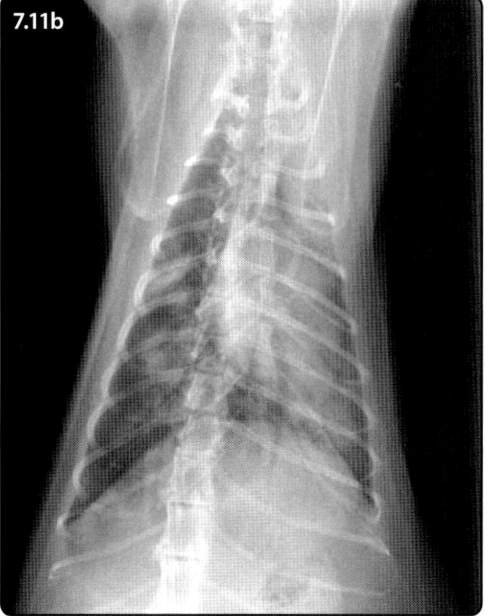

7.11a–c. Neurogenic pulmonary edema. Figures 7.11a, b are another radiographic depiction of neurogenic pulmonary edema. Once again, note the dorsal caudal distribution of the alveolar infiltrate, as seen on the lateral projection. Figure 7.11c illustrates the pulmonary edema from a dog that died from neurogenic pulmonary edema.

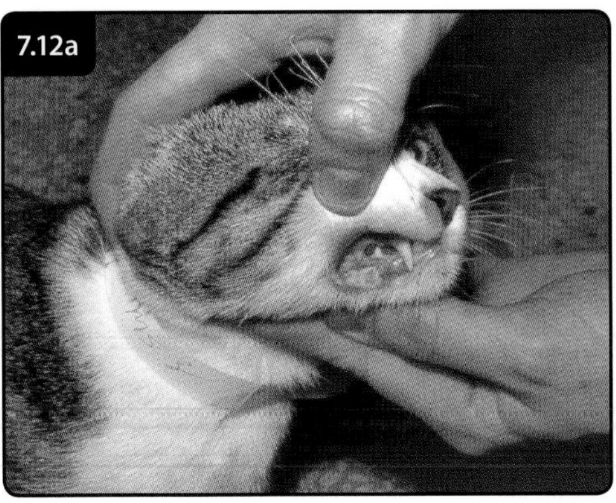

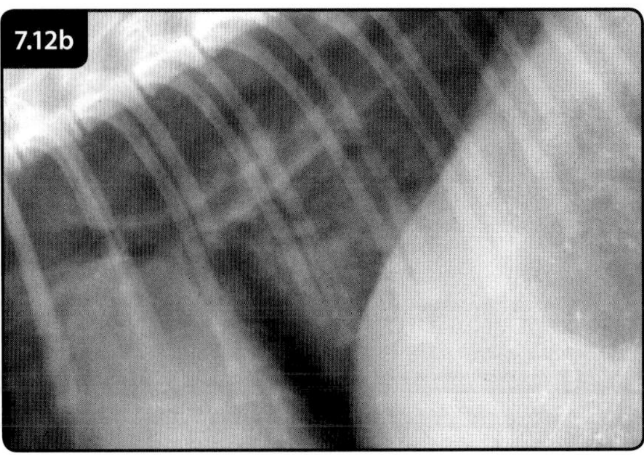

7.12a, b. Neurogenic pulmonary edema due to electric cord bite in a cat. Note the typical electrical burn involving this cat's labial commissure. Oral lesions from electric cord bite can involve the lips, tongue, and/or hard palate. The lateral radiograph provides a closer look at the dorsal caudal lung pattern.

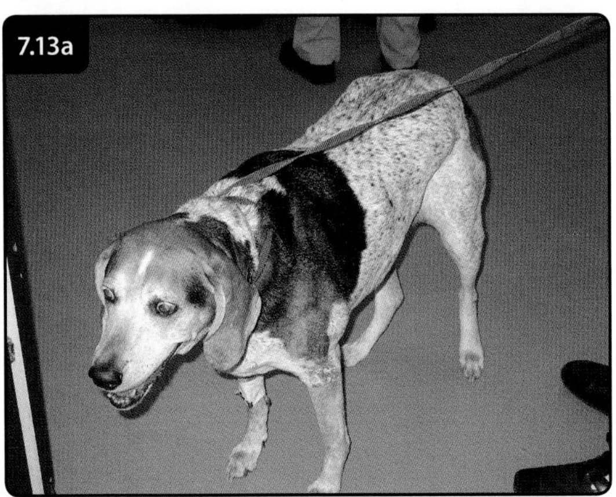

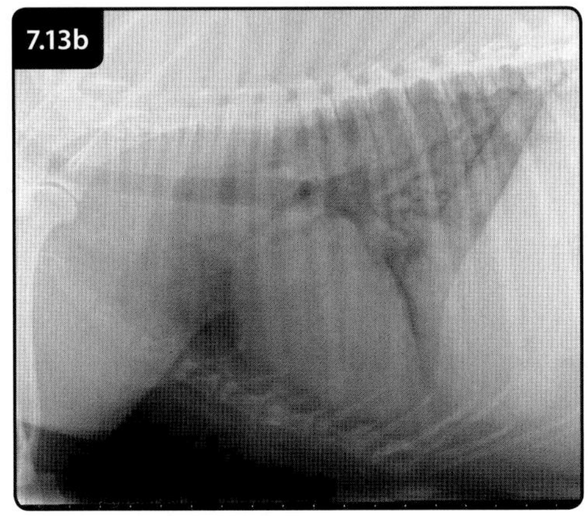

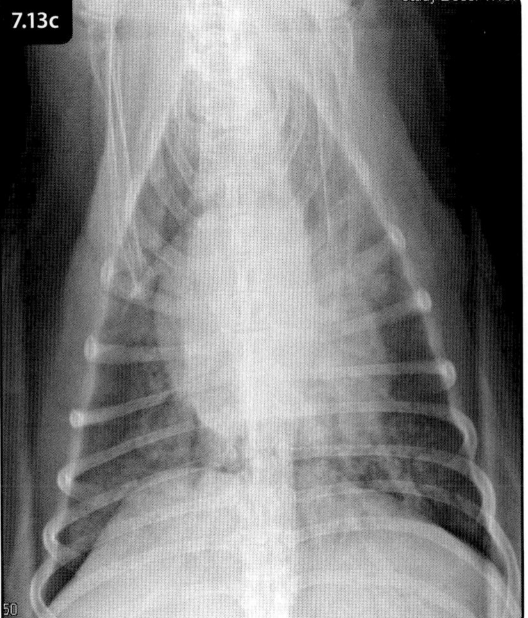

7.13a–c. Postictal neurogenic pulmonary edema. This dog was examined as a respiratory emergency case for neurogenic pulmonary edema. The cause was unknown at the time, but the thoracic radiographs were typical, and the dog responded to symptomatic treatment with oxygen supplementation and furosemide. The dog's history did not suggest any known seizures, but seizures were eventually witnessed several months later.

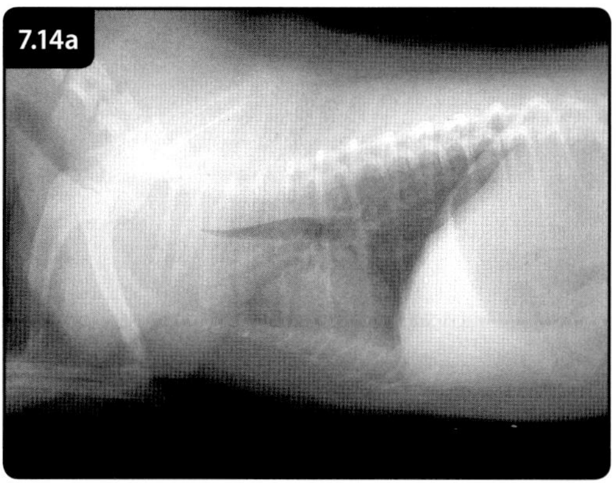

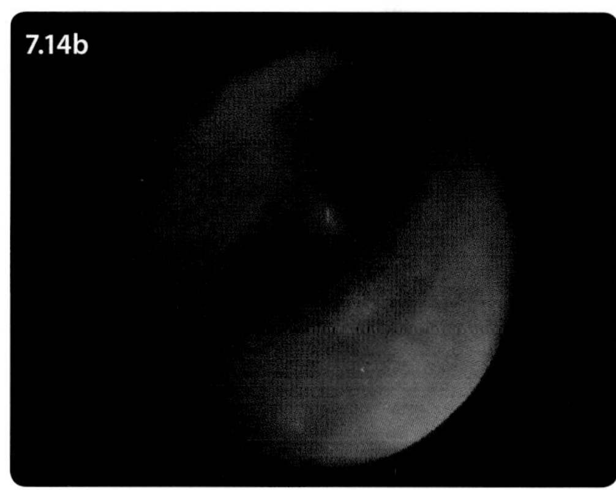

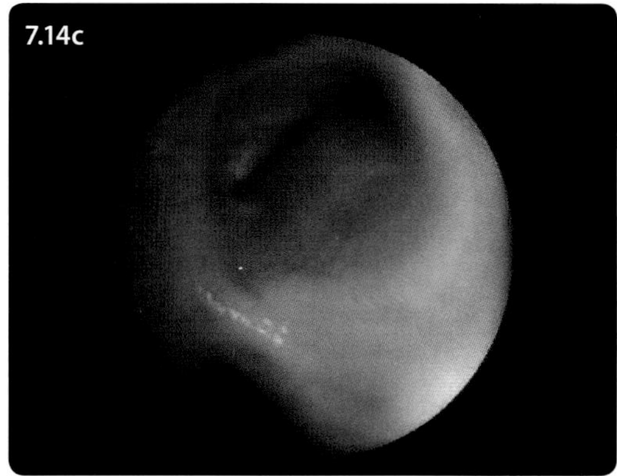

7.14a–c. Collapsed trachea. The lateral thoracic radiograph (Figure 7.14a) shows a severe collapse in the thoracic tracheal segment. Figures 7.14b, c show collapse of the major bronchi. Animals with collapsed bronchi and a collapsed trachea are usually difficult to manage with a tracheal stent because the bronchial abnormalities can persist and cause a continued problem for the dog despite the use of a tracheal stent, thus allowing for palliation of the signs at best.

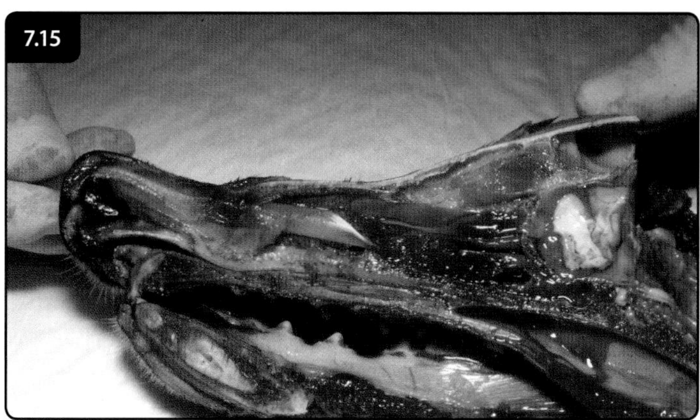

7.15. Traumatic nasal turbinate biopsy. This teaching cadaver model shows a 'cutting catheter' being used to biopsy the nasal turbinates. This technique will collect a larger tissue sample compared with using an endoscopic gastric biopsy forceps, which is considerably less traumatic and less likely to cause marked hemorrhage associated with the procedure.

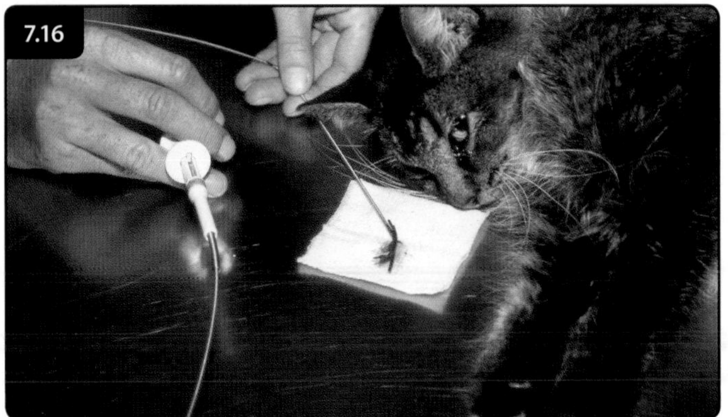

7.16. Nasal foreign body removal using a gastroscopic biopsy forceps. This cat had severe sneezing, which prompted the clinician to pass the forceps into the nasal cavities in search of foreign material, which in this case was a blade of grass. The same forceps can be used to biopsy the nasal mucosa, as discussed above.

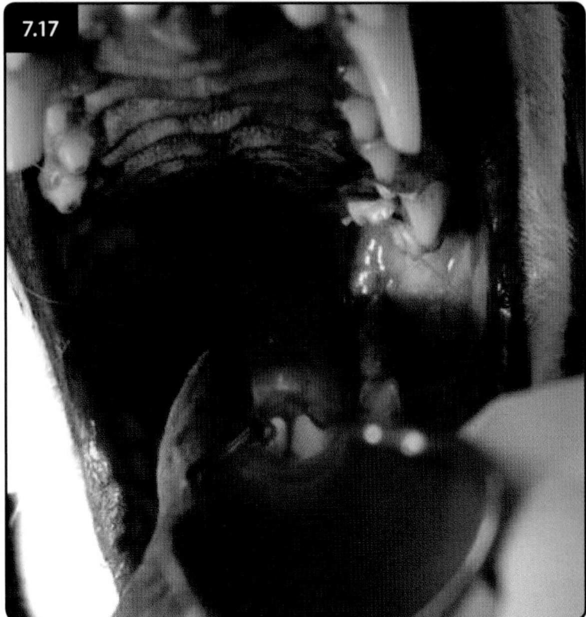

7.17. Laryngeal paralysis. This condition is frequently associated with heat exhaustion and commonly occurs in the larger dog breeds such as the Labrador Retriever. Smaller breeds of dogs and cats can also be affected. It is caused by dysfunction of the laryngeal muscles or the recurrent laryngeal nerve. Affected animals have a characteristic loud sounding inspiratory stridor associated with tremendous efforts to breathe. Diagnosis is made by inducing light anesthesia and observing the abducted position of the laryngeal arytenoid cartilages and vocal folds, as illustrated. Treatment entails sedation (if needed), glucocorticoids for laryngeal swelling, oxygen, and relieving any accompanying hyperthermia. The surgical laryngeal tie-back procedure provides a more definitive treatment, although it can predispose the patient to recurrent aspiration pneumonia postoperatively.

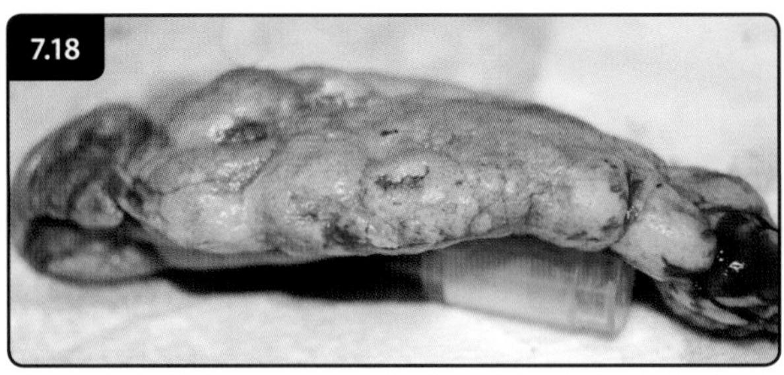

7.18. Lung bullae and spontaneous pneumothorax. This condition is usually asymptomatic until a bulla ruptures and causes spontaneous pneumothorax. The dog will present as a respiratory emergency with decreased lung sounds and increased percussion sounds on the involved side. Chest aspiration using a cannula and syringe is often unrewarding, and better reduction is achieved with chest tube insertion and continuous chest suction. This procedure is only for temporary assistance to the patient. Thoracotomy and lobectomy of the bullae affected lungs are always needed in order to provide definitive treatment.

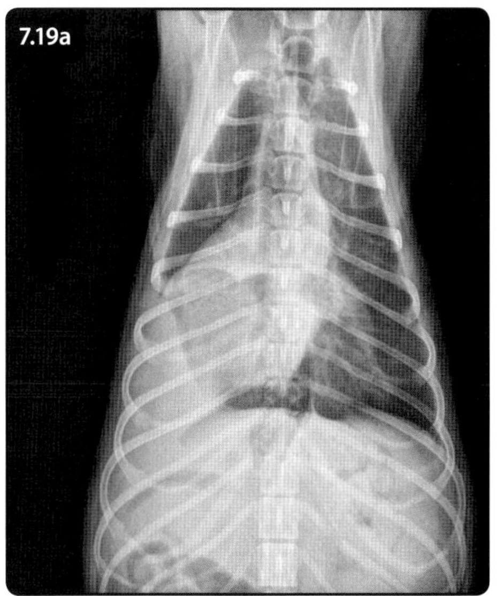

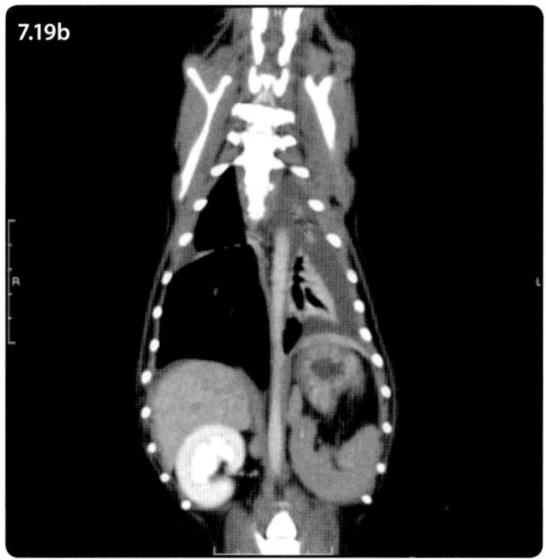

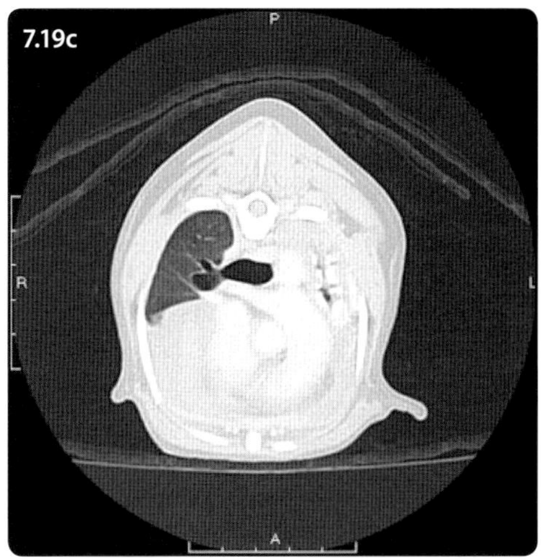

7.19a–c. Lung torsion. Figure 7.19a is a dorsoventral radiograph showing a right caudal lung lobe torsion. Many of these cases have an ipsilateral pleural effusion, but this might not be present in all cases. Figures 7.19b, c, from a different dog, are CT images of a left-sided lung torsion.

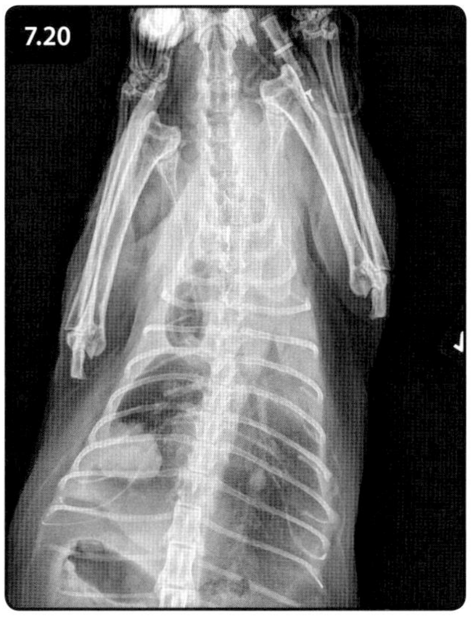

7.20. Lung tumor with metastasis. This is a dorsoventral radiographic view of a dyspneic cat showing pleural effusion and a large mass in the caudal right lung lobe and a nodule involving the left caudal and possibly the left cranial lung lobe.

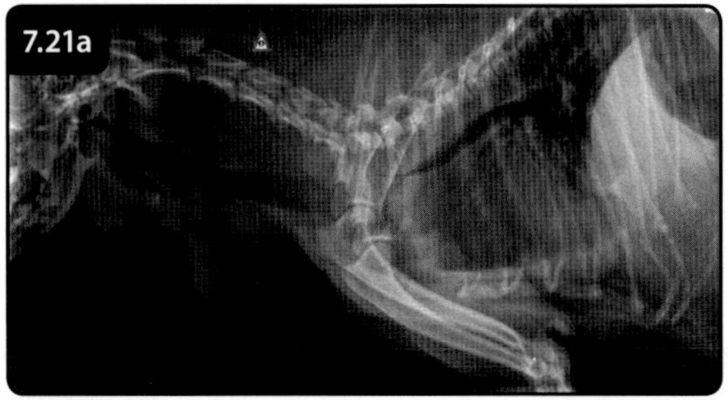

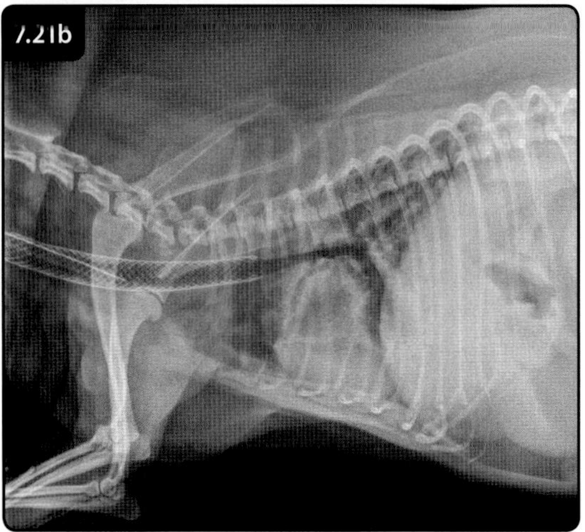

7.21a, b. Tracheal collapse radiographs before and after stent placement. The tracheal stent has brought respiratory relief for many dogs with severe tracheal collapse. The stent is placed endoscopically. It might not benefit dogs with collapse of the main stem bronchi, and it can migrate after its insertion. However, when it does work well, it brings new life to dogs that would have succumbed to airway compromise. Figure 7.21a illustrates severe tracheal collapse, while Figure 7.21b shows remarkable improvement to the proximal trachea, but there is still some collapse in the distal trachea.

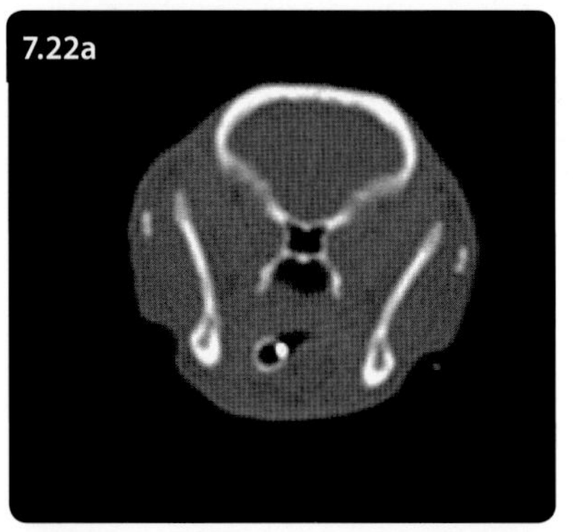

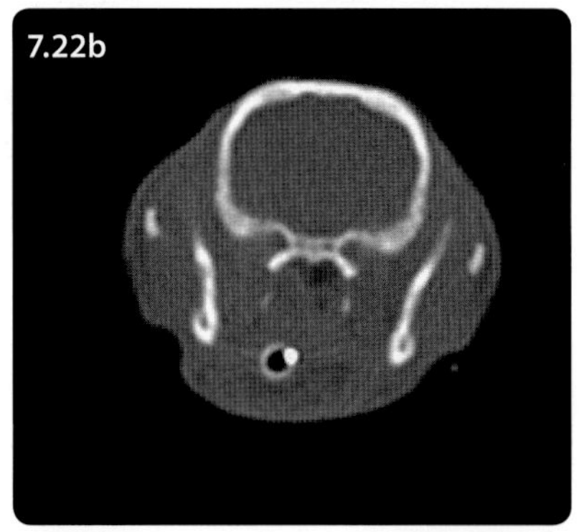

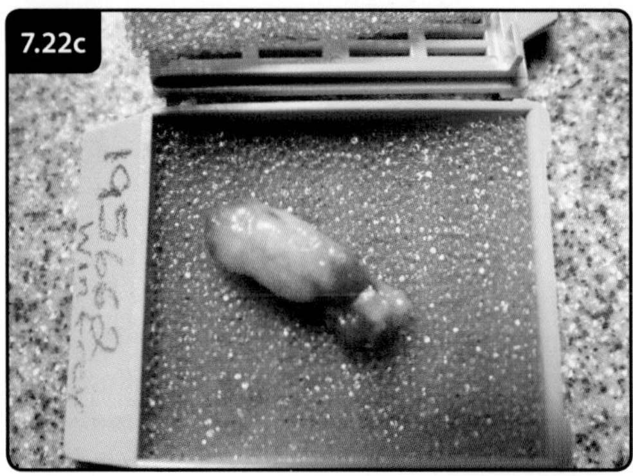

7.22a–c. CT scan of a nasopharyngeal polyp in a cat. The CT images (Figures 7.22a, b) show a partially occluded and almost complete occlusion of the nasopharynx in this young cat. Nasal tumors would be in the differential diagnosis list but the young age favored a nasopharyngeal polyp. Figure 7.22c shows the extracted polyp.

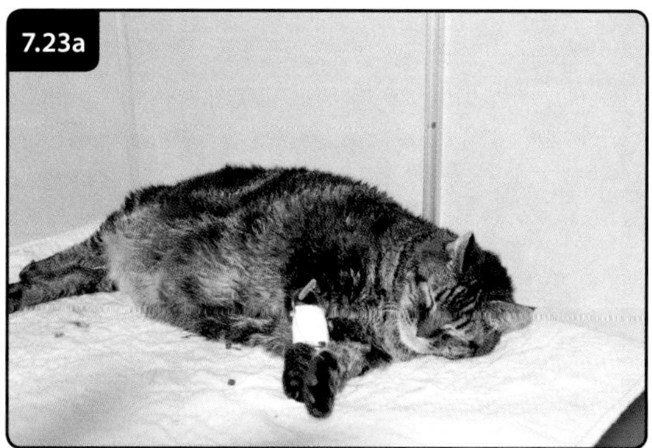

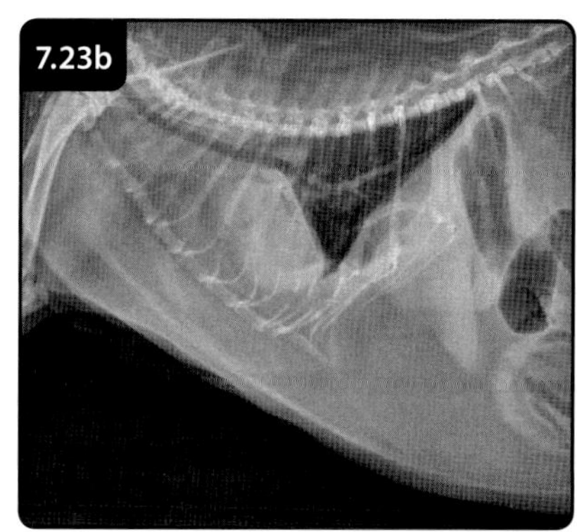

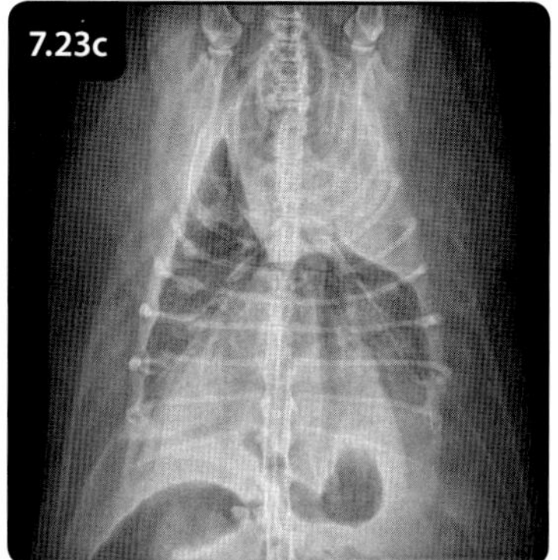

7.23a–c. Pickwickian syndrome in a cat. Named after the Charles Dickens literary character Mr. Pickwick, this condition is also known as obesity hypoventilation syndrome. In small animals, the term is used to describe obese animals who subjectively have exaggerated respiratory effort without actually measuring the ventilator parameters. The morbid obesity impairs the ability to ventilate adequately, causing the patient to become hypoxemic and hypercarbic. This cat's excess body fat is evident grossly and radiographically.

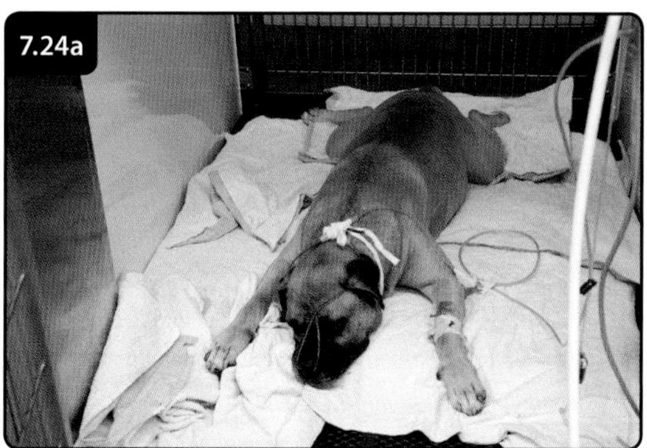

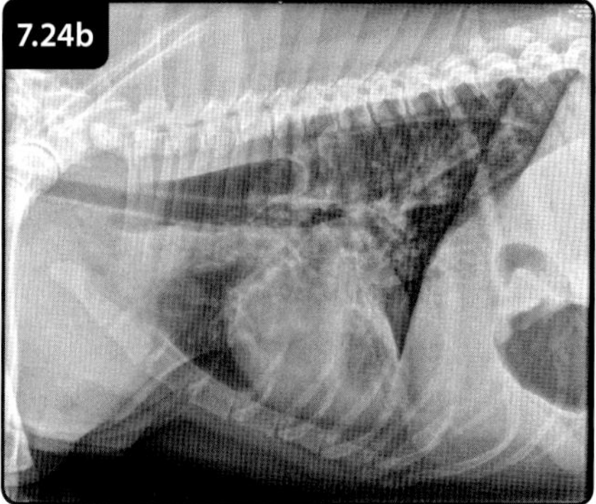

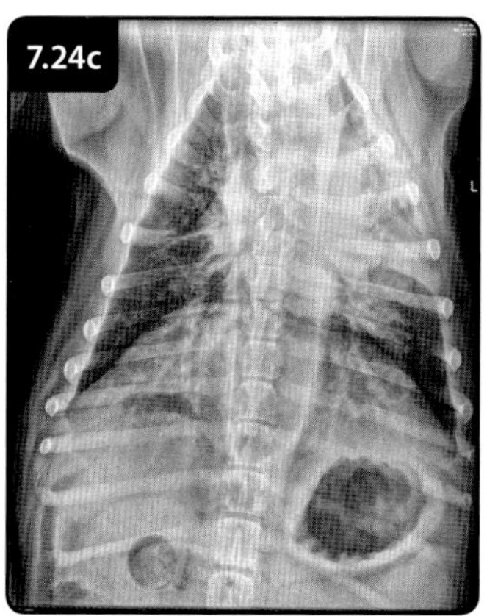

7.24a–c. Megaesophagus and aspiration pneumonia. This dog has severe neuromuscular weakness with a megaesophagus and aspiration pneumonia. The differential diagnosis can include any of the numerous causes of impaired neuromuscular junction transmission including myasthenia gravis, certain venomous snake, spider, and tick envenomations, diffuse neuropathy and its various causes, and, more rarely, hypothyroidism. Treatment would entail managing the primary disease in addition to the respiratory complications. In the two radiographs, the left cranial lung lobe is particularly affected.

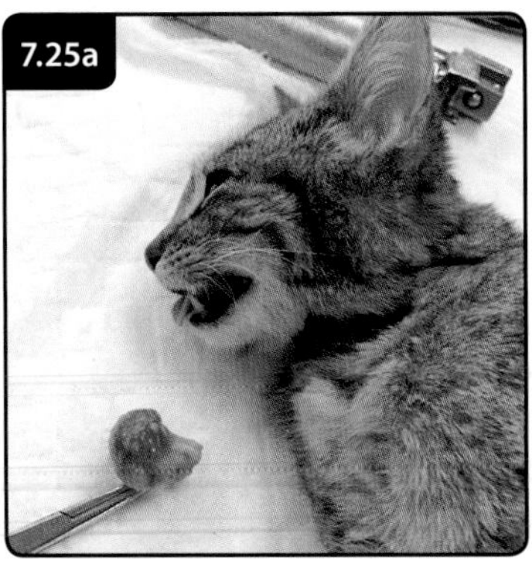

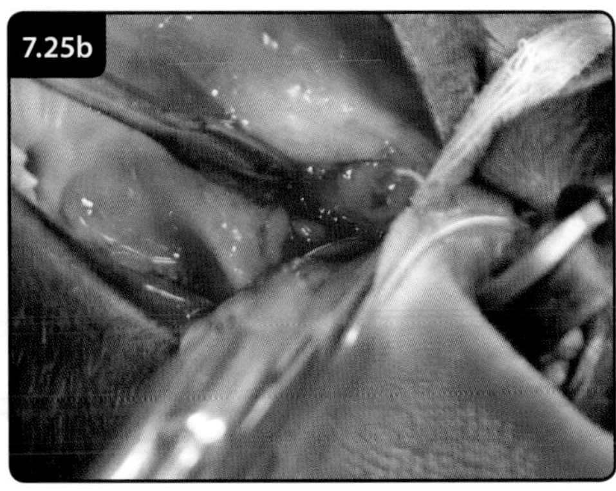

7.25a, b. Nasopharyngeal polyp. This disorder of young cats can cause a variety of signs depending on the location of the polyp. This image of a young cat (Figure 7.25a) was taken shortly after it died from massive upper airway occlusion before a bypass airway could be established. Figure 7.25b shows a polyp being isolated from the tonsillar crypt. Treatment is by surgical excision.

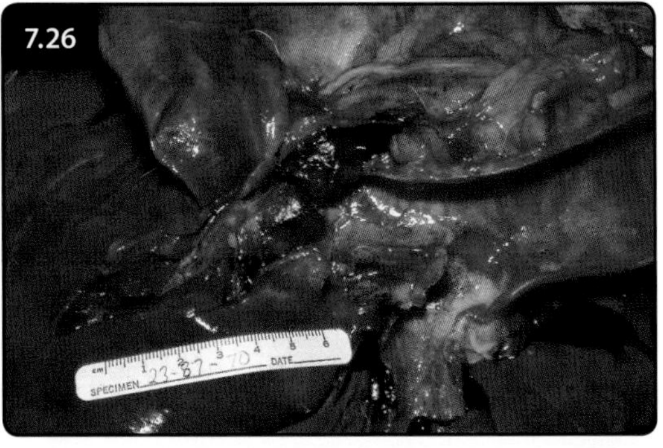

7.26. Pulmonary thromboembolism. A large pulmonary thromboembolus or thrombus is a major threat to life because of the major ventilation–perfusion mismatch it causes in the lungs. It can occur for a number of reasons including hypoalbuminemia, heartworms, foreign body such as a migrating catheter, and various medical conditions that favor a prothrombotic tendency such as Cushing's disease. Shown is a large pulmonary artery thrombus that formed in a dog with severe renal glomerular disease and proteinuria. Treatment is very difficult due to the location of some of these thrombi and the advanced stage underlying disease. Attempts for surgical removal are heroic and often meet with failure. Thrombolytic treatment using drugs such as tissue plasminogen activator can be associated with uncontrollable bleeding.

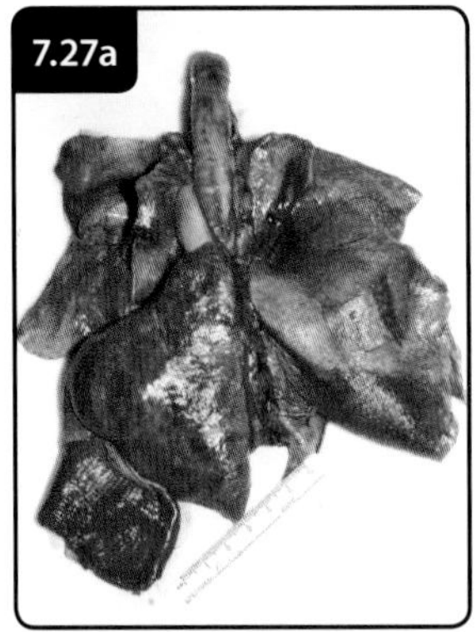

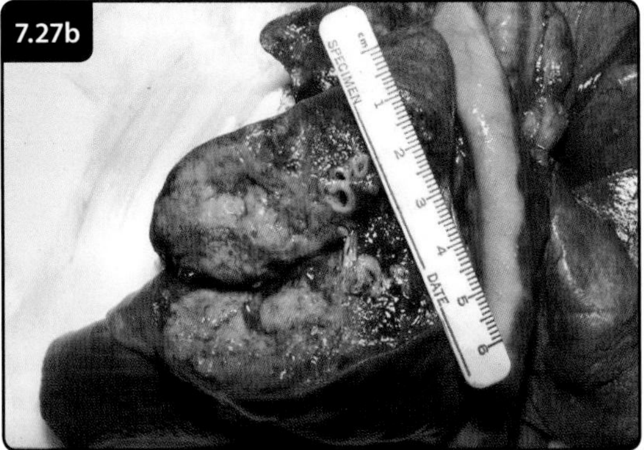

7.27a, b. Primary pulmonary adenocarcinoma. This postmortem specimen of a left caudal lung lobe tumor is from a dog that had exercise intolerance and weight loss. The hyperpnea associated with this lesion caused the dog to have respiratory alkalosis, which was characterized as an increased blood pH and a low TCO_2.

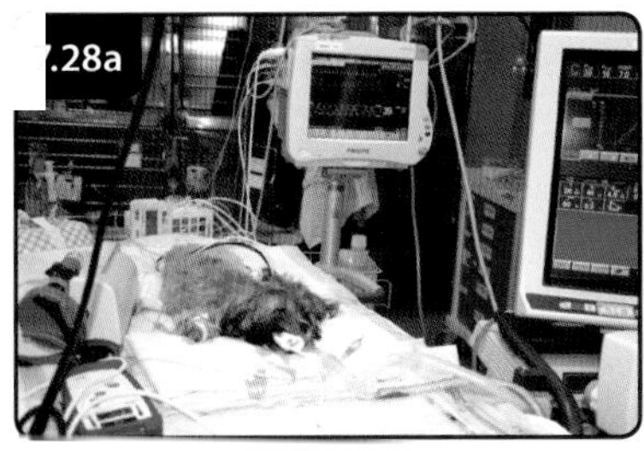

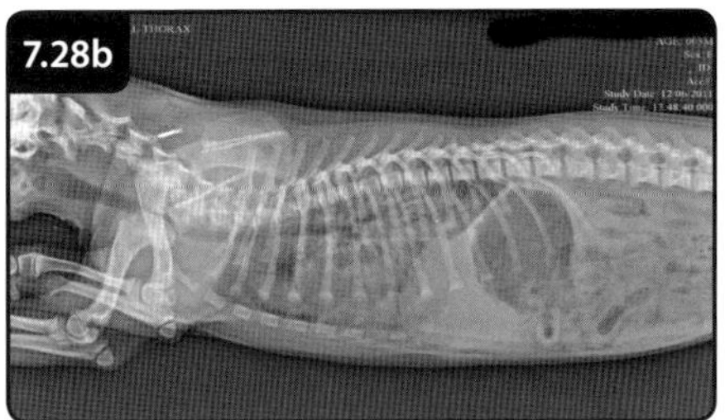

7.28a, b. Puppy choke and acute respiratory distress syndrome (ARDS). This puppy was found choking on a toy followed by labored respiration. On examination, there was marked dyspnea and harsh lung sounds. The radiograph shows a diffuse 'white out' typical of ARDS, which led to the puppy's anticipated demise.

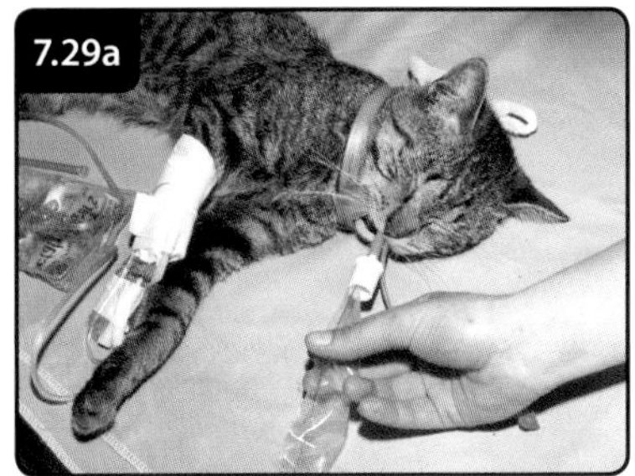

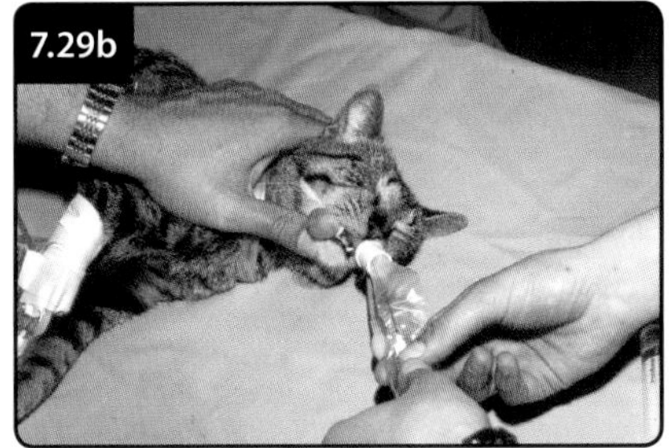

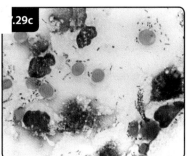

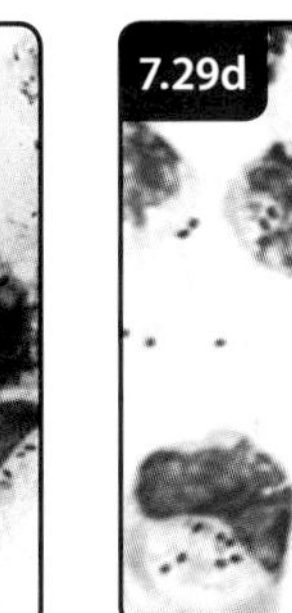

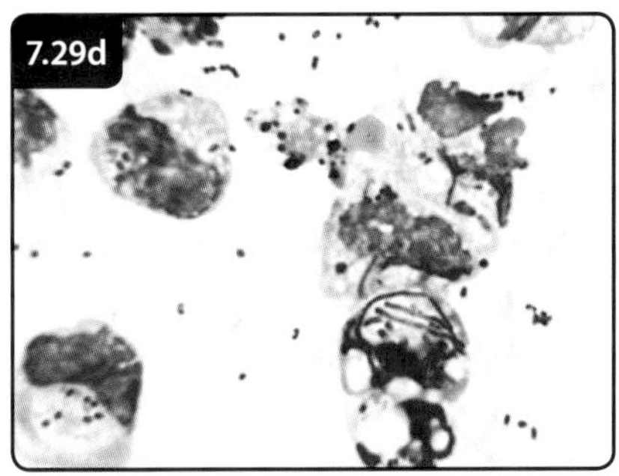

7.29a–d. Tracheal wash in a cat. Figures 7.29a, b illustrate a tracheal wash technique in a cat using a short-acting anesthetic such as propofol, an endotracheal tube, a long catheter containing a stylet, a syringe, and sterile saline. The entire procedure can take less than 2 minutes if everything is planned well. The actual fluid volume that is flushed down the catheter is 3–5 ml, which is rapidly manually aspirated and collected in the syringe. The specimen is immediately brought to the laboratory for cytocentrifugation and cytology. Figures 7.29c, d show the samples of a septic exudate containing toxic neutrophils with bacteria in their cytoplasm as well as free bacteria in the solution.

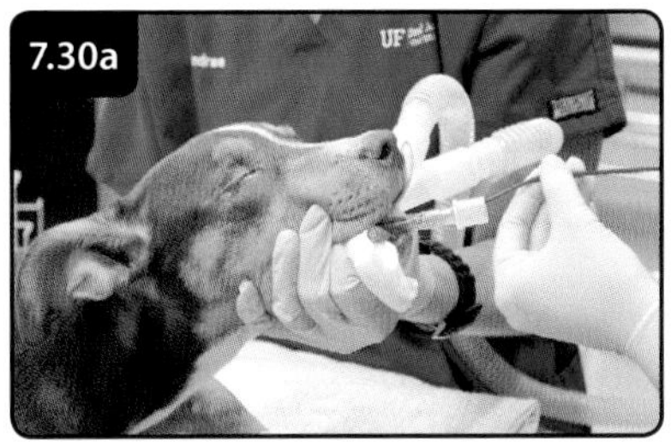

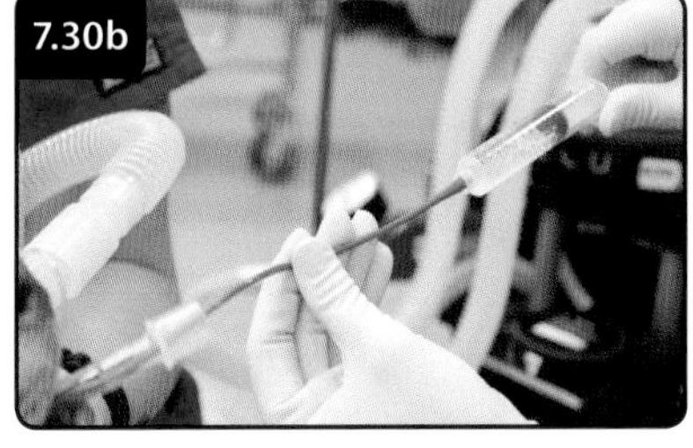

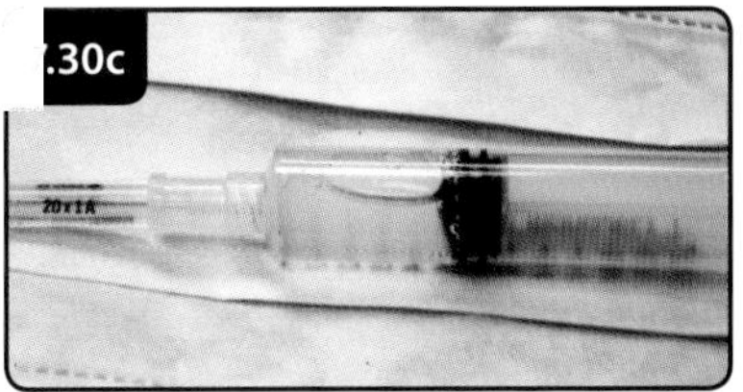

7.30a–c. Tracheal wash in a dog. This is the same technique as described above except that a brown rubber feeding tube is used in place of a cannula and stylet. For a larger animal, the amount of flush solution can be increased to 10–15 ml, as shown in the images. A positive yield is evident by the flocculent material in the syringes (Figures 7.30b, c).

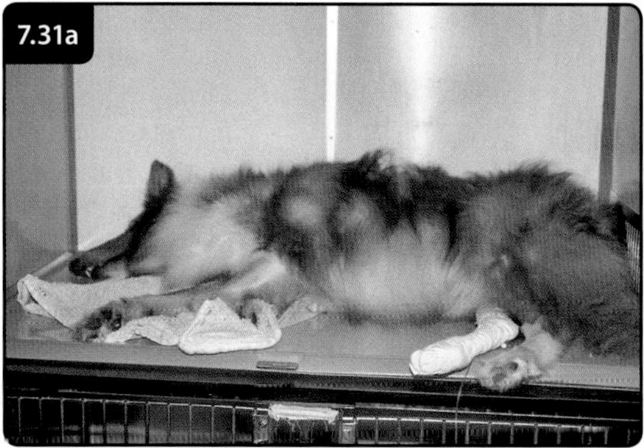

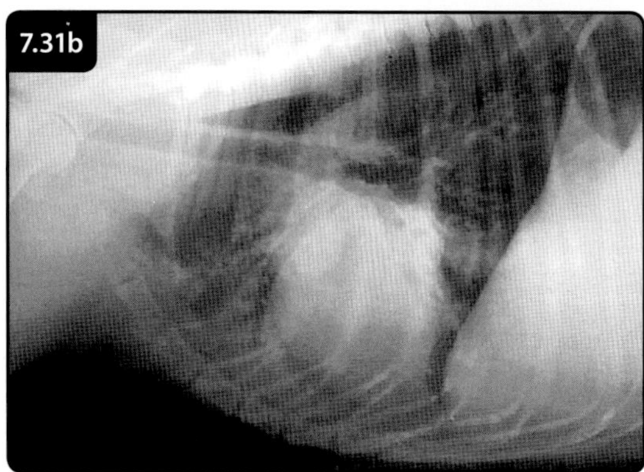

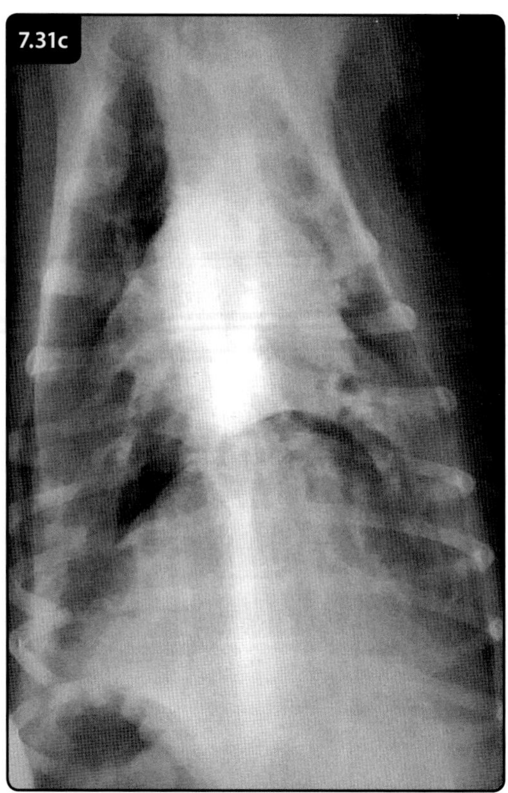

7.31a–c. Smoke inhalation in a dog. Smoke inhalation is a potentially catastrophic insult to the victim, as shown in this laterally recumbent Collie. The dog's comatose state is a grave sign that can result from hypoxemia, increased blood levels of carbon monoxide, and the inhaled chemicals that can accompany this condition. The lung pathology is often compounded by acute respiratory distress syndrome (ARDS), which is usually followed by death. The thoracic radiographs (Figures 7.31b, c) show extensive lung involvement. Complications can include ARDS and bacterial pneumonia, and if the patient survives, it can suffer from chronic lung disease (bronchiectasis, fibrosis, chronic bronchitis). This dog never regained consciousness and subsequently died.

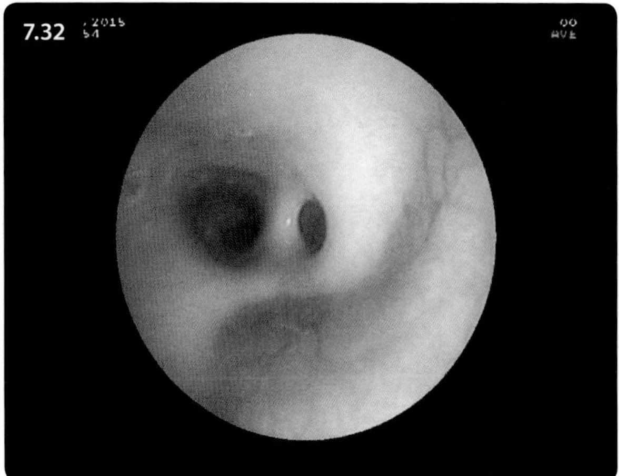

7.32. Bronchoscopic appearance of suppurative bronchopneumonia. Bronchoscopy is indicated for pneumonia patients that do not respond to prior treatment for pneumonia. The procedure might detect a foreign body or mass lesion occluding the pathologic bronchus and allows for selective sampling of bronchial secretions for cytology and culture and sensitivity.

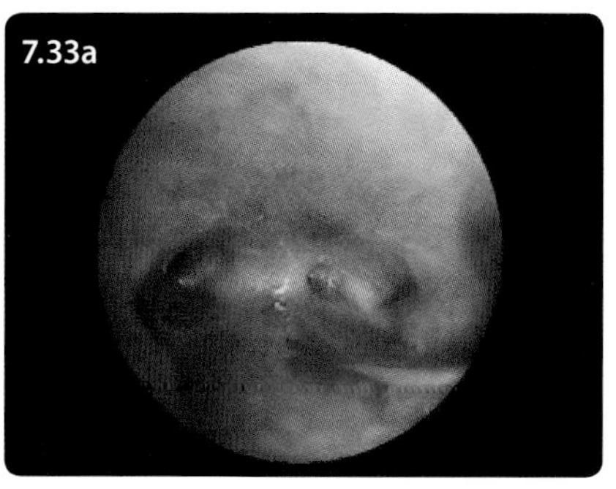

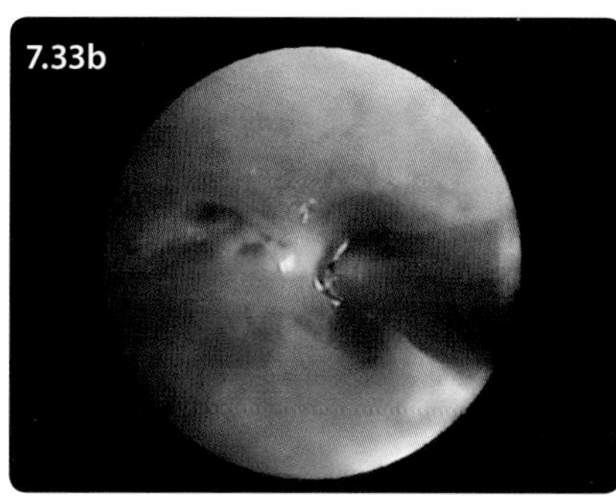

7.33a, b. Opening stenotic choanae. The nasal cavity choanae can obstruct as a result of inflammation or from an overlying mass such as a tumor. While under general anesthesia, a flexible scope is inserted behind the soft palate for a retrospective view of the nasal cavity, as shown in these images. Figure 7.33a shows the inflamed and occluded openings. Figure 7.33b shows the passage of the flexible forceps through the membrane causing the occlusion. The procedure might require repetition.

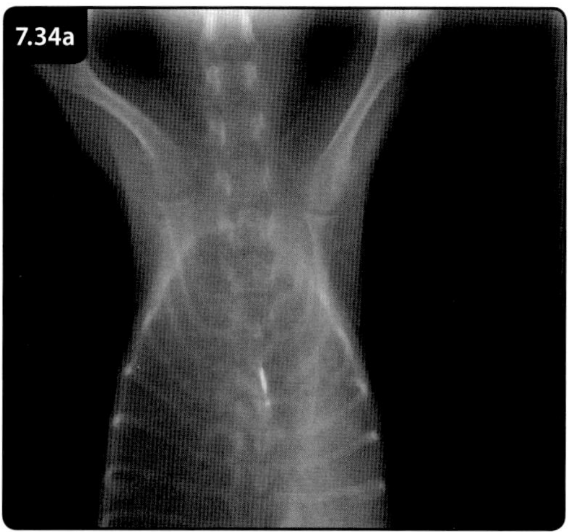

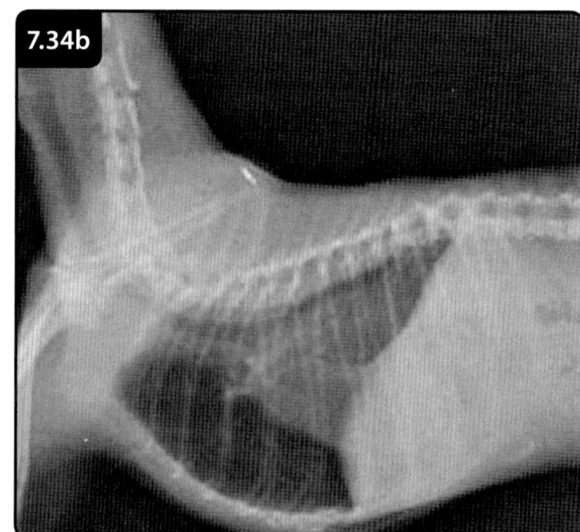

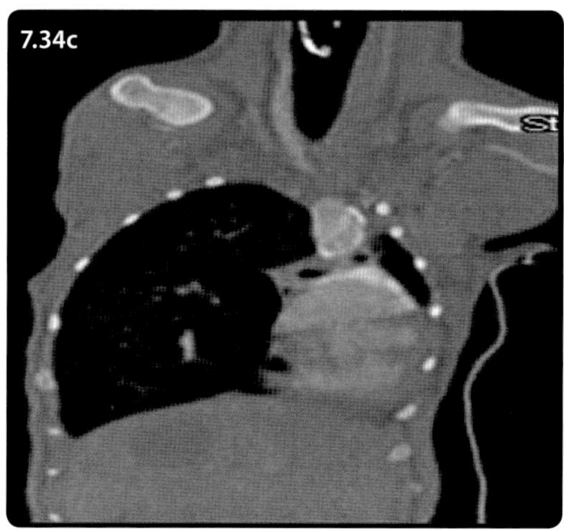

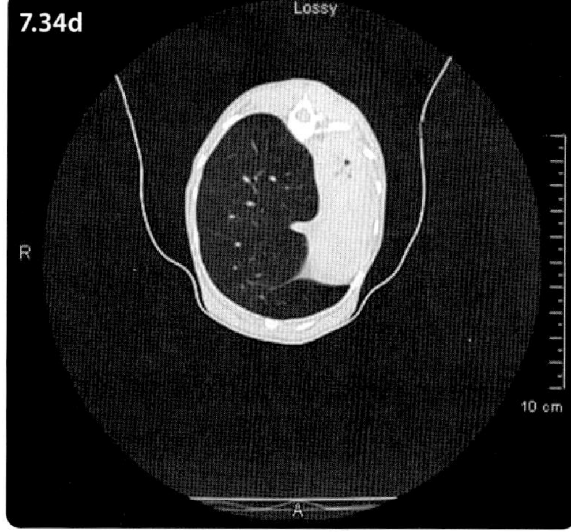

7.34a–d. Pulmonary atresia. These images depict a congenital pulmonary disorder known as pulmonary atresia. Note the displacement of the heart on the plain radiographs and the absence of the left lung lobes on the CT images.

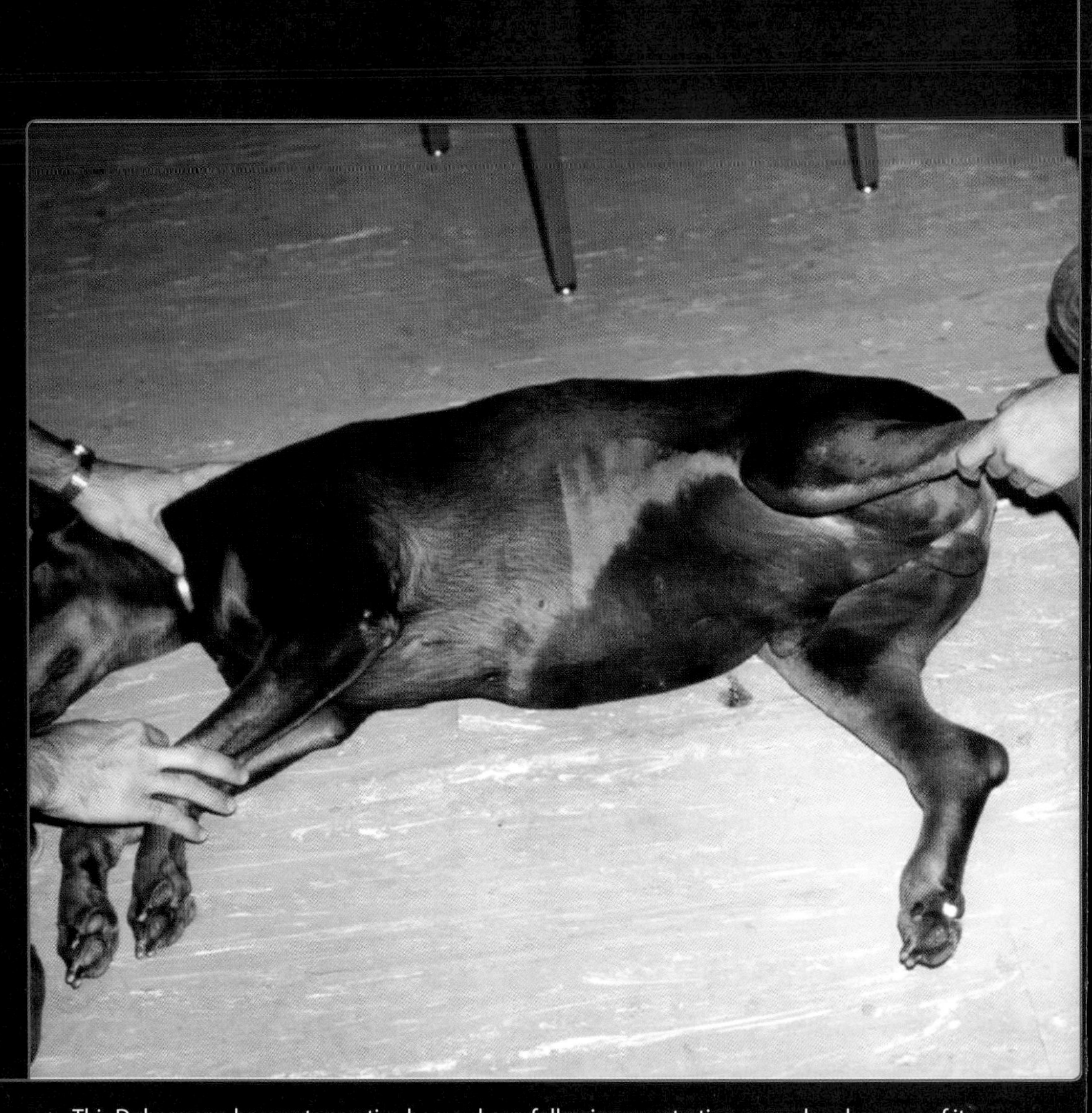

▲ This Dobermann has postoperative hemorrhage following a castration procedure because of its undiagnosed von Willebrand's disease.

8

Hematology and hemostasis disorders

HEMATOLOGY comes from the Greek word *haimatos*, meaning blood. There is no medical disorder that does not impact on the hematopoetic system, thus allowing varying amounts of information to be derived from a complete blood count. Hematologic disorders can be primary, as seen with immune-mediated hemolytic anemia, immune thrombocytopenia, or leukemia. They can also play a major role as a secondary disorder, which can reach life-threatening proportions, as seen in the hemostasis disorder known as disseminated intravascular coagulation.

Today, most hematology interpretation is done by a clinical pathologist, but primary clinicians can still derive much useful information themselves, as seen with their ability to recognize macroagglutination, detecting hemoglobin in serum, and, sometimes, surprisingly discovering abnormal cells such as schizonts, reflecting primary disorders elsewhere in the body. Examples of such abnormalities are illustrated in the following images.

8 Hematologic disorders

- Unclotted blood in clot tube – consider coagulopathy.
- Thrombocytopenia plus anemia – causes pale petechiae.
- Fulminant intravascular hemolysis: anemia, hemoglobinemia, hemoglobinuria, weakness, depression, +/- vomiting, then icterus.
- Owner can use urine dipsticks to detect hemeprotein for early signs of recurrent hemolysis.
- Fleas plus thrombocytopenia – cause 'lots of' lumbosacral petechiae.
- Low WBCs, low RBCs, low platelets – rule out bone marrow suppression and always obtain a thorough drug history.
- A normal bleeding time ensures adequate platelet hemostasis, a normal platelet count does not.

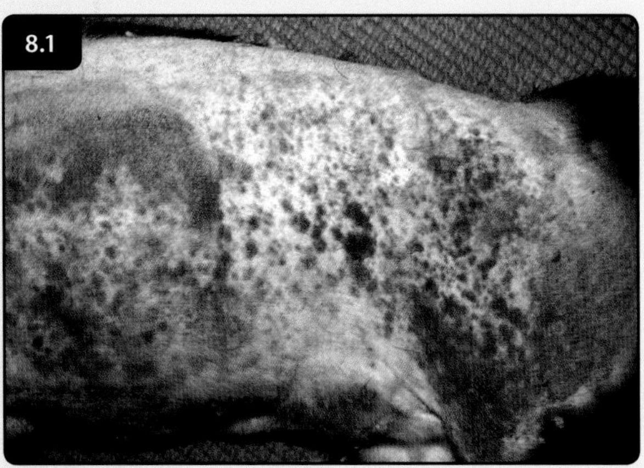

8.1. Anemia. The diffuse petechiations and ecchymoses on this cat were associated with pancytopenia caused by feline leukemia virus (FeLV) bone marrow suppression. This form of FeLV infection is fatal. The skin was shaved after the cat was euthanized in order to demonstrate the skin hemorrhages.

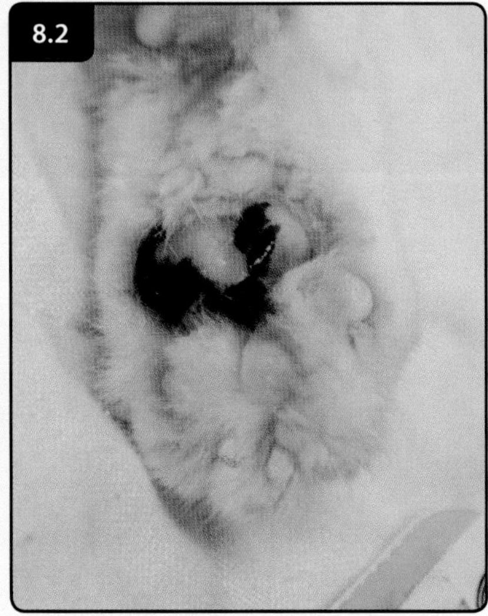

8.2. Marked pallor. The severe anemia in this cat was clearly evident by the marked pallor of its paw pads. Pallor can also occur with peripheral hypoperfusion, so objective criteria such as measuring the packed cell volume are needed to accurately assess the patient.

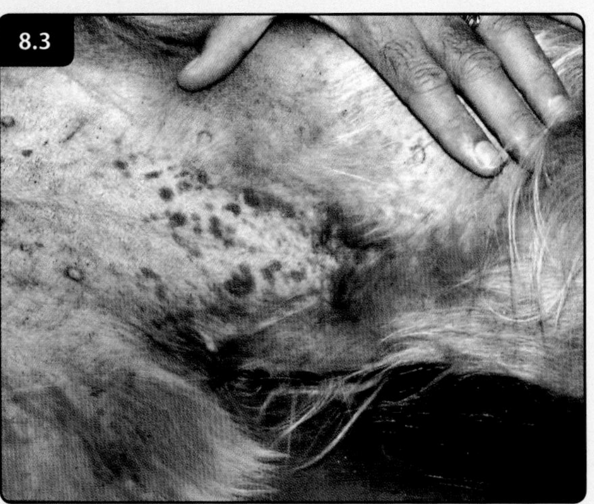

8.3. Petechiae and ecchymoses. Petechiae and ecchymoses are classic signs of thrombocytopenia, but they can also occur with vasculitis and a normal platelet count and platelet function. This dog had disseminated intravascular coagulation-associated petechiae and ecchymoses.

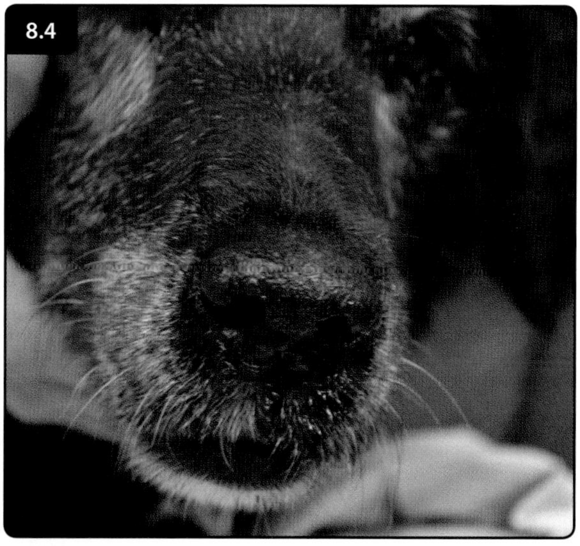

8.4. Epistaxis. Epistaxis can be caused by systemic coagulopathy, systemic hypertension, or by local pathology in the nasal cavity. Unilateral signs are usually associated with local pathology such as foreign bodies, growths, and superficial vessel abnormalities, including trauma.

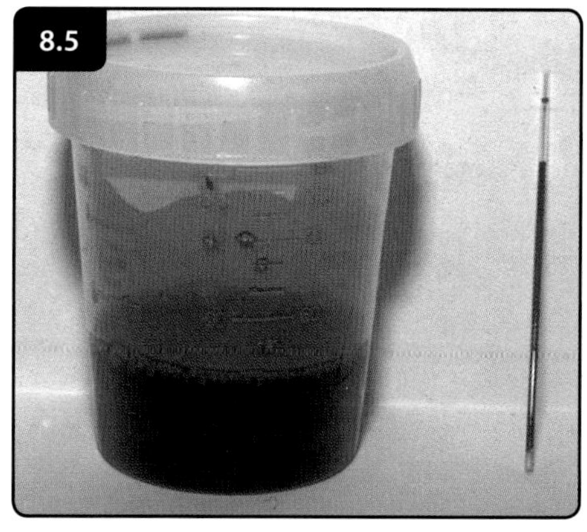

8.5. Hemoglobinemia and hemoglobinuria. These samples show hemoglobinuria and hemoglobinemia from a dog with hemolysis. The hemolysis can be caused by autoimmune red blood cell destruction, blood parasites, toxins and venoms, and congenital red blood cell enzyme deficiencies.

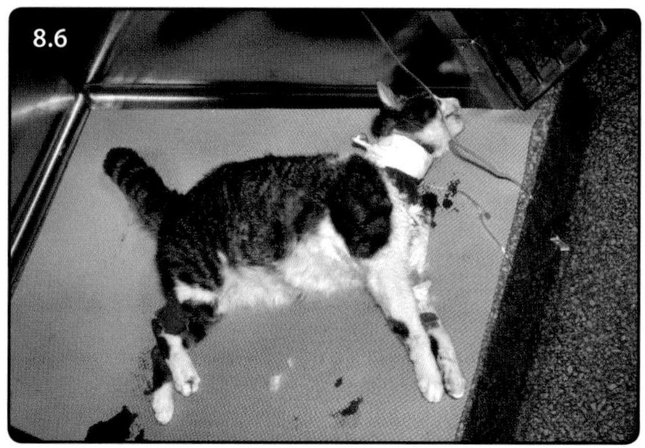

8.6. Disseminated intravascular coagulation (DIC). Animals that begin to bleed from venipuncture sites are in severe peril because of their coagulopathy. This cat had died from its DIC.

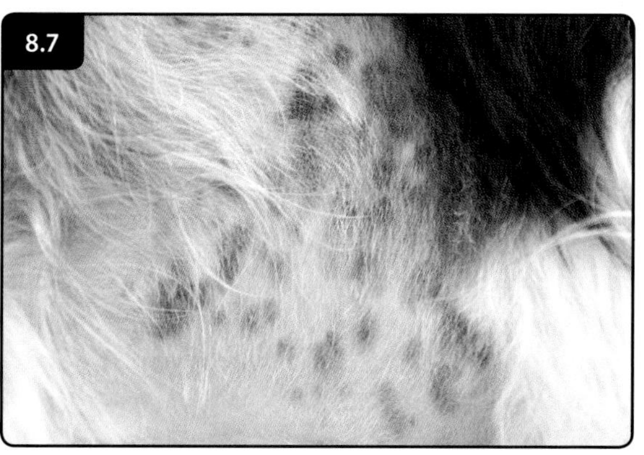

8.7. Petechiae and icterus. The petechiae in this dog are accompanied by icterus. Dogs with progressive liver disease can become coagulopathic and become affected with either acute or chronic disseminated intravascular coagulation.

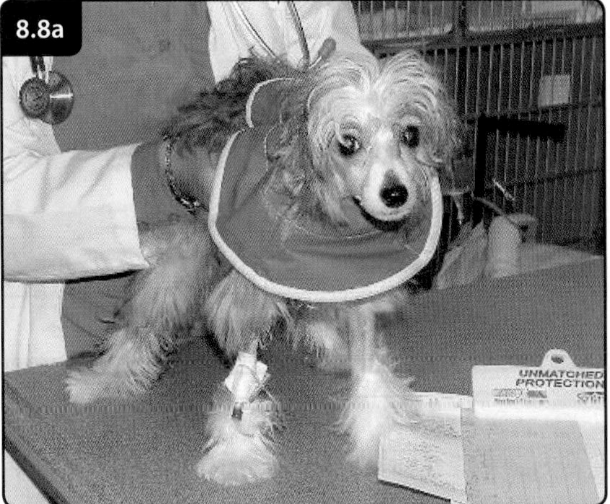

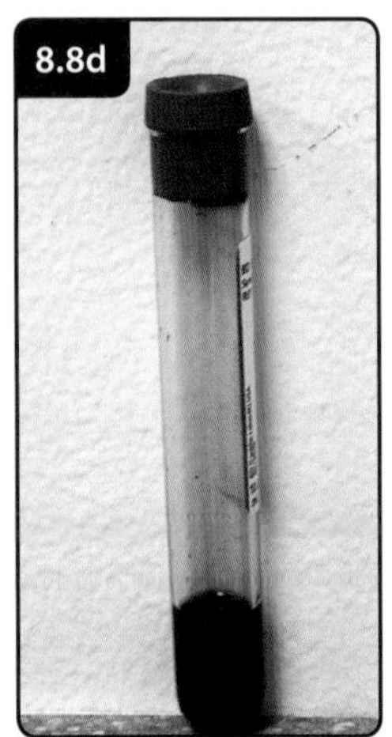

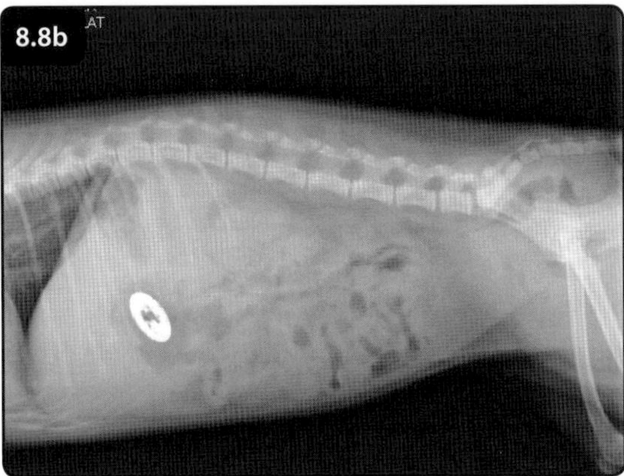

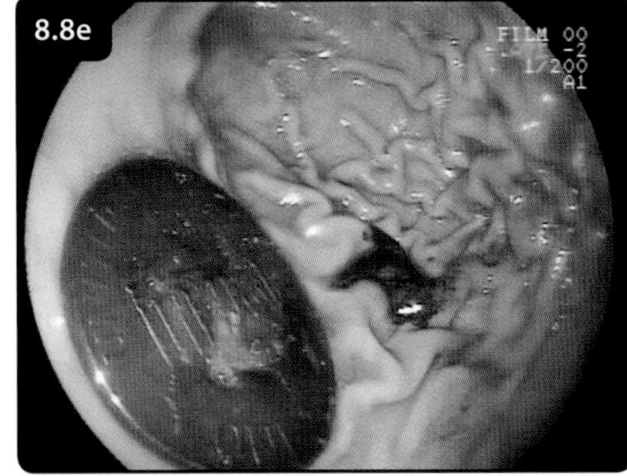

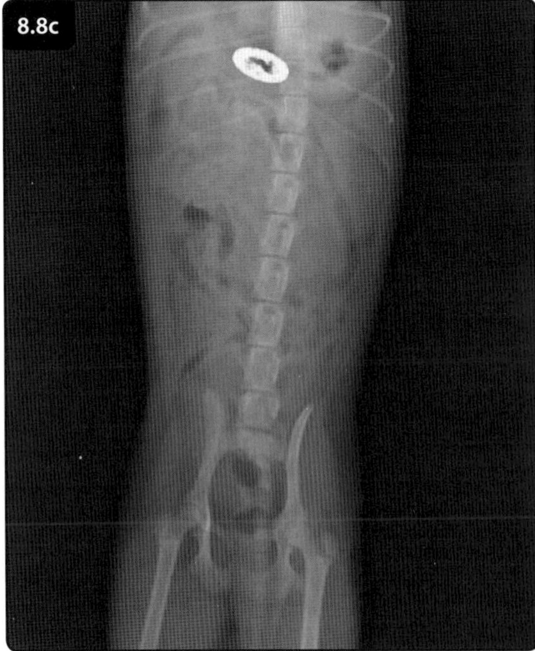

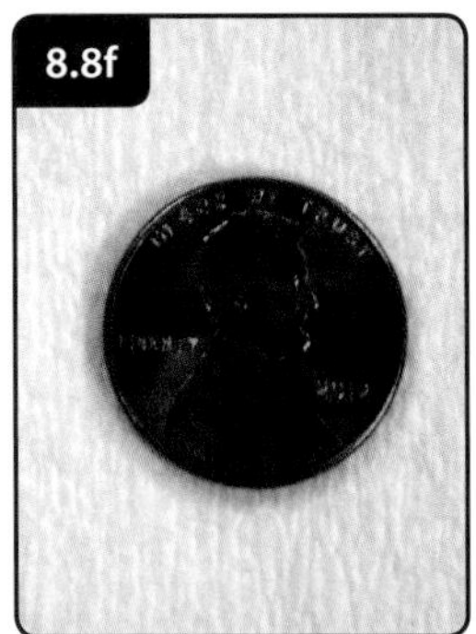

8.8a–f. Zinc intoxication. The zinc intoxication in this dog occurred after it ingested a penny. Pennies manufactured after 1982 contain zinc and copper. The zinc causes hemolysis, which is apparent in the blood tube. The abdominal radiographs depict the ingested gastric foreign body. The endoscopy image, from a different dog with a similar diagnosis, identified the foreign body as a penny. The hemolysis subsided after removal of the coin.

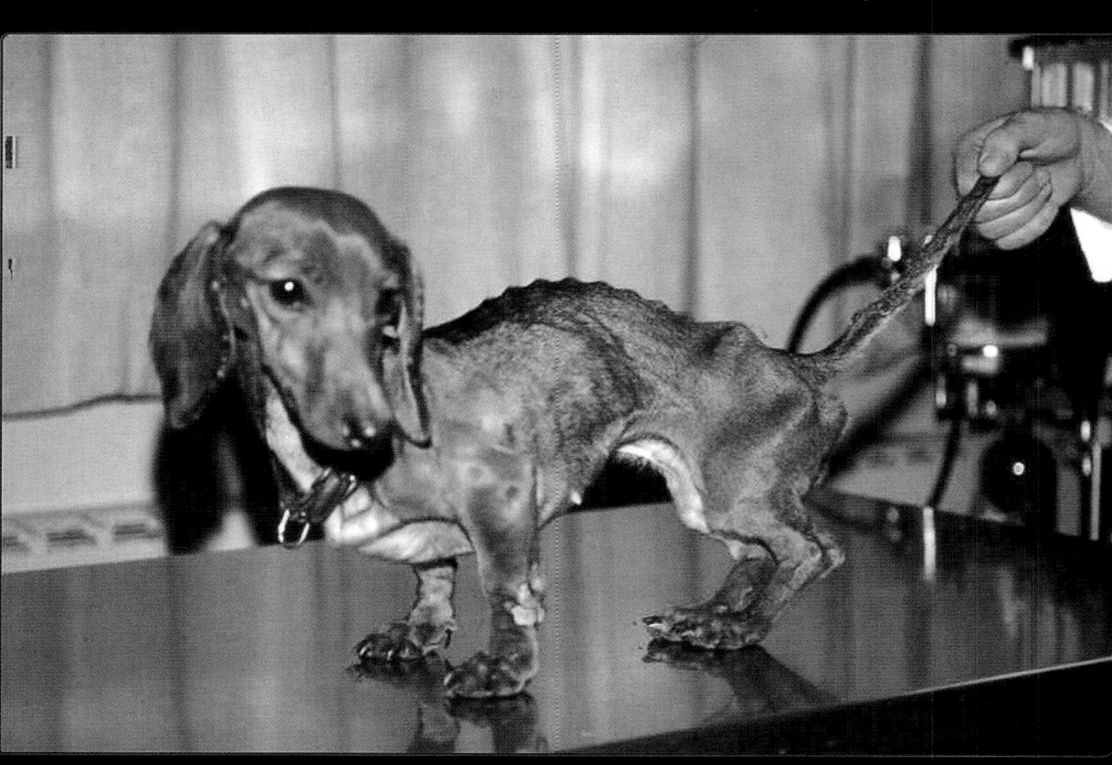

▲ This emaciated Dachshund has untreated exocrine pancreatic insufficiency.

9

Gastrointestinal disorders

GASTROENTEROLOGY is derived from the Greek words *gaster*, meaning stomach or belly, *enteron*, meaning intestines, and *logos*, meaning reason. Gastroenterologic disorders comprise a number of syndromes that are commonly seen in practice. Many are easily diagnosed, while others can be amongst the most difficult diagnostic challenges. Although gastroenterology refers to the stomach and the intestines, the discipline also includes disorders of the pancreas and liver, thus causing it to have a respectable volume in any of today's textbooks of medicine.

Most experienced clinicians begin their evaluation of the gastrointestinal (GI) tract with a thorough history and physical examination. The history should inquire about any vomiting and diarrhea, and the details of these abnormalities should be provided. A thorough dietary history is also important. The routine medical work up entails a complete blood count; a serum chemistry panel including serum electrolyte levels; fecal examination for evidence of parasites; and various specialized tests such as trypsinogen-like immunoassay, pancreatic lipase immunoassay, vitamin B12 serum concentration, and several others that can be found in any of the standard textbooks. Diagnostic imaging commonly involves radiography, abdominal ultrasonography, and endoscopy. It is essential for the clinician to biopsy any tissues when the diagnostic evaluation offers that opportunity. The images that follow illustrate the diverse pathology and the means of diagnosing many of the disorders that involve the GI system.

9 Gastrointestinal disorders

- GI obstructions – main sign is vomiting.
- Causes of coffee ground vomitus: gastric ulcers (primary/secondary), uremic gastritis.
- Melena causes: upper GI lesion, thrombocytopenia.
- Melena detection – "Let your finger do the walking".
- Elevated BUN plus normal creatinine – consider upper GI bleed, especially if kidney can concentrate urine.
- Bile in vomitus signifies pyloric patency.
- The lower the obstruction, the more feculent the vomitus.
- Never let the sun set on a linear foreign body intestinal obstruction.
- Look for pancreatic pathology when the right kidney is easily visible on a radiograph.
- Look under the tongue in any vomiting cat (and dog).

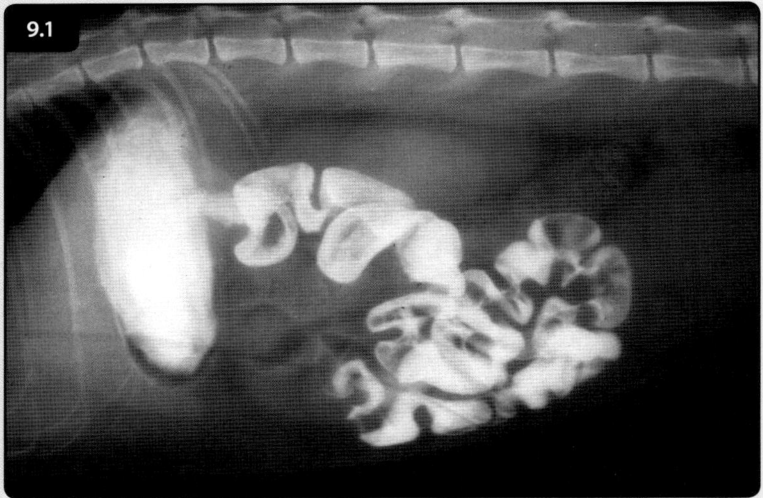

9.1. Barium study showing an intestinal linear foreign body. This lateral radiograph of a cat was taken 3 hours after a barium swallow. It shows intestinal plication (gathering) and delayed gastric emptying because of a linear foreign body obstruction. These patients typically will vomit, have anorexia, and do not pass a stool. Surgical delays are accompanied by worsened patient status and eventual bowel perforation. Treatment calls for first rehydrating the patient to correct hypovolemia and any serum electrolyte abnormalities, and then plan for surgery soon thereafter.

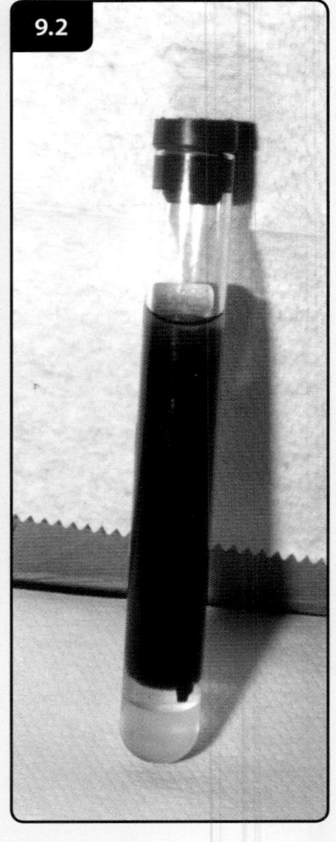

9.2. Hemoconcentration from hemorrhagic gastroenteritis. Notice how much volume the cellular fraction occupies in the blood tube from hemoconcentration. These patients suffer from acute hemorrhagic diarrhea and loose a disproportionate amount of plasma and water compared with red blood cell loss from their vascular space.

9.3. Free gas in abdomen. This ventrodorsal radiograph in a dog depicts free gas shown as a gas cap in the right diaphragm region (arrow). Free gas is a normal postoperative finding and requires close to a week to disappear. Outside of this particular setting, the presence of free gas in the abdomen constitutes grounds for an immediate surgical exploratory in search of a gastric or bowel perforation. Cytology on a fluid sample taken by fine needle aspiration of the abdomen will usually show a septic exudate.

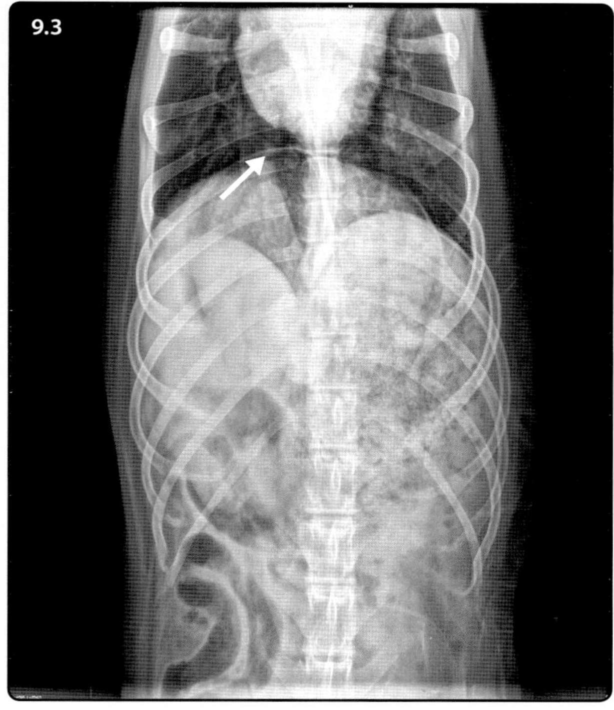
9.3

9.4. Hiatal hernia. This lateral abdominal radiograph shows the stomach herniating up the esophagus through the esophageal sphincter. This is shown as a fluid density in the distal esophagus. These patients often have considerable esophageal reflux and reflux esophagitis. They are medically treated with antacid drugs and sucralfate. Today most of these patients are corrected surgically using a gastropexy technique.

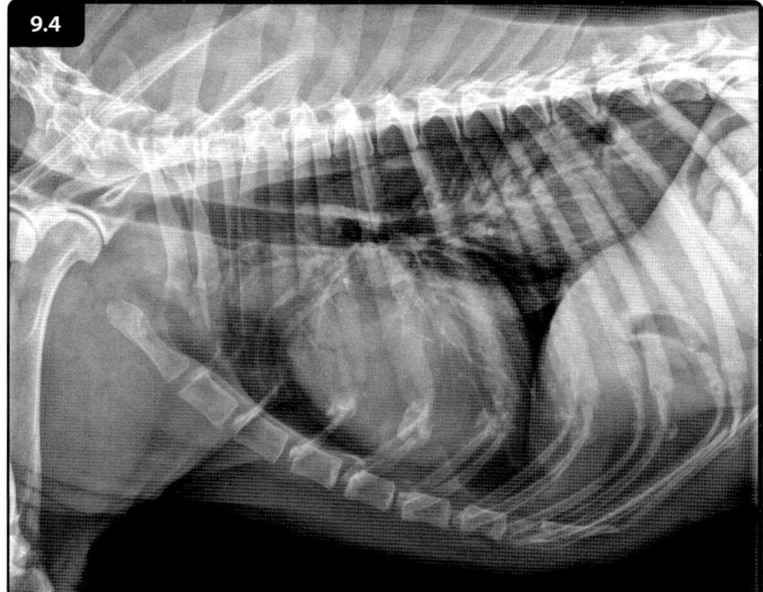
9.4

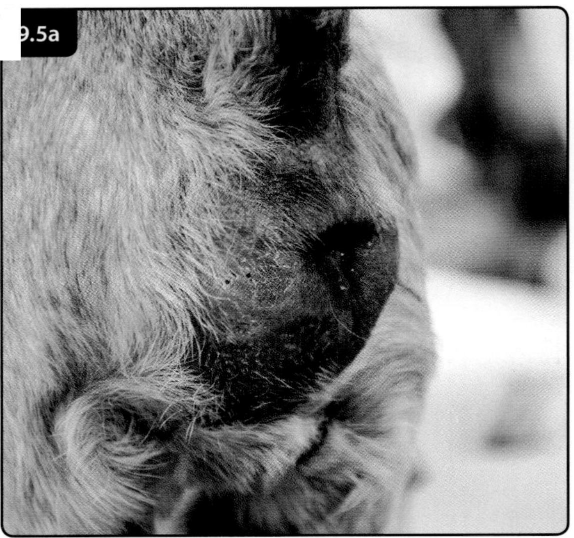

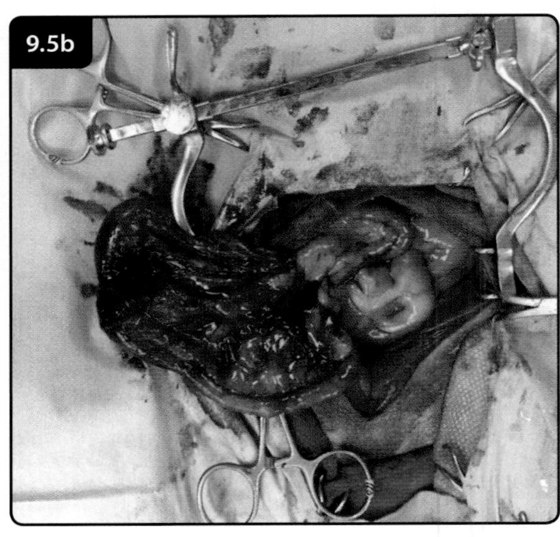

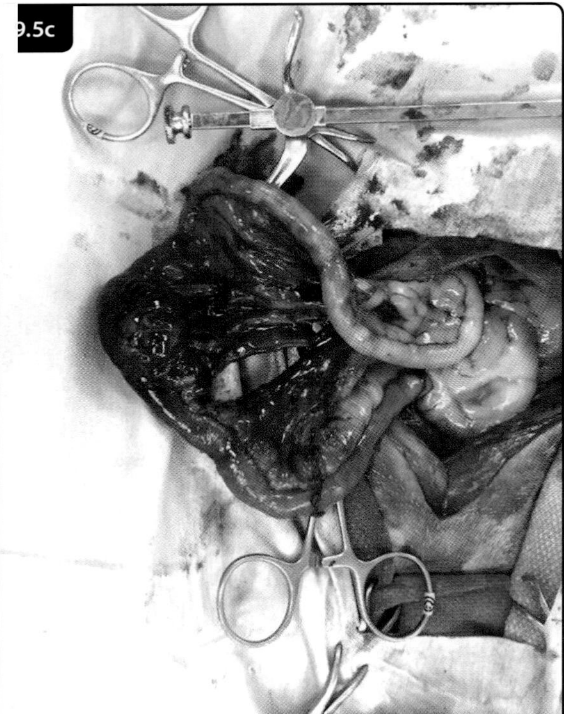

9.5a–c. Perineal hernia with bowel entrapment. This dog presented with loss of appetite and restlessness. The perineal swelling was warm and sensitive to touch. These signs precluded any fine needle aspirate tissue sampling. Surgery showed a section of devitalized bowel that required resection and anastamosis. Bulging perineal hernias can also contain the urinary bladder, which will be conspicuously absent on abdominal palpation. Organ entrapments such as these require emergency surgery to avoid further patient compromise.

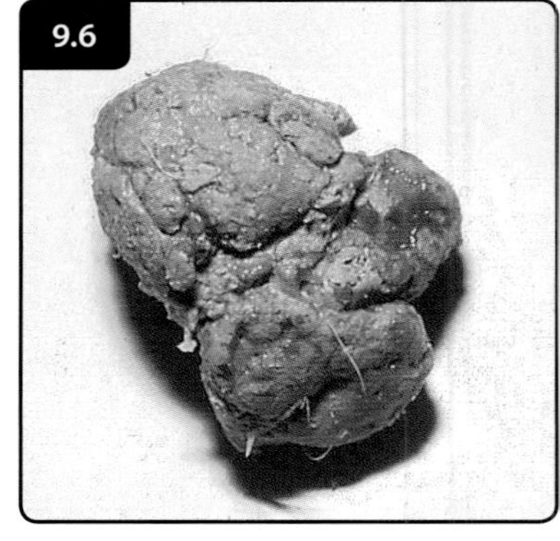

9.6. Acholic stool. This stool is light colored because it lacks bile salt pigments (stercobilins), caused by either bile duct obstruction or failure of their production in the liver. This is further explained in the chapter on liver disorders. This is rarely reported in dogs and cats, but it can occur, as shown in this figure.

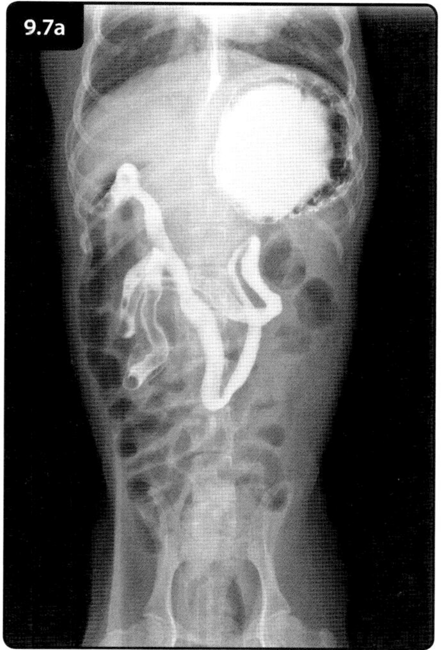

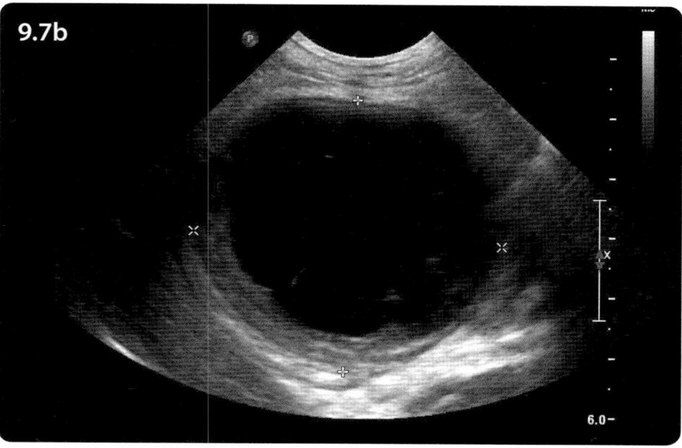

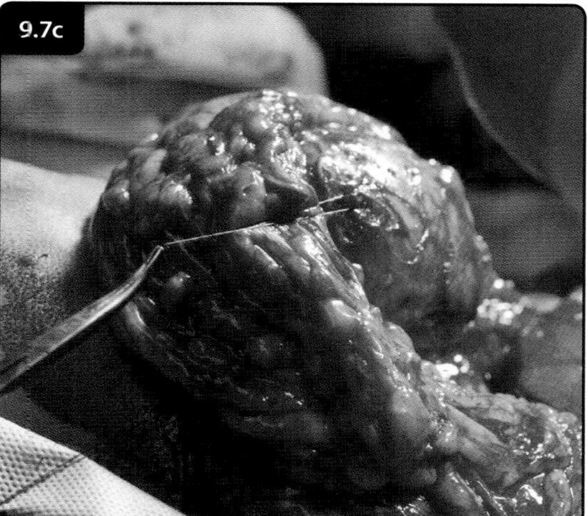

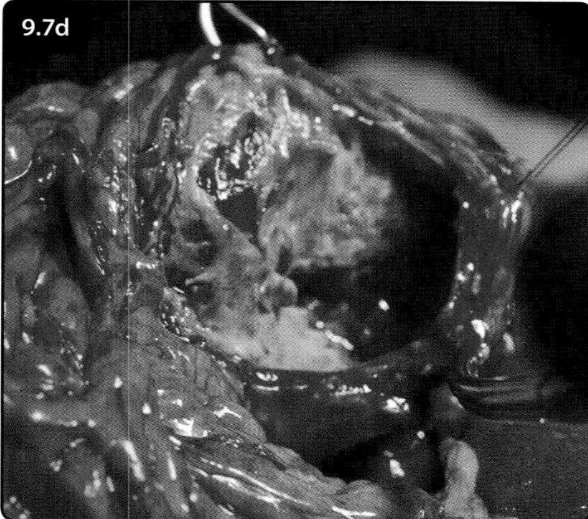

9.7a–d. Pancreatic pseudocyst. This condition occurs rarely in dogs with acute pancreatitis. It appears about 2 weeks after the acute disease and will reach variable sizes. It can appear as a space-occupying mass on the radiograph (Figure 9.7a) and cause vague abdominal discomfort. Most pancreatic pseudocysts are sterile, but some can become secondarily infected. Figure 9.7b shows a rather large ultrasonographic hypoechogenic mass associated with the pancreas, which was verified at surgery as a cyst-like structure associated with this dog's pancreas (Figures 9.7c, d). The mass was incised and drained and then marsupialized and packed with omentum.

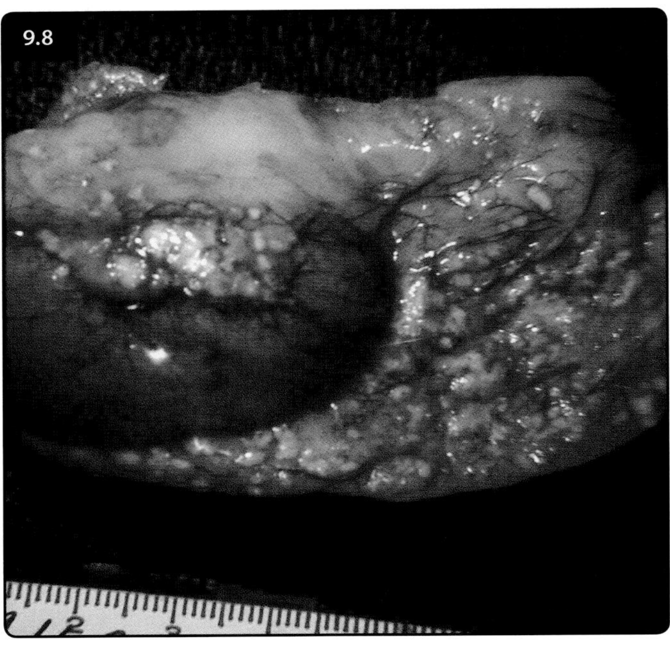

9.8. Saponification with acute pancreatitis. This image is from a dog that died from acute pancreatitis. Shown is the saponification (calcium soap formation) of the perirenal fat, which occurs as a result of lipolytic enzymes escaping from the inflamed pancreas into the abdominal cavity. The saponification process can even occur in the thorax if the enzymes settle in that particular part of the body. This kind of lesion is only associated with acute pancreatitis. The calcium soap deposits will disappear with time.

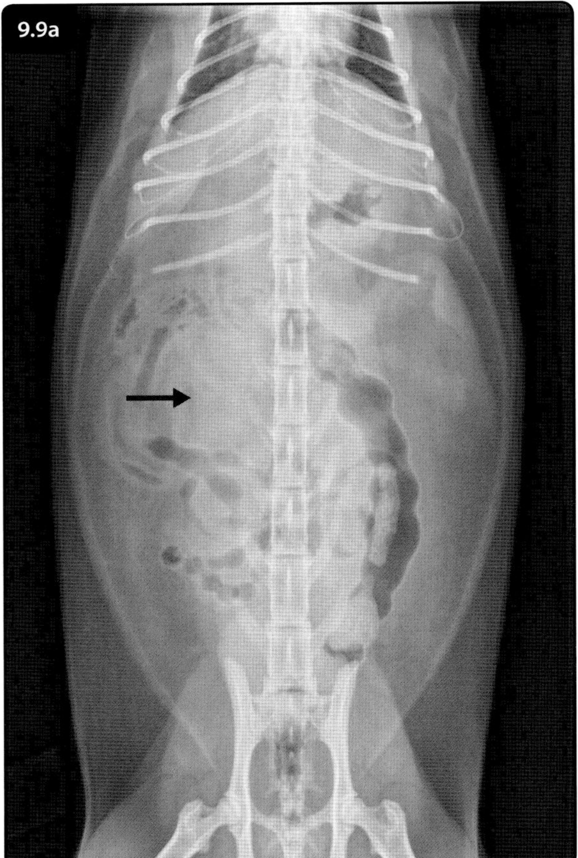

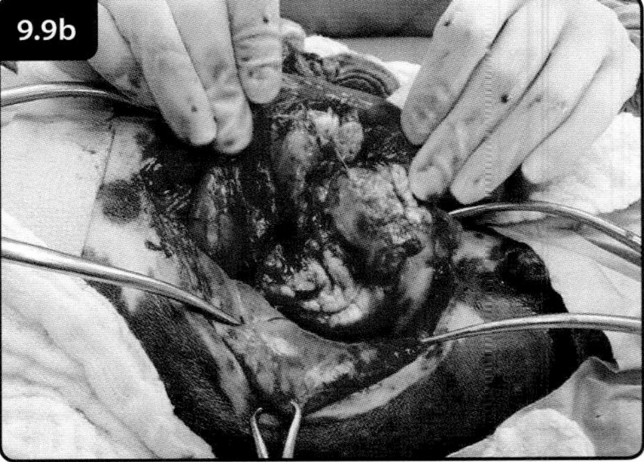

9.9 a, b. Postoperative acute pancreatitis. This dog went to surgery for insulinoma resection. The postoperative period was complicated by acute pancreatitis, which occurred after surgical manipulation of the pancreas. This complication should be anticipated in all patients that have pancreatic surgery. If it does occur, the pancreatitis should be looked upon as a major medical complication, although most cases will survive with adequate medical treatment. Figure 9.9a is a ventrodorsal abdominal radiograph that clearly shows the right kidney (arrow), a finding that is often seen in dogs with acute pancreatitis. The dog went back to surgery where acute pancreatitis and many abdominal adhesions were diagnosed (Figure 9.9b).

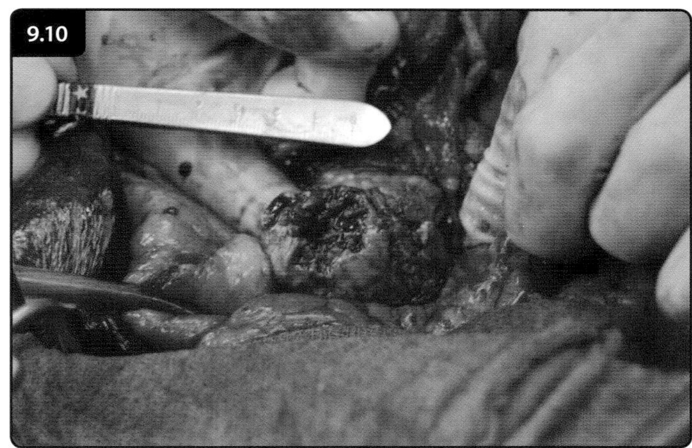

9.10. Pancreatic abscess. This lesion can be present in the pancreatitis patient 1–2 weeks after the initial acute signs. In veterinary patients, we use the term loosely because the puss-filled cavity is usually not surrounded by a fibrous wall. Surgical resection is the usual technique employed. The omentum is usually brought over to cover the retained segment. The abscess can be infected, most commonly by gram-negative bacteria, so the appropriate antibiotic should be used in these patients.

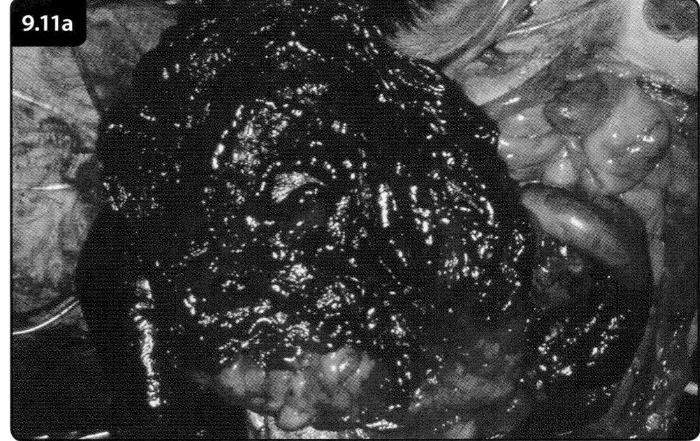

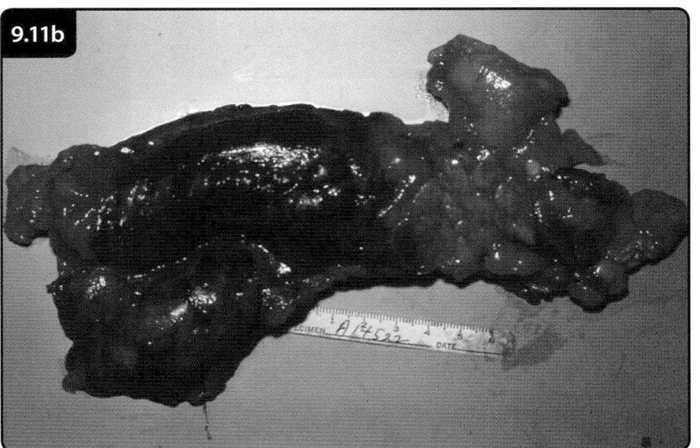

9.11a, b. Vascular infarction associated with acute pancreatitis. These surgical images were from a dog that presented as an abdominal emergency that soon went to surgery after it was stabilized in the intensive care unit. The omentum (Figure 9.11a), the pancreatic lymph node, and most of the pancreas (Figure 9.11b) were black in color because of regional infarction caused by the prothrombotic action of acute pancreatitis and the systemic inflammatory response syndrome. The vascular supply to the duodenum was also compromised, which led to the dog being euthanized.

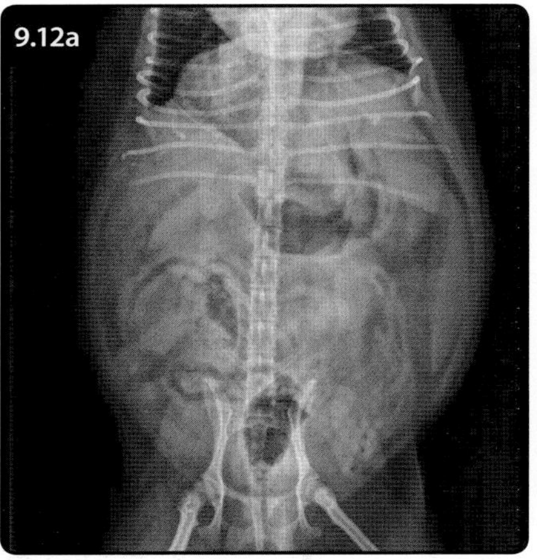
9.12a

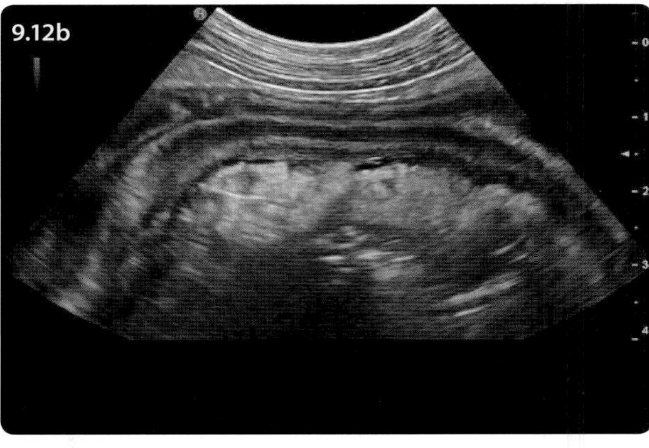
9.12b

9.12a, b. Radiographic findings with acute pancreatitis. The ventrodorsal view shows a clear outline of the right kidney, which the author has repeatedly seen with acute pancreatitis. This appearance might be due to abdominal adhesions moving bowel out of the way and so visualizing the right kidney, which is rarely visible in normal dog abdominal radiographs. There is also a loss of serosal detail because of abdominal fluid accumulation from the accompanying acute peritonitis. The abdominal ultrasound image clearly shows the hyperechoic pancreas, which is associated with localized calcium soap deposition.

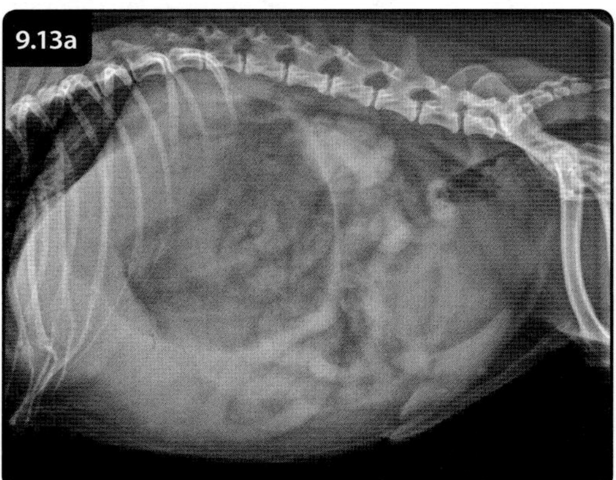
9.13a

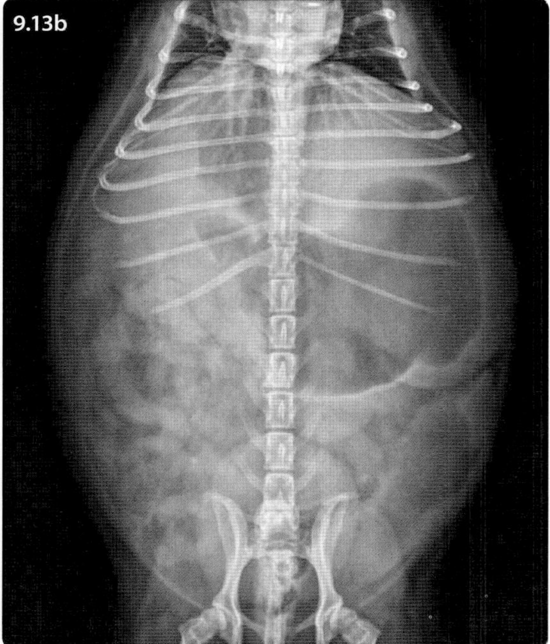
9.13b

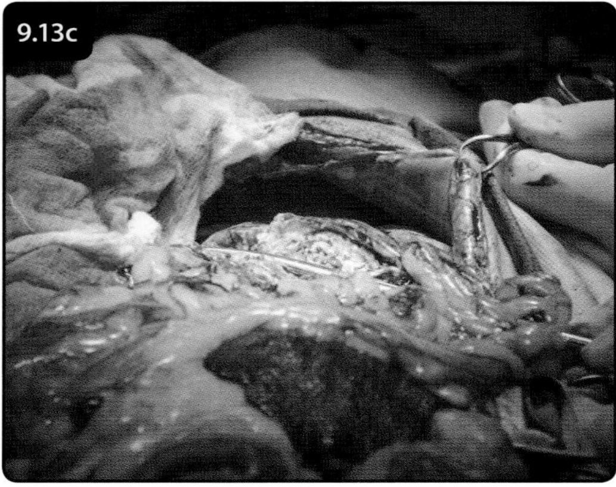
9.13c

9.14. Fine needle aspiration and cytology in pancreatitis. This procedure in Case 9.13 above yielded a serosanguineous sterile exudate with neutrophils and amorphous debris.

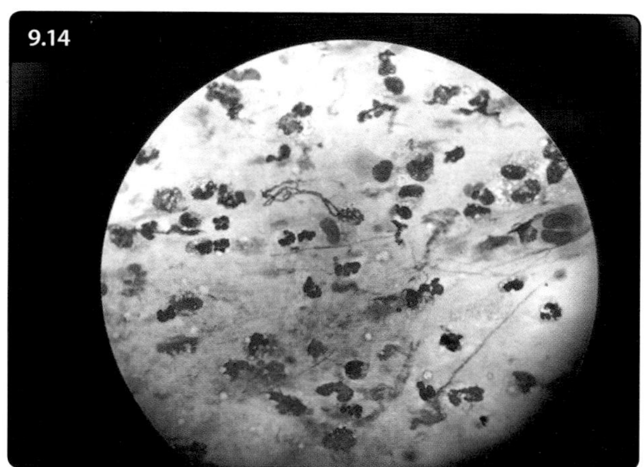

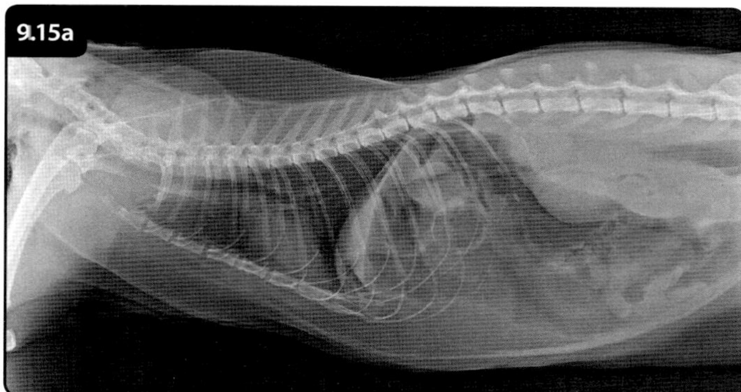

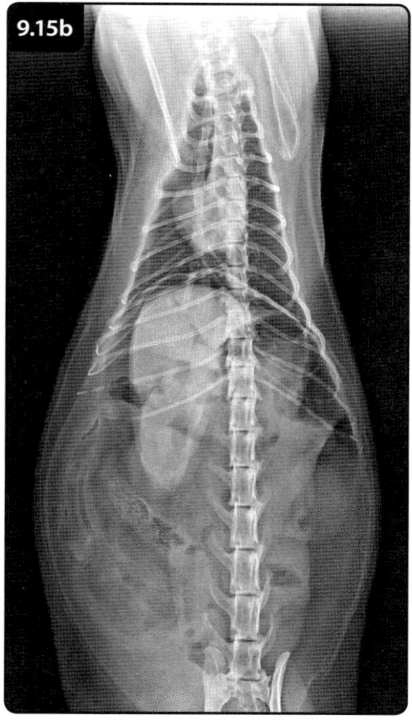

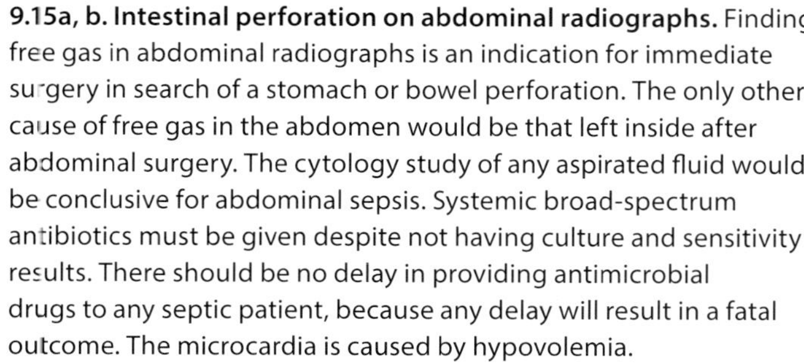

9.15a, b. Intestinal perforation on abdominal radiographs. Finding free gas in abdominal radiographs is an indication for immediate surgery in search of a stomach or bowel perforation. The only other cause of free gas in the abdomen would be that left inside after abdominal surgery. The cytology study of any aspirated fluid would be conclusive for abdominal sepsis. Systemic broad-spectrum antibiotics must be given despite not having culture and sensitivity results. There should be no delay in providing antimicrobial drugs to any septic patient, because any delay will result in a fatal outcome. The microcardia is caused by hypovolemia.

9.13a–c. Acute pancreatitis with phlegmon radiographs. The lateral and ventrodorsal views show a gas-filled distended stomach, loss of serosal detail, and a fluid density in the cranial right abdomen in the pyloric region. The distended stomach is the result of a paralytic ileus that accompanies the peritonitis; the latter also causes the loss of serosal detail. The fluid mass is in the area where the right limb of the pancreas would normally lie. Figure 9.13c shows the phlegmon formed by the acute pancreatitis. This is a serious complication that has a very guarded prognosis. There is no surgical remedy for this problem because the abdominal viscera are aggregated into one large inflammatory mass and dissection would likely injure the involved organs. Surgical irrigation, insertion of a jejunostomy feeding tube, and meticulous postoperative care would be the only possible treatment.

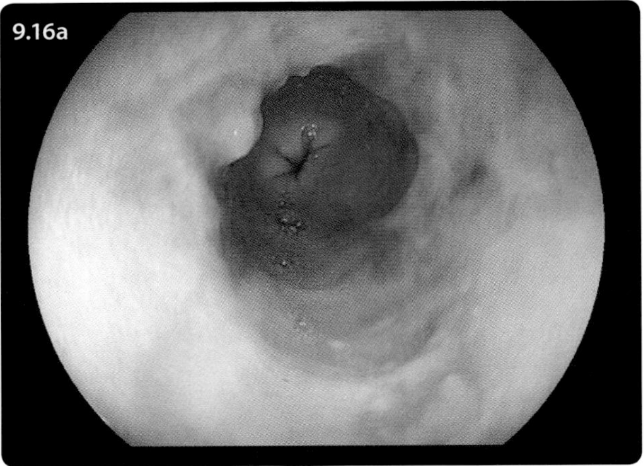

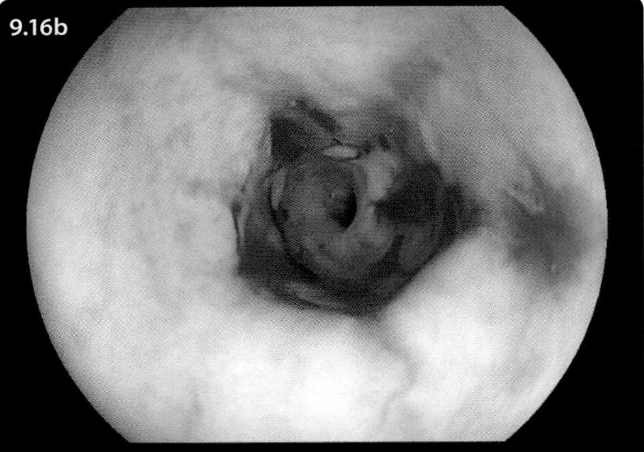

9.16a, b. Esophageal stricture. Figure 9.16a shows a constricted esophageal lumen during esophagoscopy. This lesion can develop from irritating oral antibiotics, such as doxycycline and clindamycin, foreign bodies and tumors, and episodes of acid reflux from the stomach. The characteristic clinical signs include regurgitation, retching, ptyalism, and sometimes painful posturing. Thoracic radiographs should be obtained to inspect for perforation and to assess the lungs for any aspiration pneumonia. The uncomplicated case can be successfully treated with several scheduled esophageal balloon dilatation procedures, which will gradually break down the stricture (Figure 9.16b). The procedure should be done carefully to avoid perforating the esophageal wall.

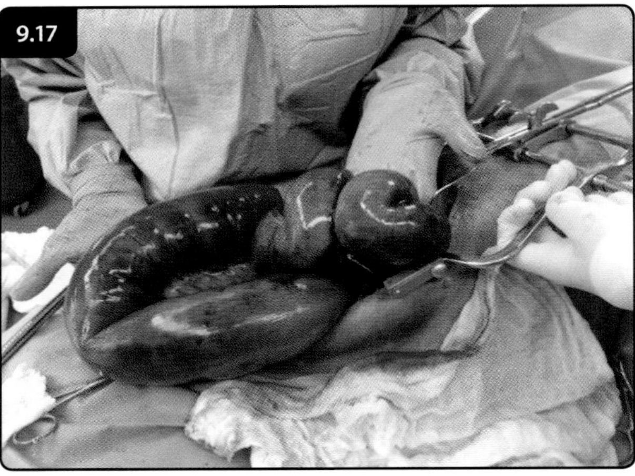

9.17. Diaphragmatic hernia and bowel strangulation. As a general rule, the larger the rent in the diaphragm the less chances for compromising the blood supply to the organs that slip into the chest cavity. However, a large volume of viscera or torsion of the herniated organs can be met with disastrous consequences such as ischemia or necrosis, as seen in this image. Generally, it is best not to untwist the involved organ, but rather to clamp, resect, and anastomose, if possible. The prognosis for the extensive hypoperfusion in the organs shown would be guarded to grave.

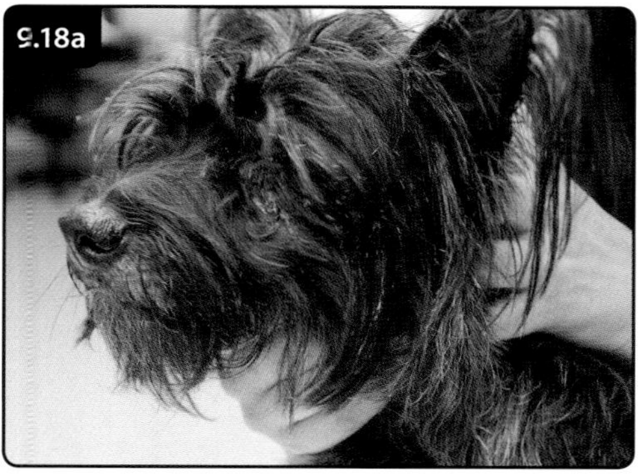

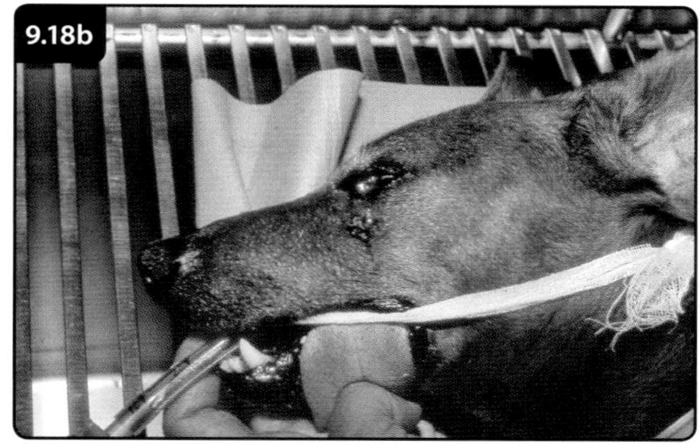

9.18a–c. Carnassial tooth abscess. A Cairn Terrier (Figures 9.18a, c) and a Dachshund (Figure 9.18b) were brought to the veterinarian when their owners noticed a draining tract under the left eye. The dogs were eating their food more slowly than usual. The location of the draining lesion is typical of a carnassial abscess that involves the upper 4th premolar tooth (Figure 9.18c). Dental radiographs are recommended in order to assess the extent of the damage. Treatment requires extracting the tooth, antibiotics, and routine wound care.

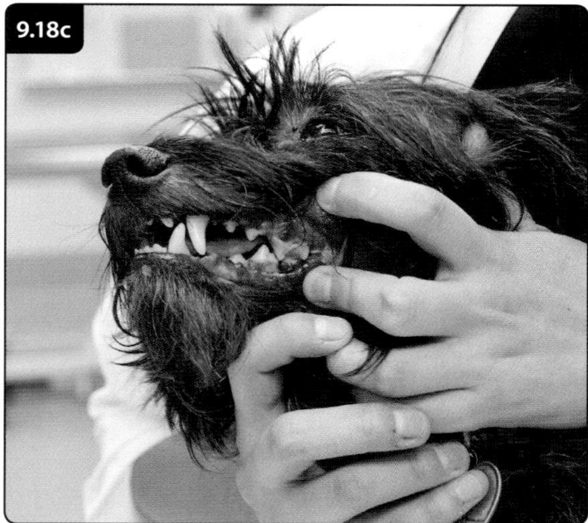

9.19. Large bowel mucus cast in a cat. The stool specimen located on the right of this image was coated with a reddish colored mucoid layer depicting colon inflammation. Colitis in the cat has several causes but despite a thorough work up in search of an etiology (e.g. parasites, diet, inflammatory bowel disease, neoplasia), some incidents are random and limited.

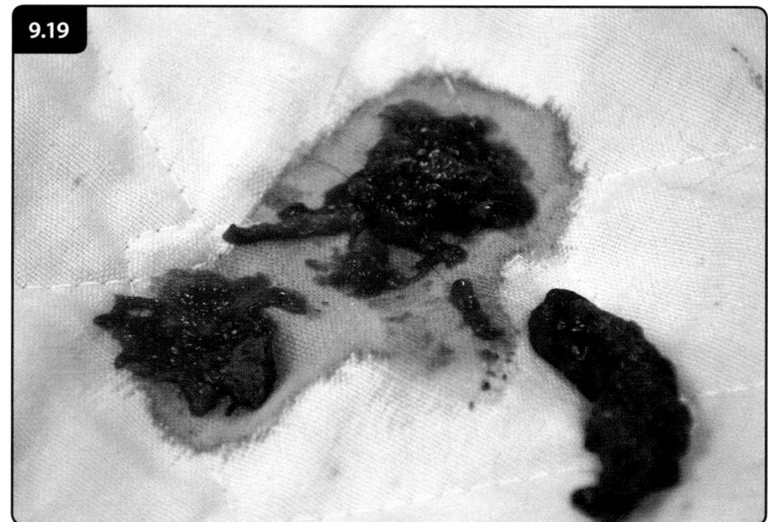

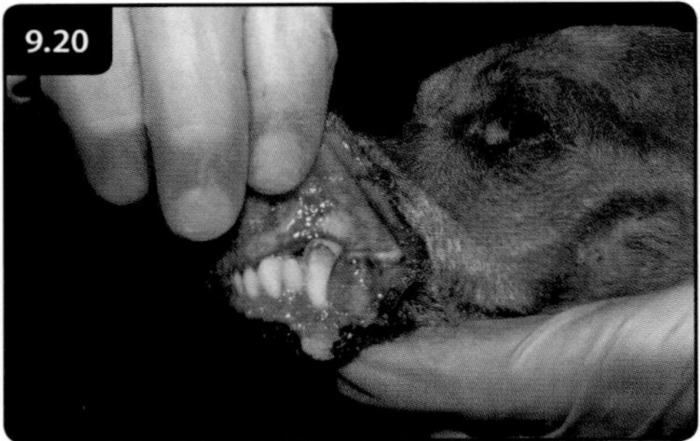

9.20. Cheilitis. Lip inflammation can occur from irritant contact or it can represent some advanced disease process such as pemphigus vulgaris, as shown in this patient that also has severe stomatitis. Treatment depends on the cause, ranging from minor cleansing to long-term anti-inflammatory drugs.

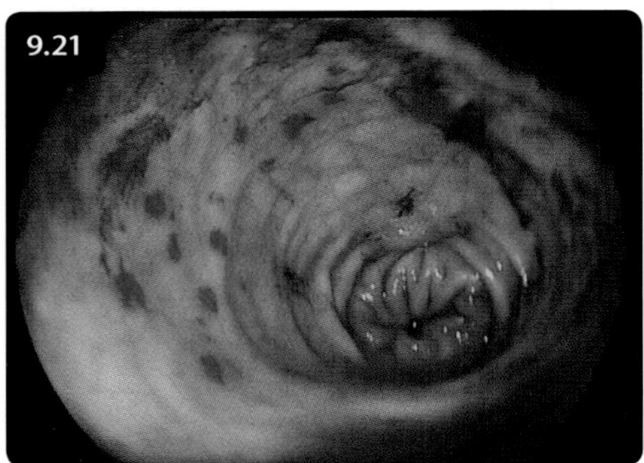

9.21. Vascular ectasia. This coloscopic view of the large bowel shows areas of vascular ectasia that were responsible for this dog's profuse hematochezia. This is a rare condition characterized by the formation of superficial dilated blood vessels that can bleed spontaneously. Several anti-inflammatory drugs were attempted but to no avail. Treatment success required colonoscopic intraluminal cauterization. (Image courtesy University of Florida Small Animal Internal Medicine Service)

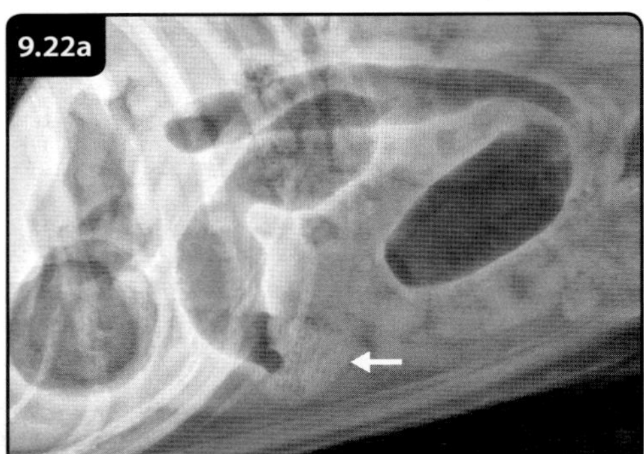

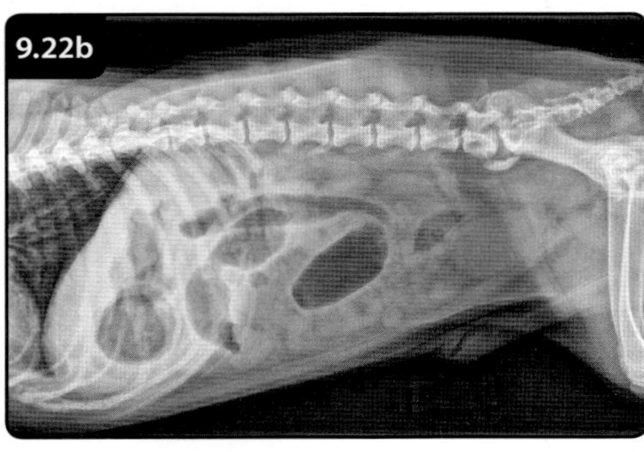

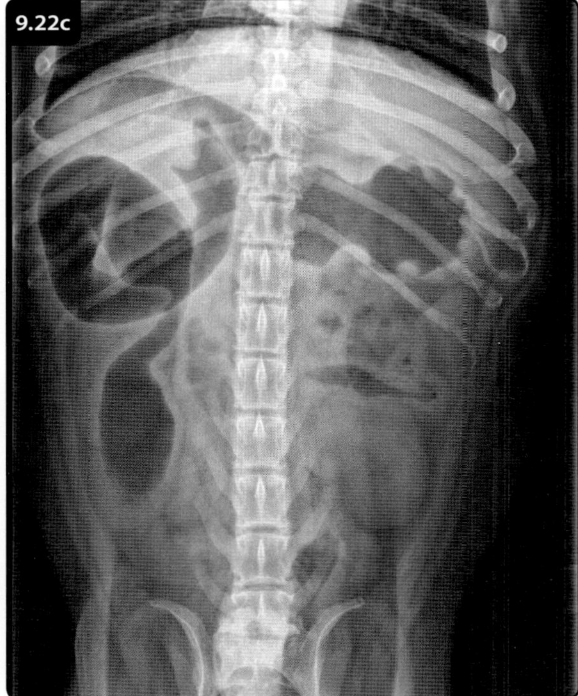

9.22a–c. Corn cob small bowel obstruction. These radiographs show an intestinal foreign body obstruction caused by an ingested corn cob. The air cells of the corn cob are visible in Figure 9.22a (arrow). The intestinal obstruction is evident by the segmental asymmetrical distended bowel loops. It is the gas pattern and gas–fluid interphases on the radiograph that characterize the bowel as being obstructed.

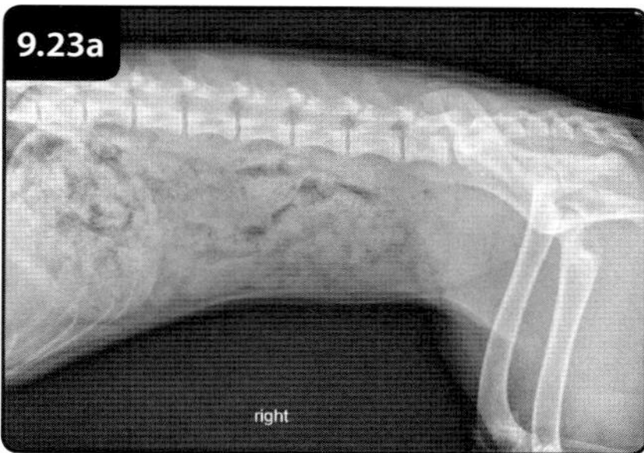

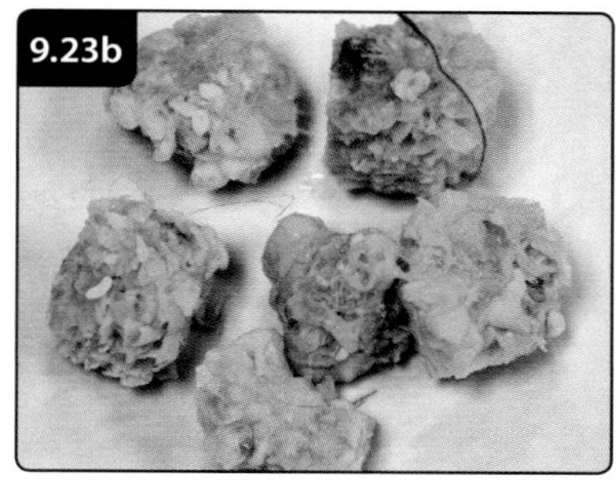

9.23a, b. Gastric corn cob foreign bodies. This lateral abdominal radiograph is from another dog that ingested many corn cobs, which are visible in the stomach. The large number of pieces and the possibility that the duodenum is involved justified a surgical exploratory to remove the foreign bodies. Figure 9.23b shows the corn cobs that were surgically removed by gastrotomy.

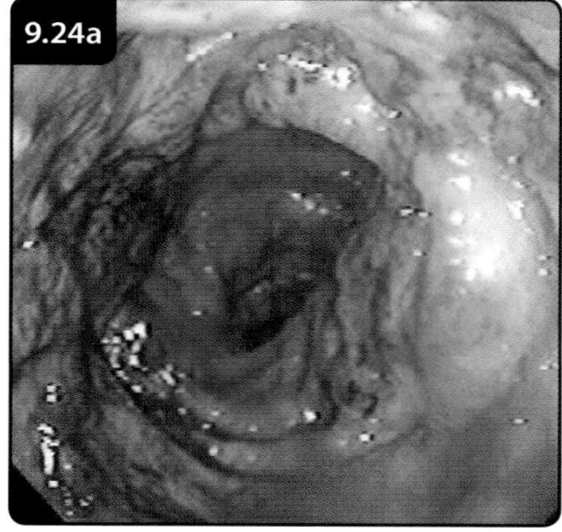

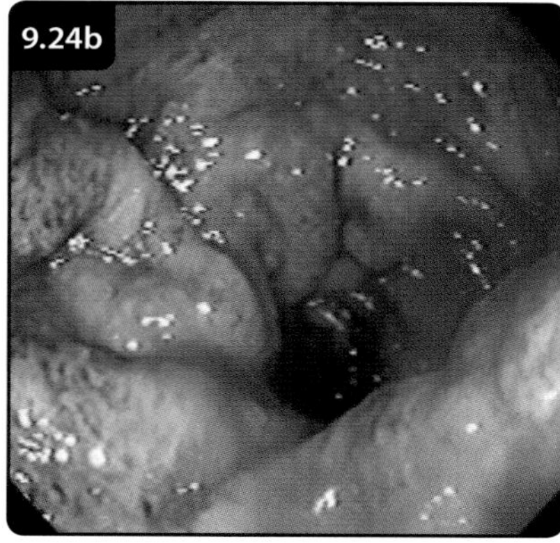

9.24a, b. Colon carcinoma. These colonoscopic images show colon carcinoma. Rectal palpation would detect bowel mucosal irregularity and thickening with luminal attenuation. Historically, such patients might have hematochezia and abnormally flattened stools. Diagnosis is made with histopathology of a biopsy specimen. Treatment would entail a partial or total colectomy, but metastasis to the liver and proximal structures is possible.

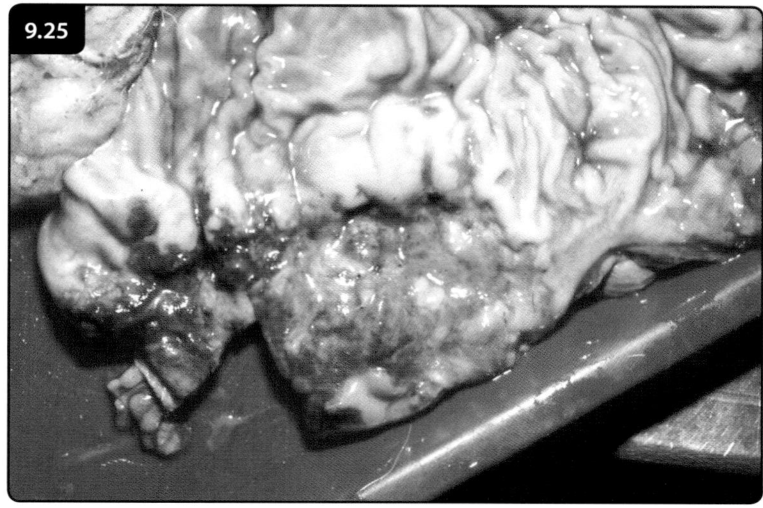

9.25. Gastric ulcer. This postmortem specimen shows a large crater ulcer of the stomach. The patient had immune thrombocytopenia and was treated with large doses of dexamethasone, which very likely caused the gastric mucosal compromise. The dog became septic and formed a thrombus that obstructed her femoral artery.

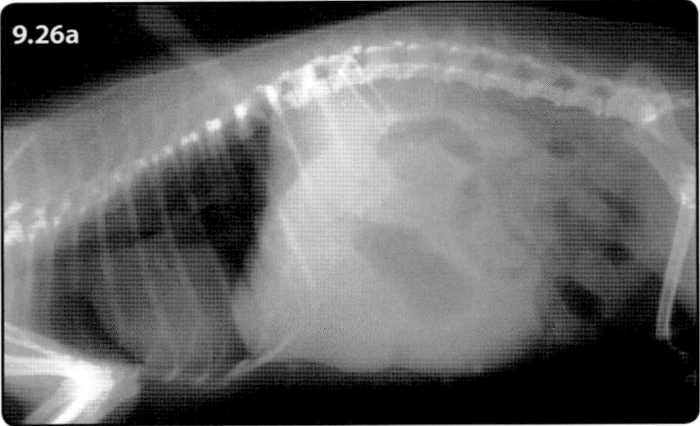

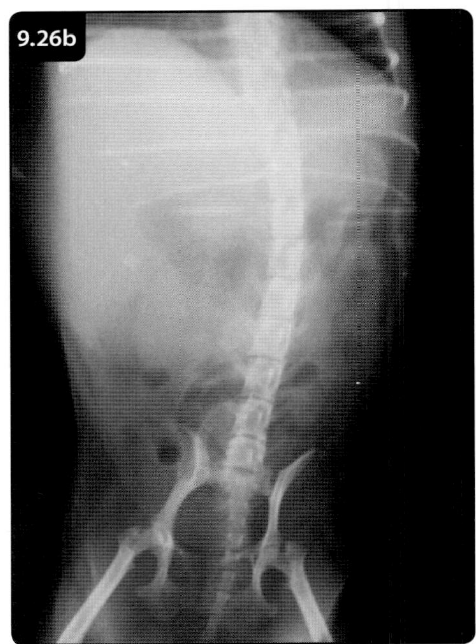

9.26a, b. Iatrogenic gastric ileus. These lateral and dorsoventral abdominal referral radiographs depict a very distended fluid-filled stomach, which was caused by the administration of a parasympatholytic drug that was given for the dog's diarrhea. Such distension caused this dog to be distressed. It was relieved by the passage of an oral gastric tube, which was used to empty the stomach. An example such as this attests to the adverse side-effects when using this type of drug.

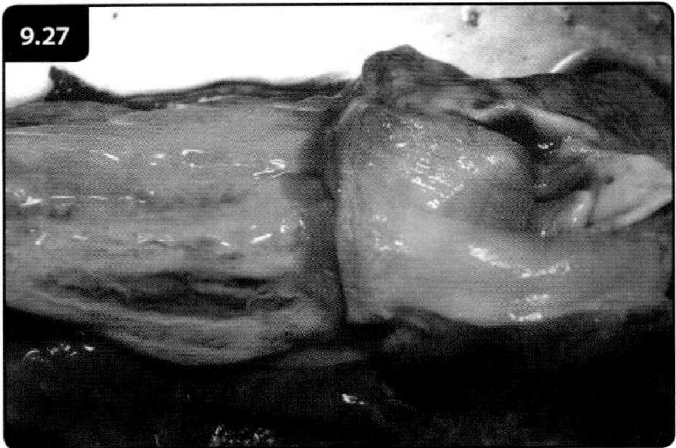

9.27. Esophageal erosion. Shown is a dog's esophagus with several large erosions. This dog was showing clinical signs of retching and was regurgitating a clear mucoid fluid. The dog's primary disease was glomerulonephropathy and renal failure. Treatment for this dog's esophageal lesions would need to consist of antacid drugs, such as H2 or proton pump inhibitors, and sucralfate.

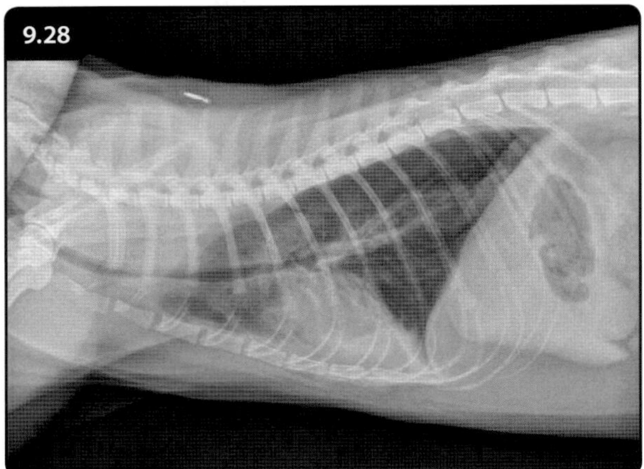

9.28. Esophageal hairball obstruction. The consequences of hairballs in the cat span the spectrum of severity. This radiograph shows the 'bad' side of that curve, as shown by the hairball foreign body obstruction in the esophagus. Note the ventral displacement of the cat's esophagus. There is also some consolidation of the middle lung lobe, which might represent an aspiration pneumonia.

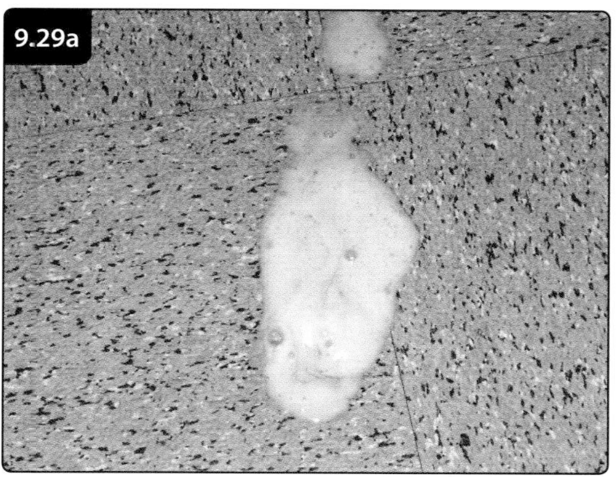

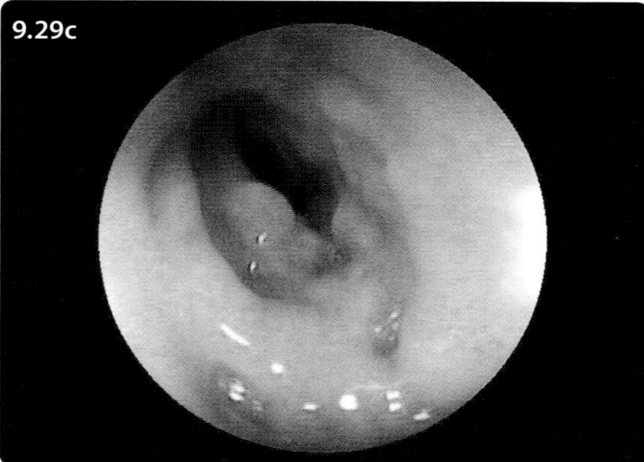

9.29a–c. Esophageal regurgitated fluid. This fluid (Figure 9.29a) is typical of esophageal reflux. The clinical sign of esophageal regurgitated fluid can accompany many conditions ranging from nausea associated with systemic disease to specific esophageal pathology. Figures 9.29b, c show the underlying cause of the reflux, as evidenced by the ulcers and stricture.

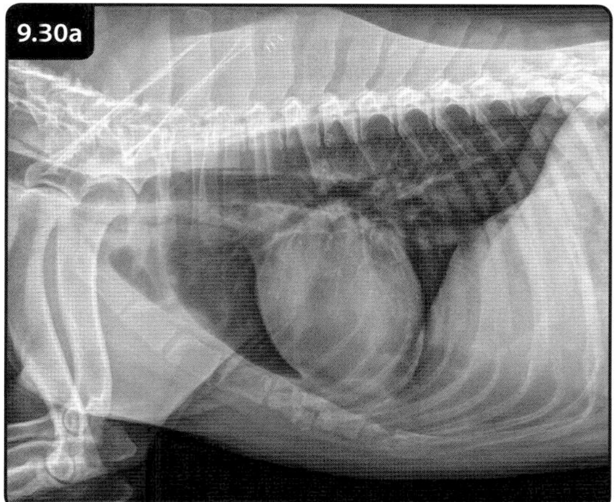

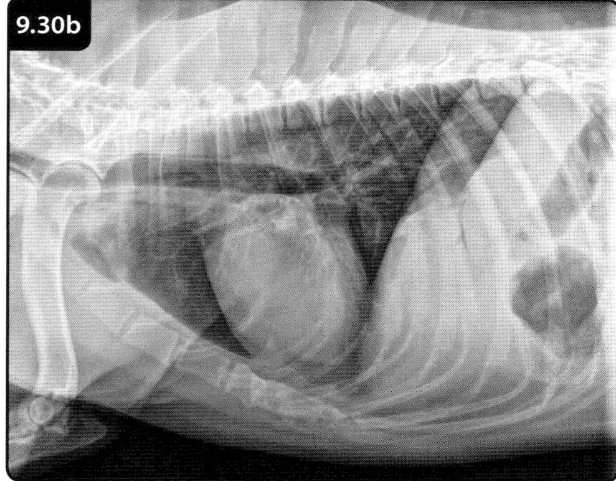

9.30a, b. Esophageal tear and mediastinal gas. These two thoracic radiographs show gas in the cranial mediastinum that was due to an esophageal tear. With the absence of pleural fluid, it was decided to treat this conservatively with sucralfate suspension. The dog recovered without consequence.

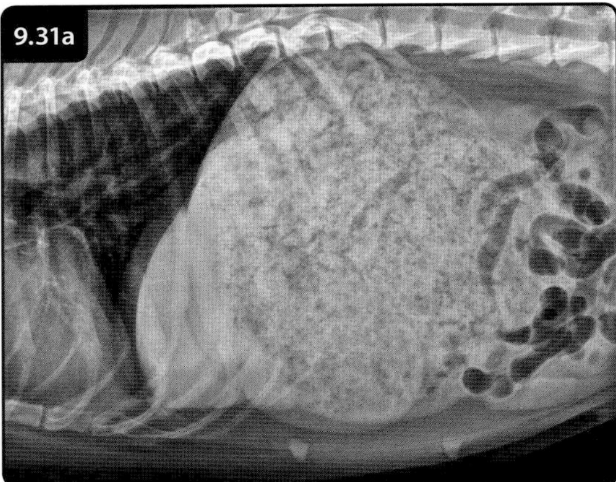

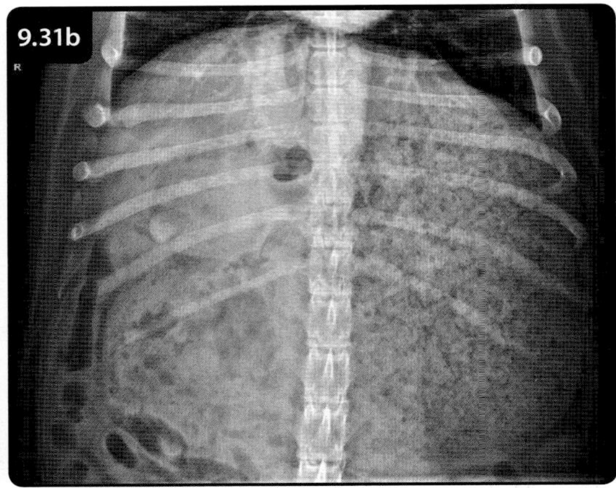

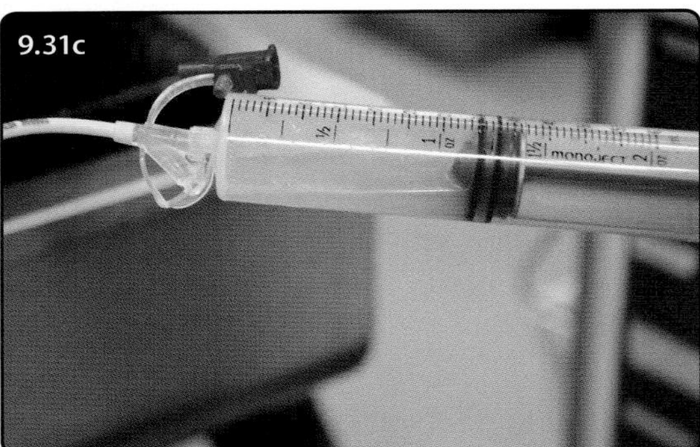

9.31a–c. Gastric dilatation. These two radiographs (Figures 9.31a, b) show that the stomach is in a normal position, but its size is very enlarged because of retained food contents. Since the dog was distressed at the time of examination, it was given intravenous crystalloid solution, anesthetized, and underwent stomach decompression using a gastric tube (Figure 9.31c). Recovery was uneventful.

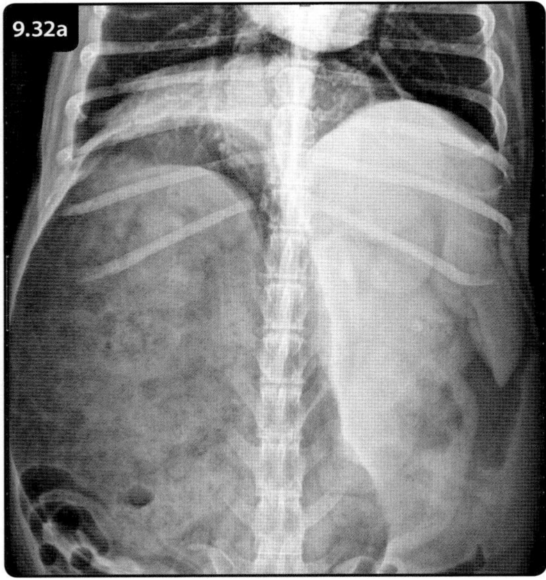

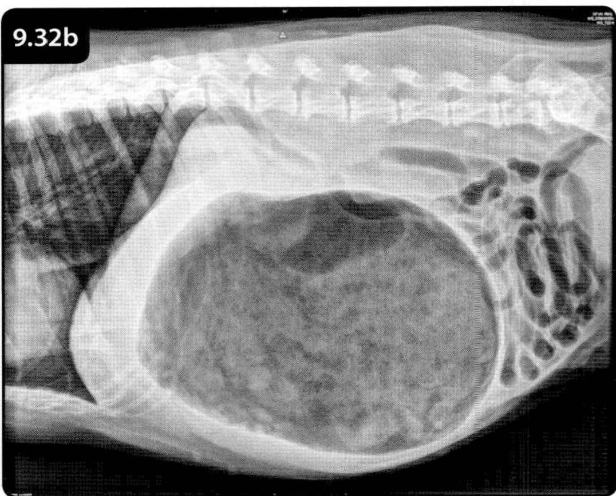

9.32a, b. Gastric volvulus. These abdominal radiographs show that the stomach is malpositioned. The fundus is displaced to the right side of the abdomen and the pylorus is not visible in the ventral abdomen. Treatment requires patient stabilization with repeated intravenous fluid boluses, gastric decompression, and surgical decompression once the hypovolemia is improved.

9.33a, b. Lymphagiectasia with lipogranuloma. These pathologic images clearly depict the mucosal and serosal features of lymphagiectasia with lipogranuloma. The linear white streaks on the serosal aspect are anomalous gastrointestinal lymphatic vessels. These same abnormalities are depicted as white vascular distensions on the mucosal aspect. The lipogranuloma is a secondary tissue change, as seen on the serosal aspect. There is no cure for this disease other than nutritional support to help compensate for the loss of protein and other nutrients through the abnormal lymphatic vessels.

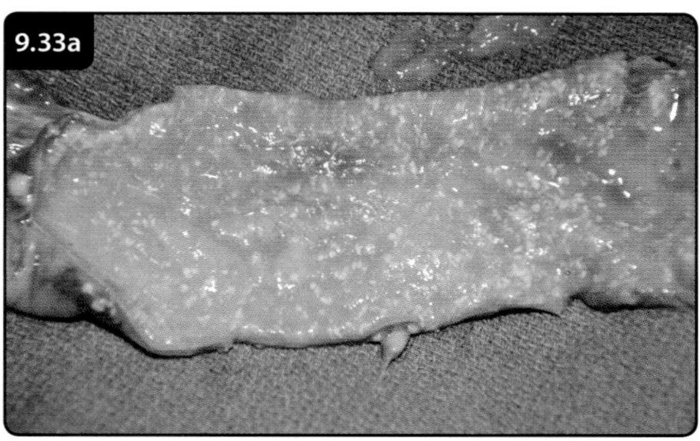
9.33a

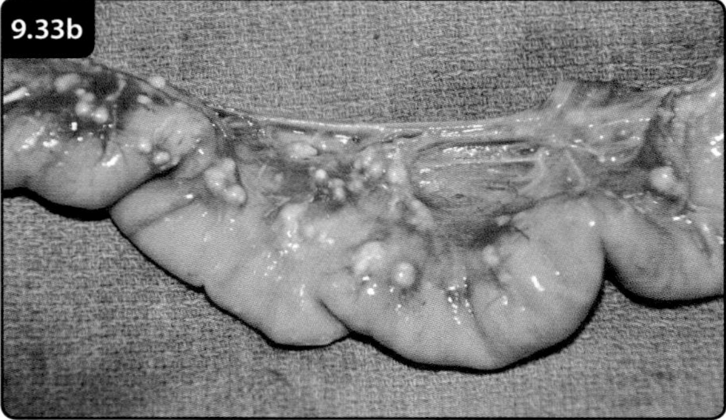
9.33b

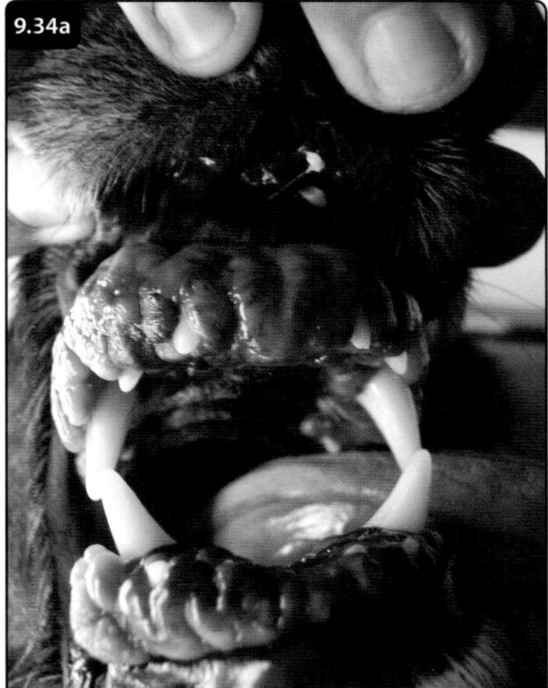
9.34a

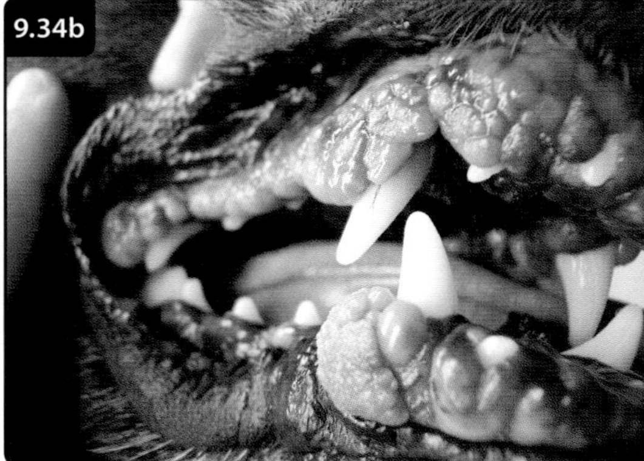
9.34b

9.34a, b. Cyclosporine-induced gingival hyperplasia. Cyclosporine is known to cause several side-effects such as vomiting, papilloma formation, anorexia, hair coat changes, and gingival hyperplasia. The diagnosis is obvious, with the supporting history noting that the lesions appeared several weeks after cyclosporine treatment had begun.

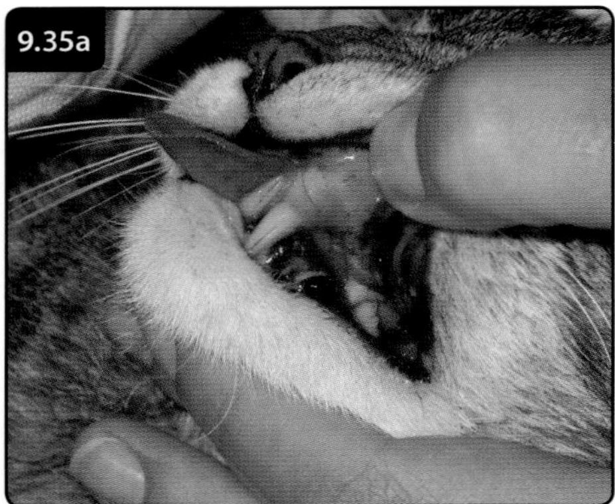

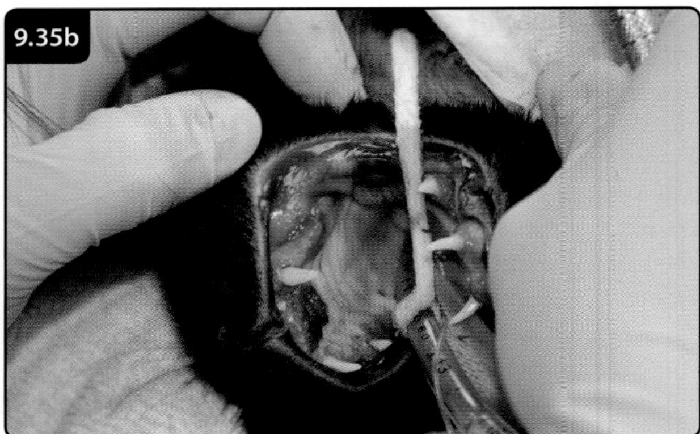

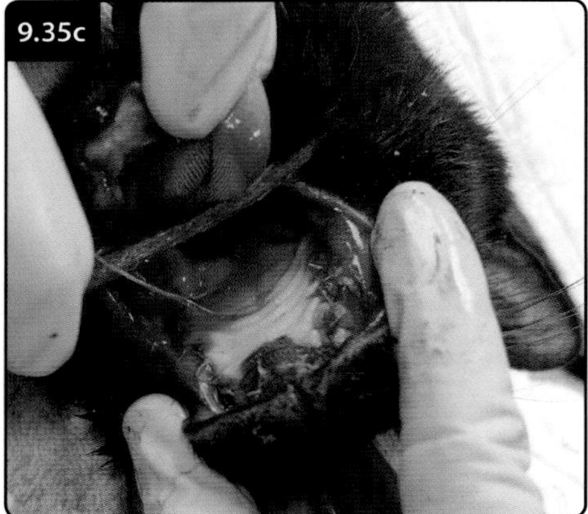

9.35a–c. Gingivitis and stomatitis in the cat. Figure 9.35a shows a limited degree of gingivitis compared with the cat in Figure 9.35b, which has very extensive inflammation. Note that the teeth appear healthy, which is often the case with this disorder. The inflammation is thought to be an immune response to the microflora that inhabit the tiny crevices of the mouth. Treatment involves a combination approach using antibiotics, anti-inflammatory drugs (glucocorticoids), and many tooth extractions, which in some cases might involve all of the teeth (Figure 9.35c).

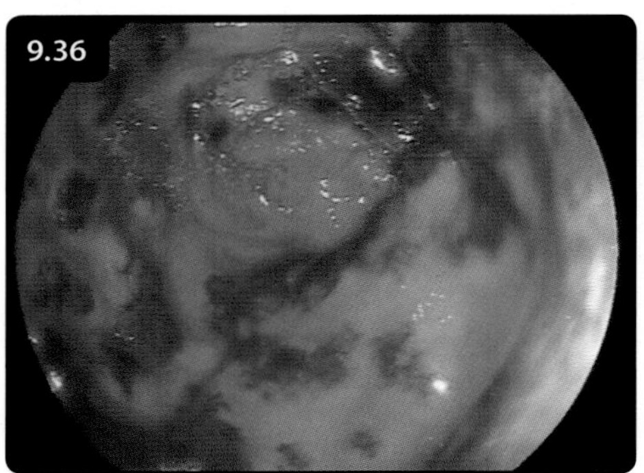

9.36. Gastric ulcers and gastritis. This endoscopic view of the stomach shows hemorrhage from inflammation and bleeding ulcers. These lesions can be associated with NSAID administration or a systemic disorder such as uremia. Treatment would entail discontinuing any offending drug, administering a proton pump inhibitor and sucralfate, and treating the underlying disorder; for example, acute kidney injury associated with leptospirosis.

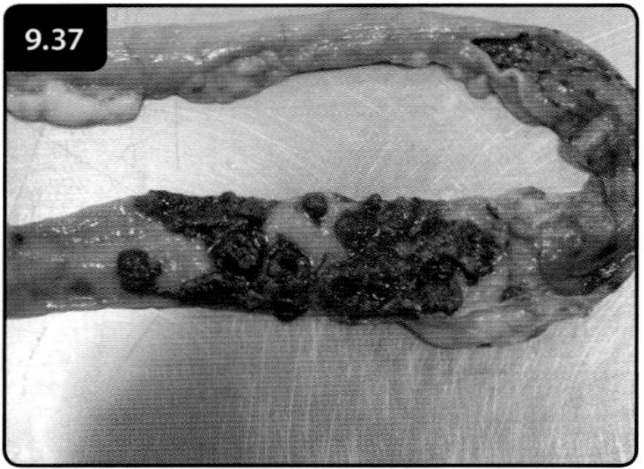

9.37. Granulomatous enteritis. This pathology specimen came from a dog that had chronic and debilitating gastrointestinal disease that led to its demise. The pathology was impressive but the etiology was never discovered. This condition will show accumulations of plasma cells and lymphocytes in the bowel mucosa much like inflammatory bowel disease, but to a much greater degree. Treatment would be specific for an identifiable cause or nonspecific using anti-inflammatory drugs with the hope for palliation.

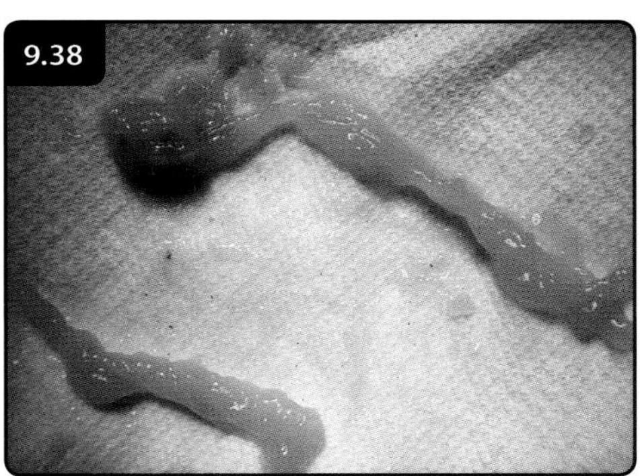

9.38. Colon mucus cast. This mucus cast exited a dog's rectum during its initial treatment phase for heat stroke. It was probably produced from the ischemia to the bowel caused by the heat stroke, and the dog was fortunate not to slough its entire bowel mucosa. It is not uncommon for patients with this condition to have hemorrhagic diarrhea as well because of the compromise in tissue perfusion and the bacterial takeover.

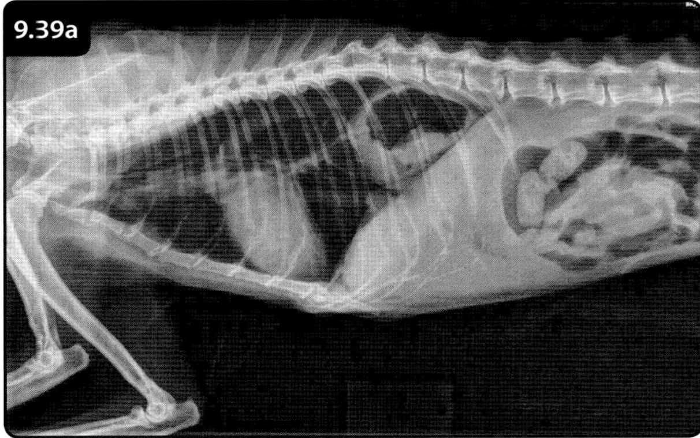

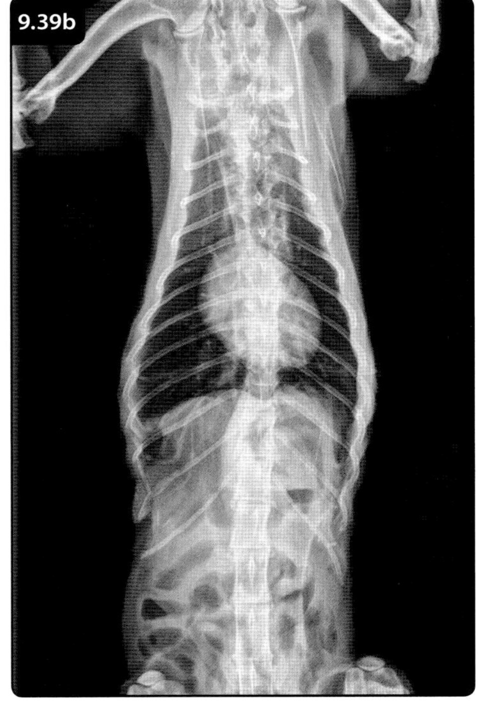

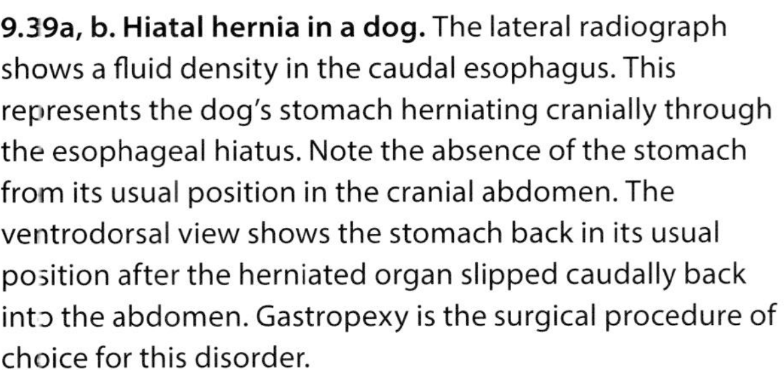

9.39a, b. Hiatal hernia in a dog. The lateral radiograph shows a fluid density in the caudal esophagus. This represents the dog's stomach herniating cranially through the esophageal hiatus. Note the absence of the stomach from its usual position in the cranial abdomen. The ventrodorsal view shows the stomach back in its usual position after the herniated organ slipped caudally back into the abdomen. Gastropexy is the surgical procedure of choice for this disorder.

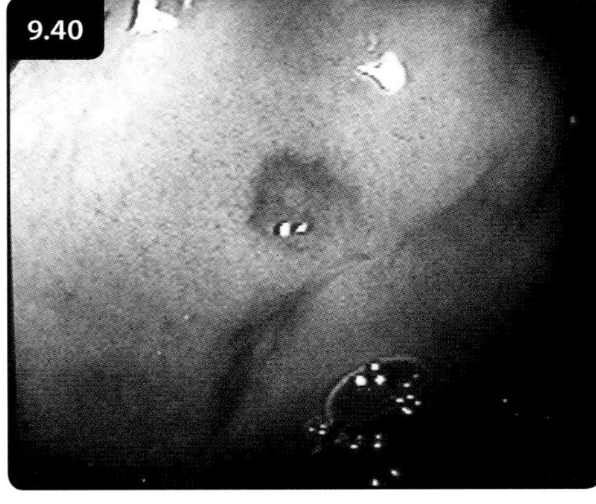

9.40. Ibuprofen-induced gastric ulceration. This gastroscopic view shows a clear view of gastric ulcers caused by this NSAID. There was no active bleeding at the time of the study, which allowed the clinician to have a clear view of the typical linear and other erosions that are produced from this class of drugs. Treatment calls for discontinuing the NSAID and providing a proton pump inhibitor drug and sucralfate treatment.

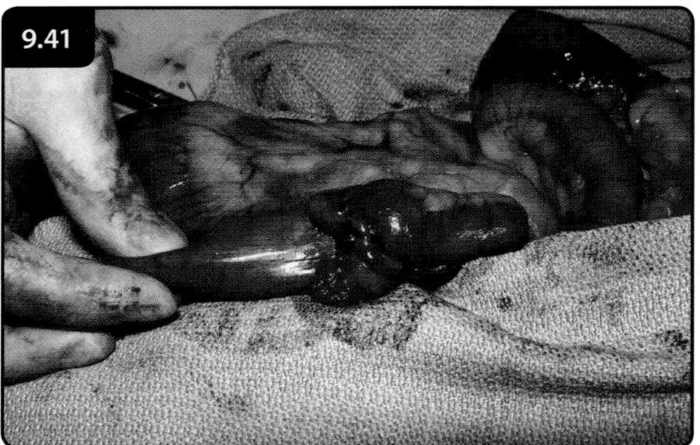

9.41. Intestinal obstruction and 'third spacing' fluids. Shown is an intestinal obstruction caused by slow-onset stricture formation from a prior surgery. The obstructed bowel segment acts as a third space within the extracellular fluid compartment, where extracellular fluid accumulates and does not exchange with the fluid in the interstitial and plasma spaces. This is the reason why parenteral fluids are usually administered at double the maintenance volume during surgery in order to keep the plasma space filled and maintain normal blood pressure.

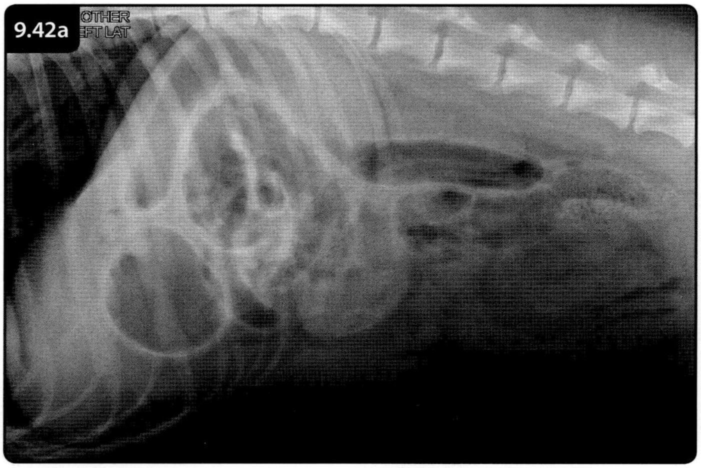

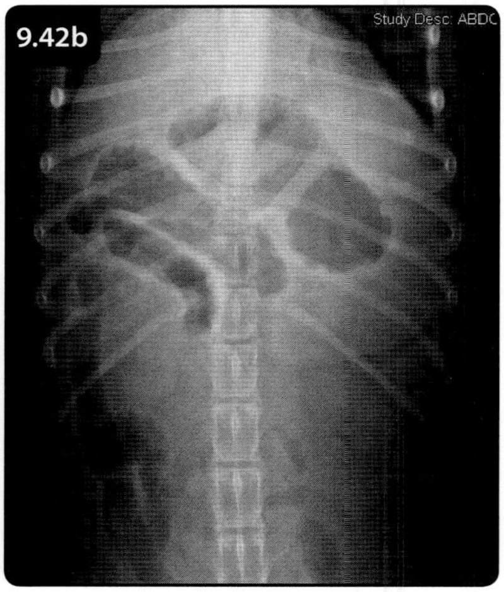

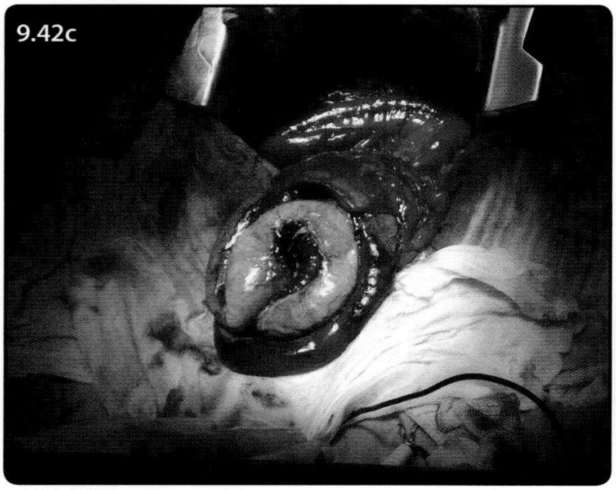

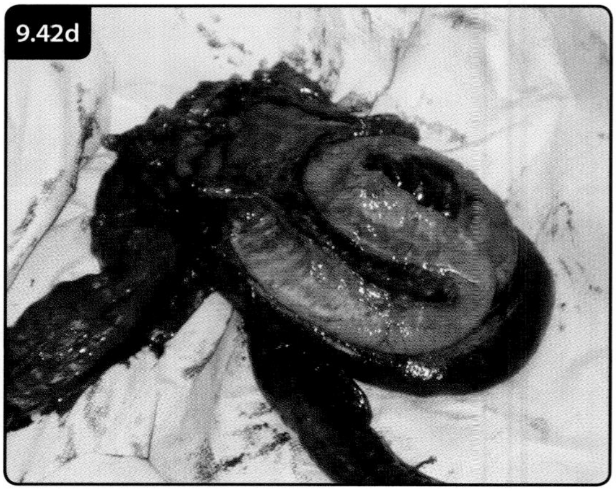

9.42a

9.42b

9.42c

9.42d

9.42a–d. Intestinal volvulus. The abdominal radiographs show segments of abnormally distended bowel and loops with gas–fluid interphases compatible with obstruction. At surgery, the jejunum was torsed and necrotic. Surgical resection of all the necrotic bowel was performed and the dog recovered without complications.

9.43. Pelvic cellulitis. The left ischial part of the pelvis has a gas pocket in the soft tissues (arrow). This finding is compatible with bite wound cellulitis and possible abscess formation. A fine needle aspirate with cytology and culture would give important information for case management. This wound should be rapidly drained and débrided in order to avoid spread of the cellulitis, which would make everything a lot more complicated. Antibiotics should be broad spectrum and modified according to the results of culture and sensitivity.

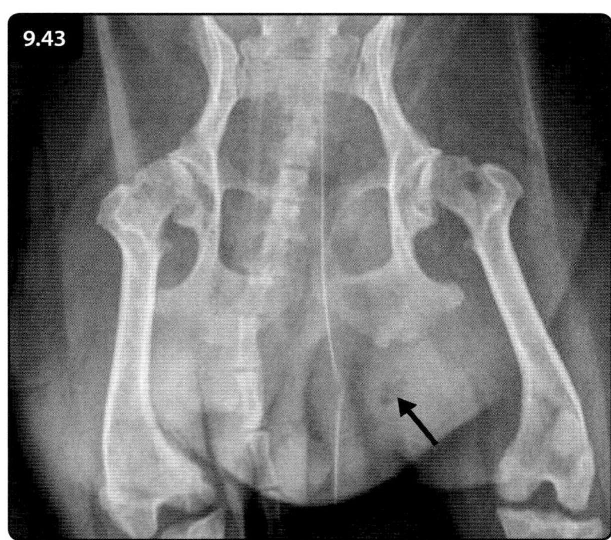

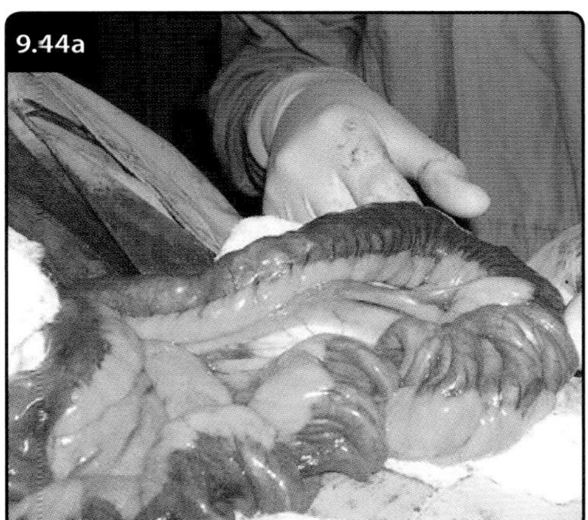

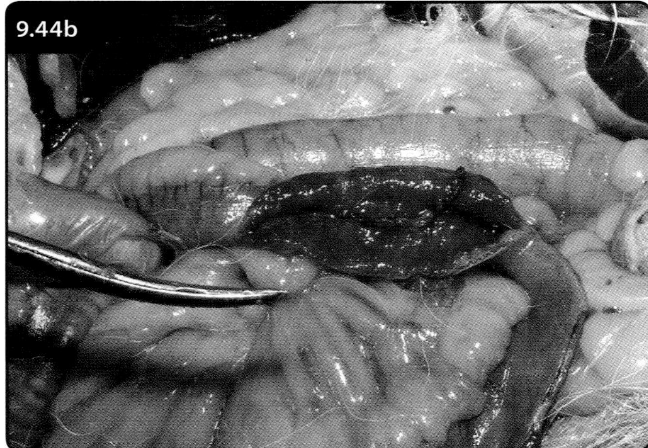

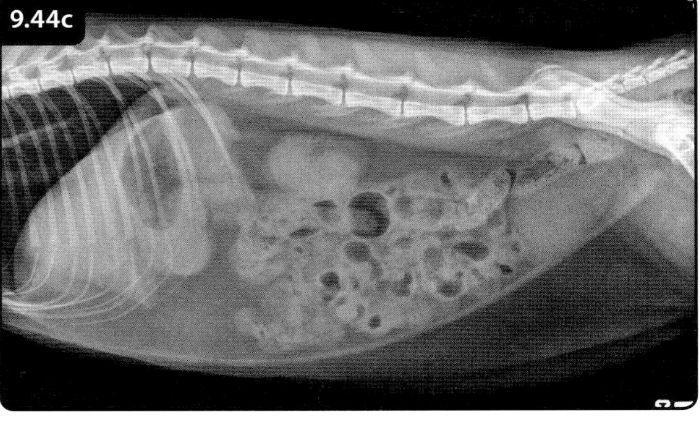

9.44a–c. Linear foreign body. Dogs, like cats, can acquire a linear foreign body obstruction following ingestion of string, sewing thread, pantyhose, and other similar objects. Diagnosis and surgery should be done as soon as possible in order to avoid perforation and sepsis. The sublingual area should be inspected for evidence of a linear foreign body in every vomiting dog and cat. The first image (Figure 9.44a) shows extensive plication in a dog at surgery, while the second (Figure 9.44b) is a necropsy view of an incised bowel loop of a dog showing that the linear foreign body lines the mesenteric border of the bowel. Figure 9.44c is a lateral abdominal radiograph of a cat with a typical linear foreign body obstruction pattern: aggregated bowel and dilated gas–fluid interphase involving the small bowel.

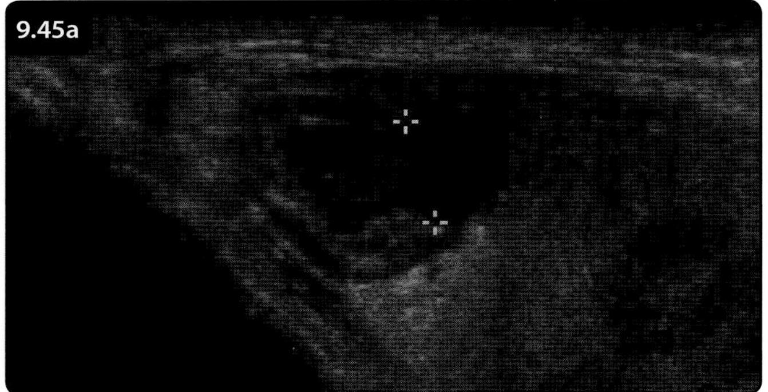

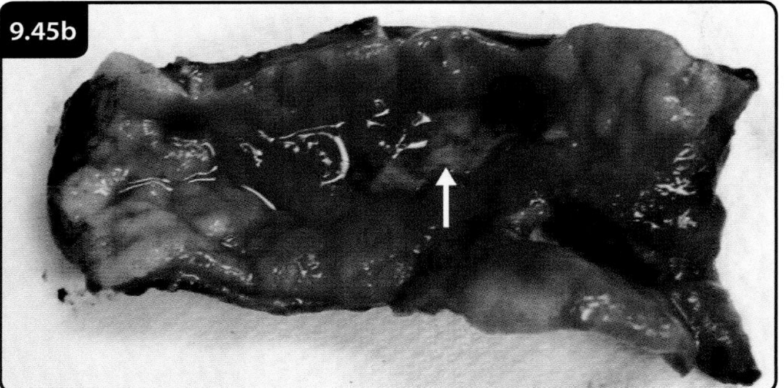

9.45a, b. Bowel ulcer with hemorrhage. Figure 9.45a is an abdominal ultrasonogram of a cat that presented to the emergency room in a collapsed state with a PCV of 9% (0.09 l/l) and gross melena. It shows an irregularity in the mucosal outline of a duodenal ulcer. The cat received a pack of red blood cells and stabilized before going to surgery. At surgery the ulcer was found to have perforated, but the omentum had sealed the leak. The resected segment, containing a large ulcer, is shown (arrow). Histopathology reported the lesion to be mild inflammation only. There was no evidence of a cancer, in particular, mast cell tumor.

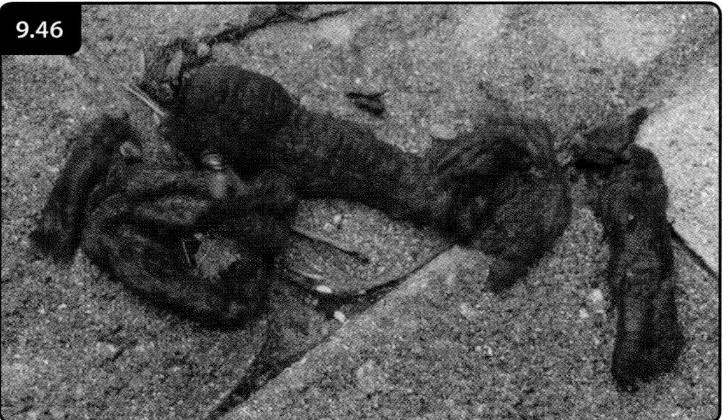

9.46. Intestinal mucosal slough. Shown is what came out of a dog's rectum during defecation while it was receiving chemotherapy treatment for intestinal lymphoma. The major concerns about this situation would be the status of the bowel mucosal defense barrier and the integrity of the bowel wall. Bowel perforation and sepsis would be disastrous for this patient, who might be immunocompromised from the anti-cancer drugs.

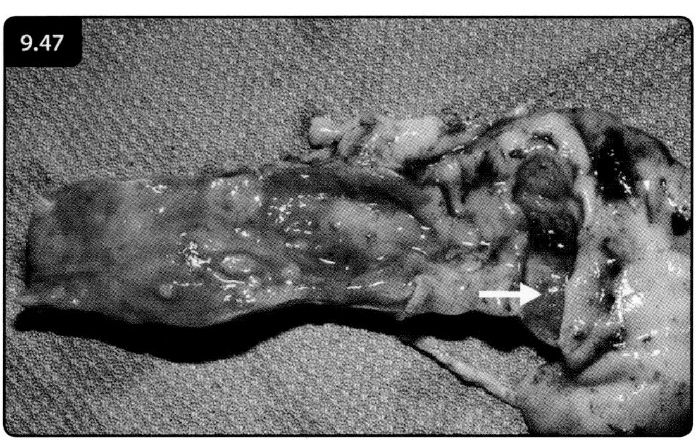

9.47. Duodenal ulcer. This section of duodenum had bleeding ulcers as a result of a mast cell tumor. Surgical resection would be indicated for ulcers as large as the one shown (arrow). Treatment for mast cell tumor usually has an unrewarding outcome.

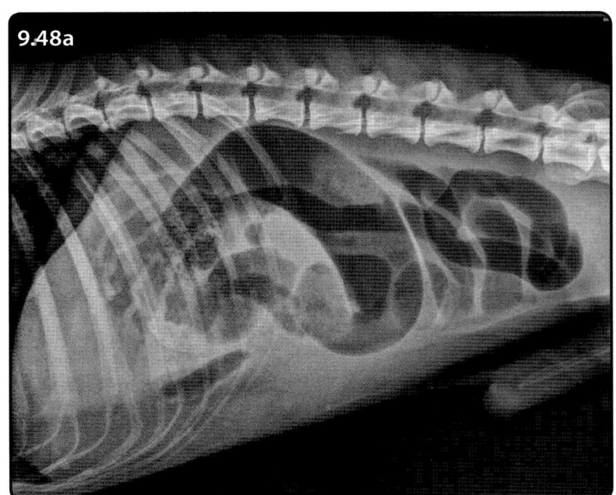

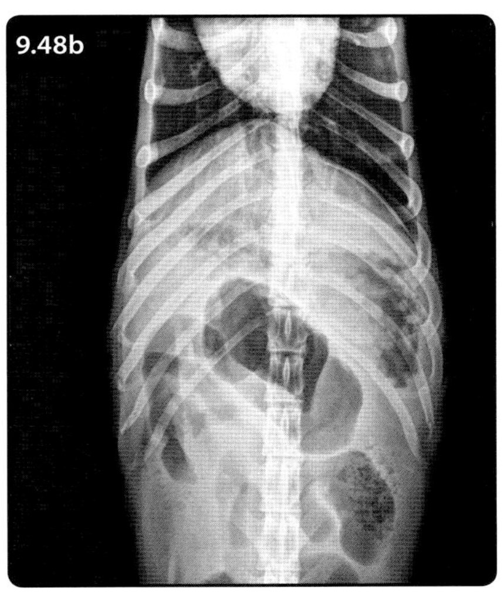

9.48a–c. Small intestinal volvulus. These lateral and ventrodorsal radiographs (Figures 9.48a, b) show very large distended bowel loops, which is compatible with intestinal volvulus. These patients are commonly markedly hypovolemic and require prompt intravenous fluid resuscitation and emergency surgery. The bowel shown in Figure 9.48c is green–black from gangrene. Prognosis is grave when such extensive amounts of tissue are involved, as in this case. The patient was euthanized during surgery.

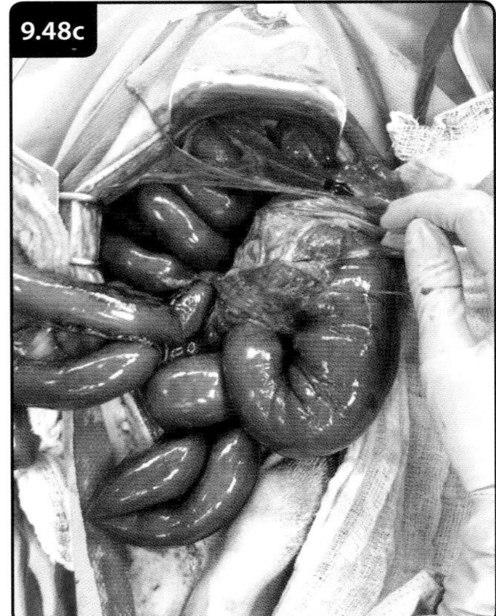

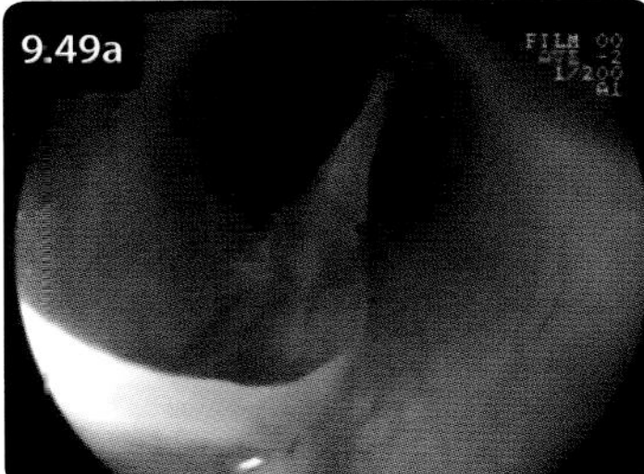

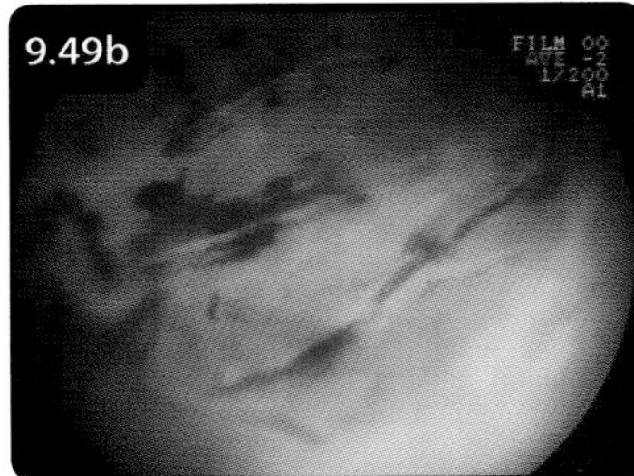

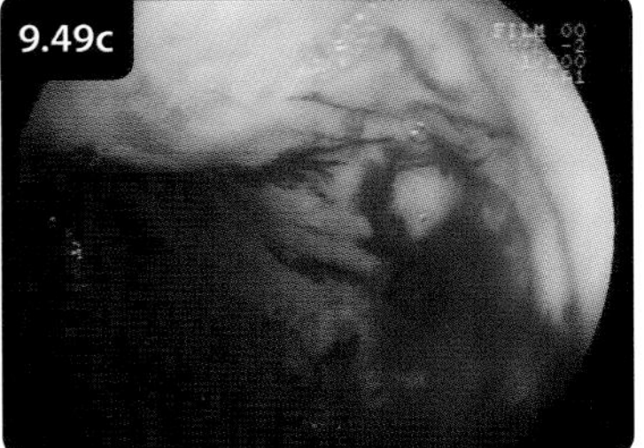

9.49a–c. Esophageal and gastric erosions. These esophagoscopy images are from a cat that had received a popular oral NSAID. The owner reported that her cat "was vomiting up its stomach". Sloughed esophgeal mucosa is shown (Figure 9.49a) together with several areas of bleeding gastric ulcers. The linear erosions are typical of NSAID-associated erosions. Treatment consisted of a proton pump antacid drug, sucralfate, and discontinuing the offending drug. The cat recovered completely with only 2 weeks of treatment.

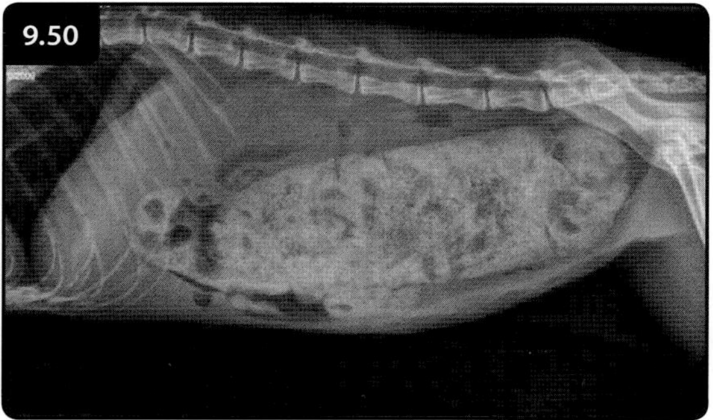

9.50. Obstipation. This condition is characterized by an inability to pass stool. It is fairly common in cats. When rock hard concretions are formed, enemas are of no avail. De-obstipation in this cat will require general anesthesia and manual breakdown of the stool mass alternated with colonic flushing with water. This procedure can often take a full hour until the colon is completely evacuated. Once empty, some cases will go on to be refractory to medical options. Full surgical colectomy is then the final solution.

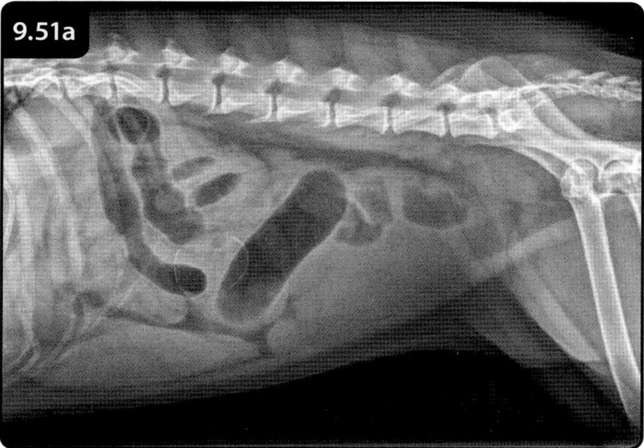

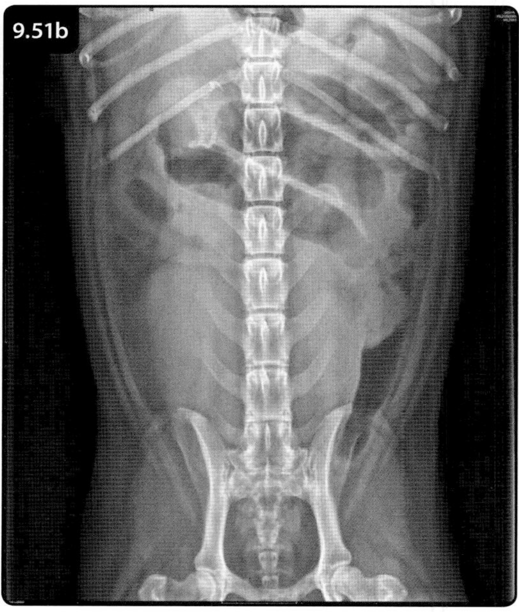

9.51a, b. Small bowel obstruction. These radiographs depict a typical small bowel obstruction as shown by the varying loops of small bowel distension and gas–fluid interphases. The obstruction can be further documented with abdominal ultrasound, but in cases such as this, plain radiographs will suffice for diagnosis.

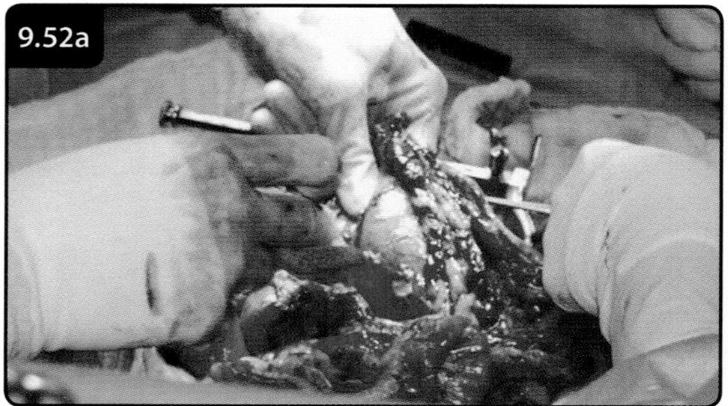

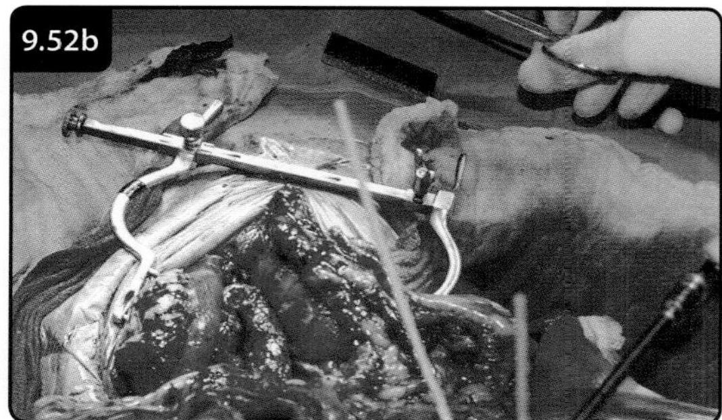

9.52a, b. Pancreatic phlegmon. Acute pancreatitis has a full spectrum of severity. If we hypothetically set the range from 1 to 10, with 10 as the most severe, then pancreatitis with phlegmon would be a 9 or 10. The aggregation of the soft tissues in the anterior abdomen impairs any type of surgical interference because it is impossible to identify the normal anatomic landmarks. The veterinary literature gives this condition a grave prognosis. The images show how difficult it is to identify the various involved tissues.

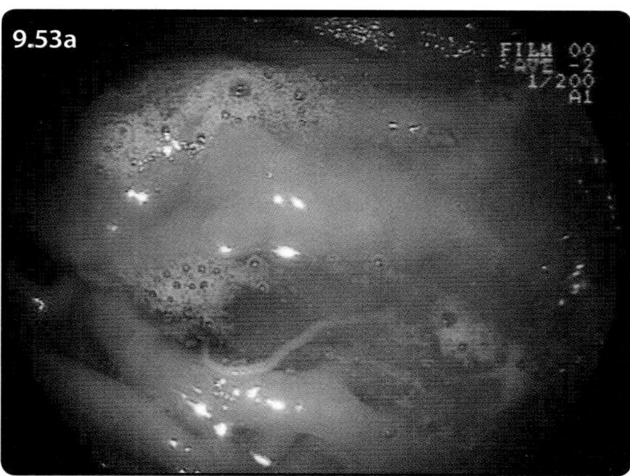

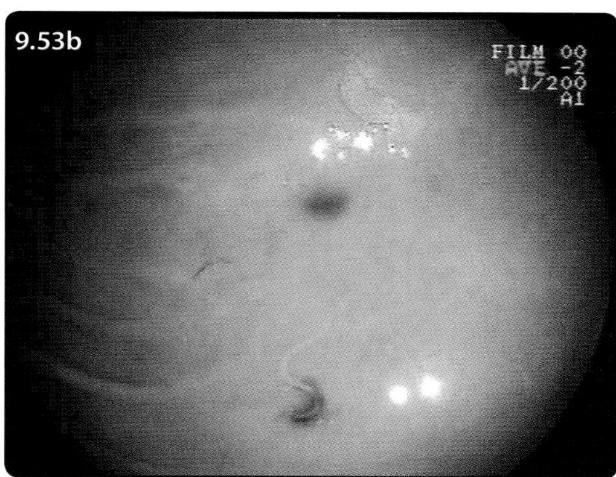

9.53a, b. *Physaloptera* spp. This is the stomach worm of the dog and cat. It is of rare incidence and the main clinical sign is periodic vomiting. The worms are small and range from 30 mm to 40 mm in length. Diagnosis is usually by chance when the animal is undergoing diagnostic gastroscopy and the worm is visualized. Treatment is best accomplished by physical extraction. Anthelminics such a pyrantel in cats and fembendazole in dogs have been used.

9.54. Pythiosis. This postmortem specimen is from a dog that was diagnosed with pythiosis. The main complaint was vomiting, as can be appreciated with the duodenum and pancreas adhered in the mass of granulation tissue. This disease offers a guarded to grave prognosis in most cases because of its refractoriness to most medications. Dogs usually acquire the visceral form from ingesting infected stagnated water, which is readily available in still bodies of water such as ponds. There is also a cutaneous form of pythiosis.

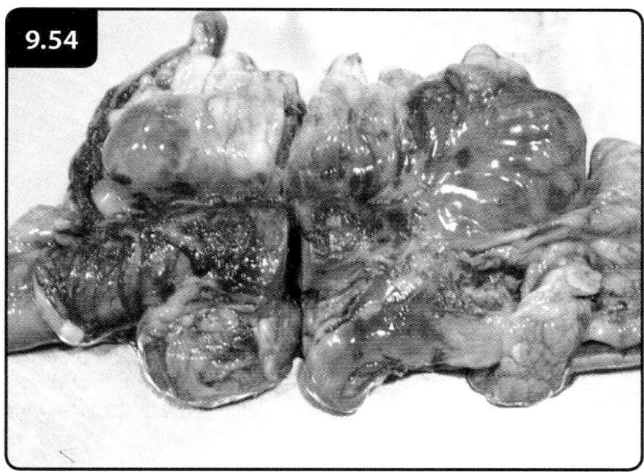

9.55. Lymphangiectasia. This condition in dogs is caused by anomalous gastrointestinal (GI) lymphatic development that is associated with a loss of body proteins causing panhypoproteinemia. The clinical signs will vary from periodic diarrhea to no GI abnormalities whatsoever. Instead, the animal is presented because of cachexia and transudative ascites. Diagnosis is made by intestinal biopsy and identifying stunted villi and dilated lymphatic vessels. Inflammatory bowel disease can also accompany the lymphangiectasia. This gastroscopic view shows many visible mucosal villi projections. In some cases the diagnosis has to await full-thickness surgical biopsy evaluation.

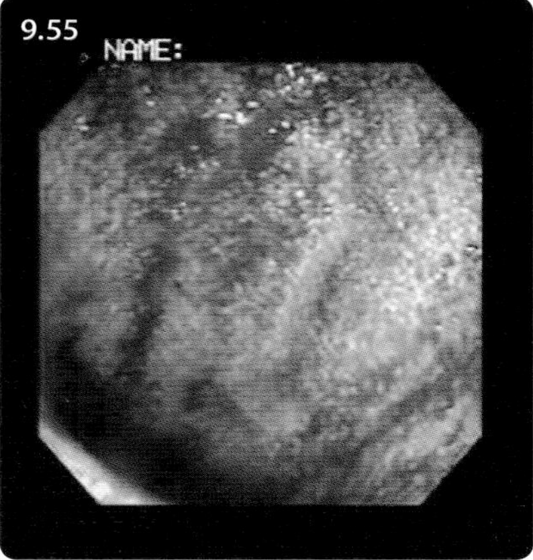

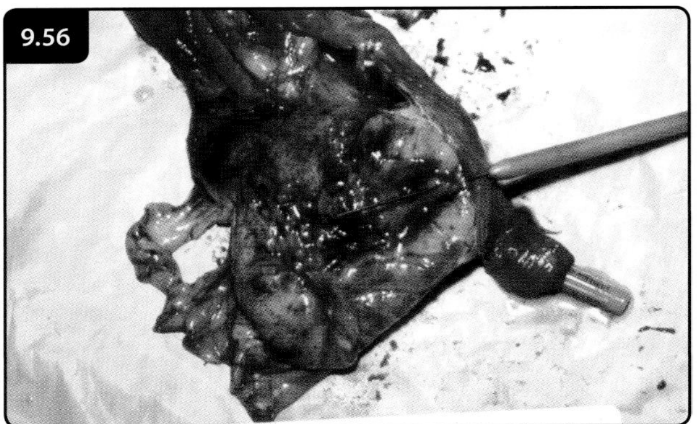

9.56. Small bowel leiomyosarcoma. This necropsy specimen comes from a dog that was examined for septic shock as a result of bowel perforation. The specimen shows a pointer going through the serosal side of the bowel loop, demonstrating the cause of the perforated bowel. Unlike bowel adenocarcinoma, which typically forms a signet ring kind of constriction of the bowel lumen, causing the animal to vomit, leiomyosarcoma might grow toward the serosal side of the involved bowel segment and possibly perforate, as shown, without causing any signs of vomiting.

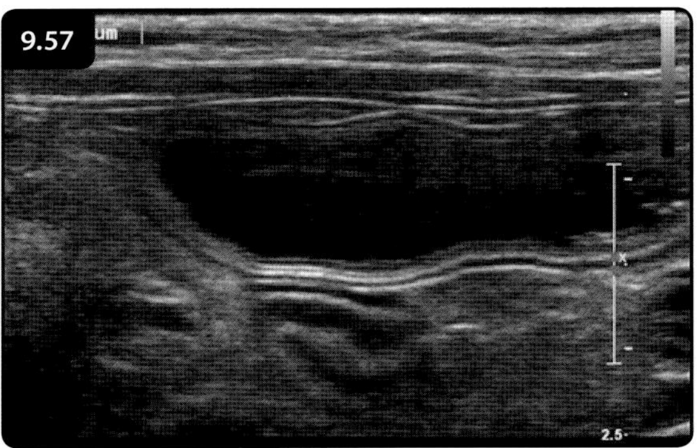

9.57. Ultrasound of small bowel obstruction. This ultrasonogram shows a dilated segment of the jejunum caused by a linear foreign body obstruction. Radiologists believe that ultrasonography has higher diagnostic accuracy compared with plain radiographs for diagnosing small bowel obstructions.

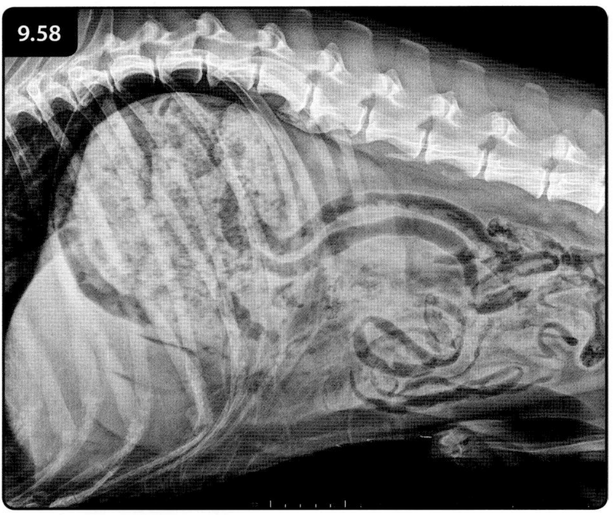

9.58. Gastric perforation radiograph. Free gas in the abdomen, as detected in this radiograph, is a sure indication for a gastrointestinal perforation if there is no recent history of the animal having abdominal surgery or laparoscopy. This lateral radiograph shows exceptional detail of the abdominal viscera, made possible by the presence of free air in the abdominal cavity. A fine needle aspirate of the abdominal fluid was septic; this prompted exploratory laparotomy, which detected a gastric perforation.

9.59a, b. Stomatitis, glossitis, and cheilitis in a dog. This dog has widespread inflammation involving all of its oral mucous membranes. The differential diagnosis for this degree of involvement includes immune-mediated disease, contact with a highly irritating substance, and systemic illness such as uremia; therefore, the medical work up should be comprehensive and include tissue biopsies. Dental disease due to a hypersensitivity to oral flora might also be the cause. If the latter is the major consideration, then total or subtotal tooth extractions might be necessary.

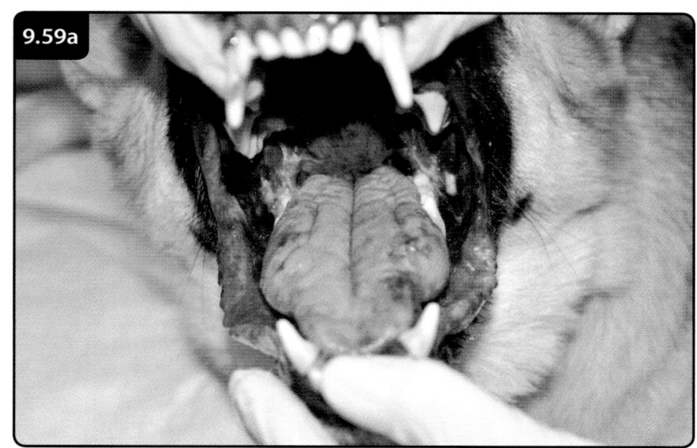
9.59a

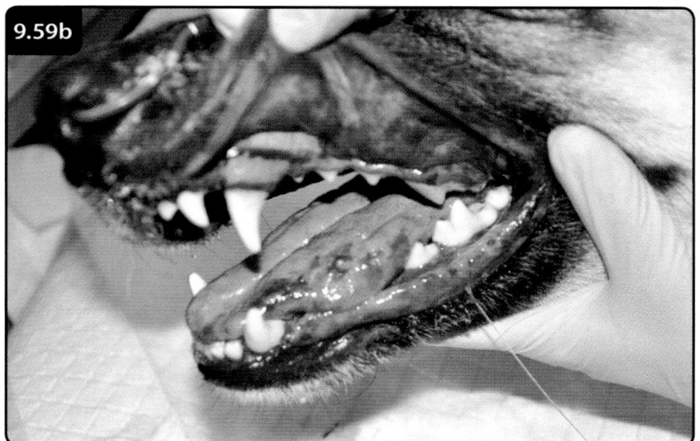
9.59b

9.60. Stomatitis in a cat. This cat has severe stomatitis that was due to hypersensitivity to its oral flora. After a major dentistry, oral mucosal biopsies and culture and sensitivities, complete serum chemistries, and a hemogram, the most likely cause was the cat's dentition. Most of the teeth were extracted, but a few were left behind. In many cases this treatment is adequate, but in others continued disease requires treatment with antibiotics and glucocorticoids. A feeding tube, as shown in this image, is sometimes necessary until the appetite returns.

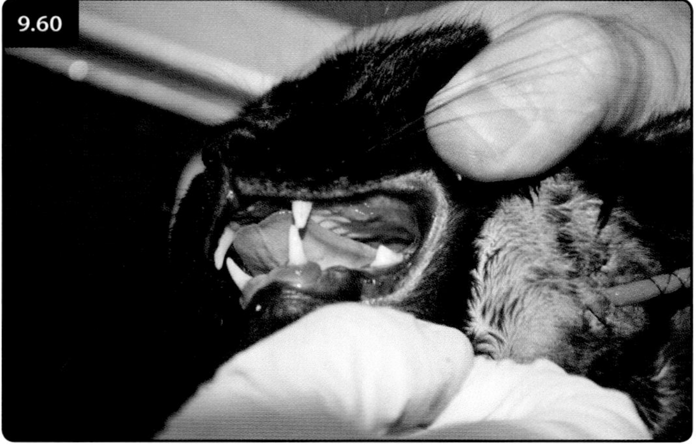
9.60

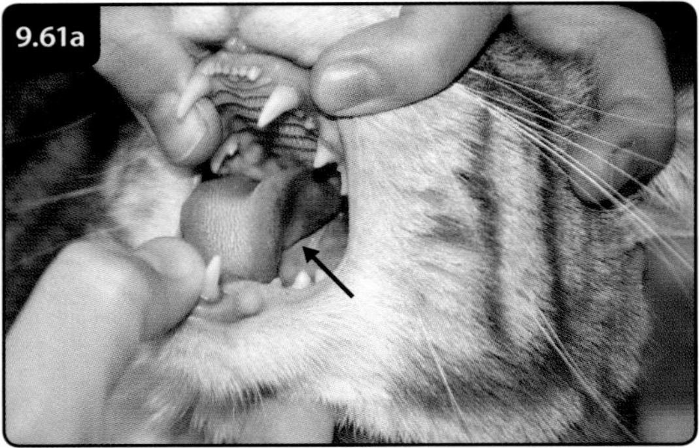

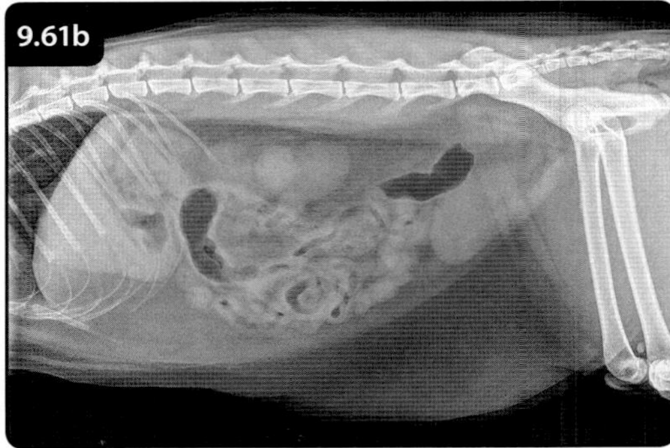

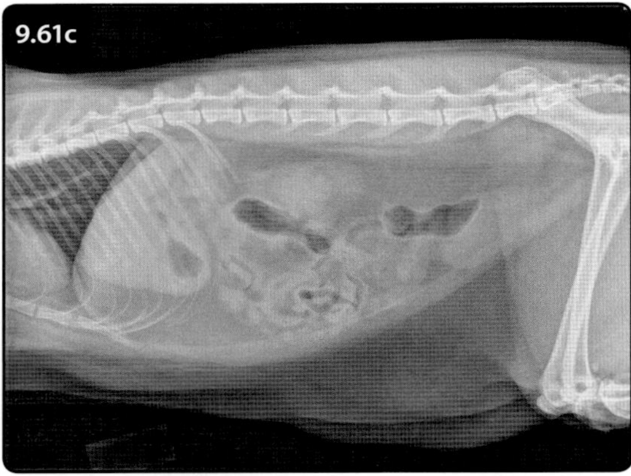

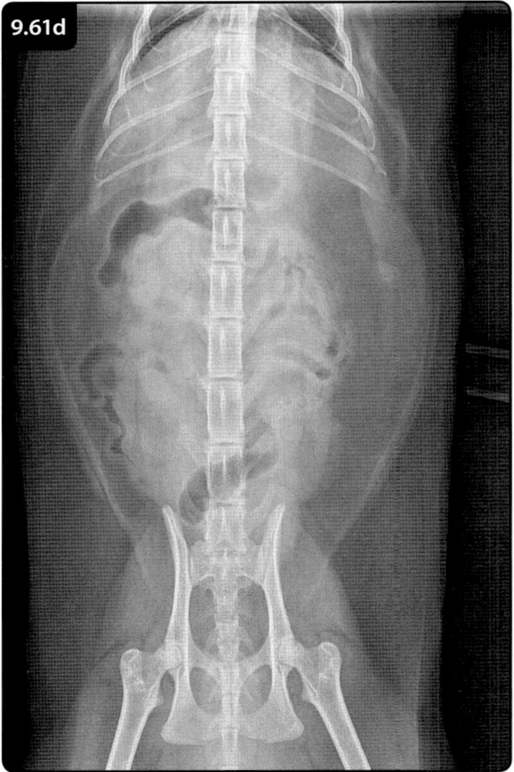

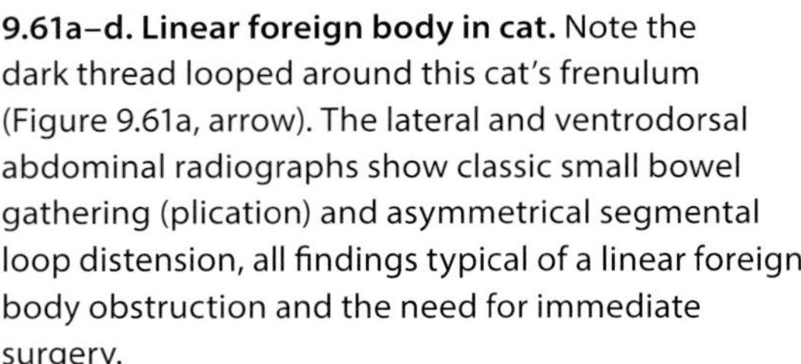

9.61a–d. Linear foreign body in cat. Note the dark thread looped around this cat's frenulum (Figure 9.61a, arrow). The lateral and ventrodorsal abdominal radiographs show classic small bowel gathering (plication) and asymmetrical segmental loop distension, all findings typical of a linear foreign body obstruction and the need for immediate surgery.

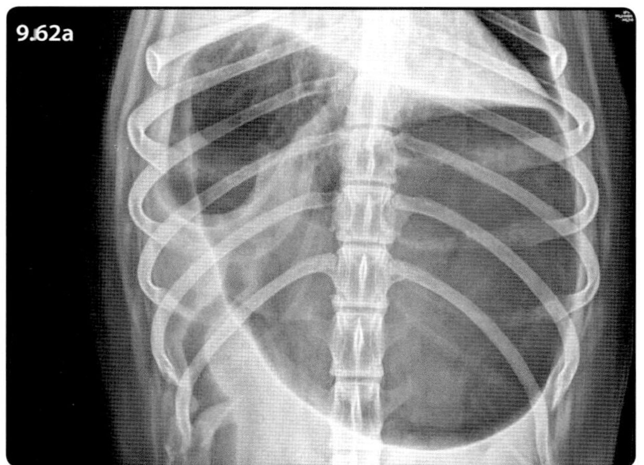

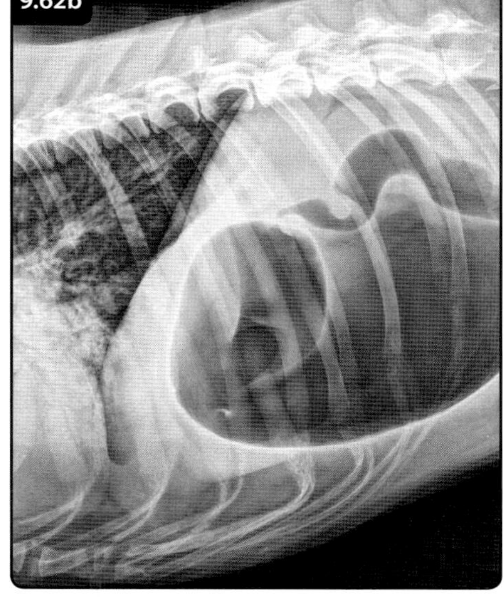

9.62a, b. Gastric dilatation in a dog: radiographic appearance. Note that the pylorus is in its normal position and the stomach is very distended with air, therefore eliminating gastric volvulus as a diagnosis. The gastric dilatation can be managed by passing a stomach tube and removing the gas. The condition will return if the inciting cause is not removed.

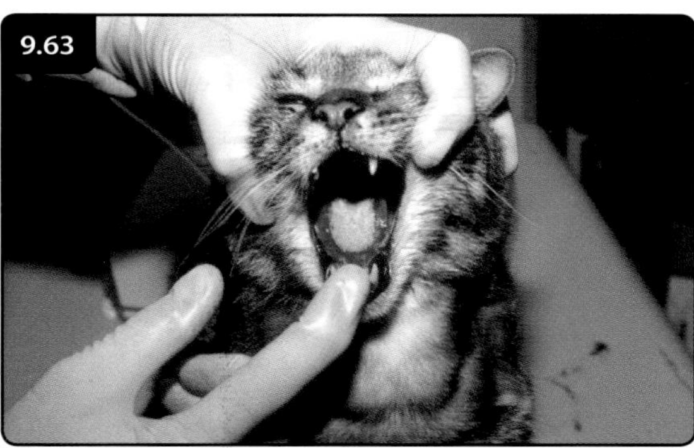

9.63. Glossitis in a cat. The circumferential ulceration involving this cat's tongue was caused by contact with an irritating antiseptic solution used to clean the cat's cage. The differential diagnosis would include infectious disease and systemic disease caused by organ failure (uremia).

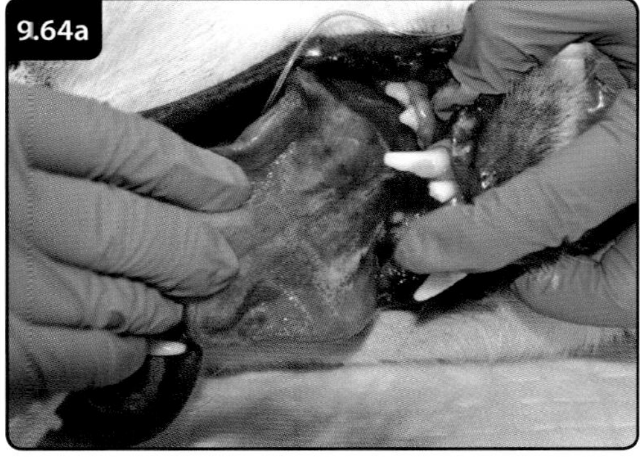

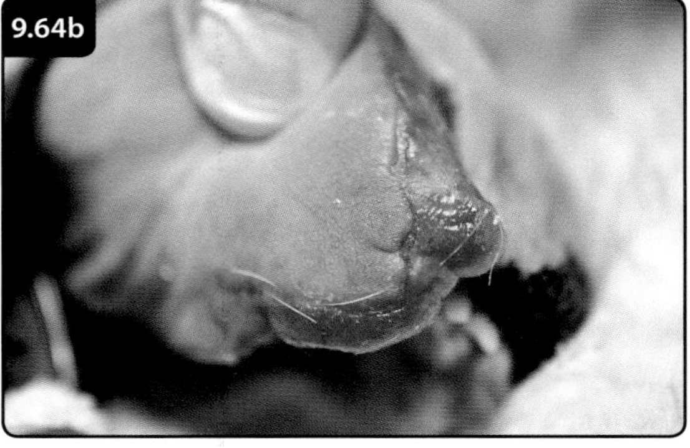

9.64a, b. Uremic glossitis in a dog. This dog's tongue is inflamed around the perimeter. There is an ulcer present as well. The medical diagnosis was kidney injury with uremic glossitis. Both acute kidney injury and chronic kidney disease can cause this disorder.

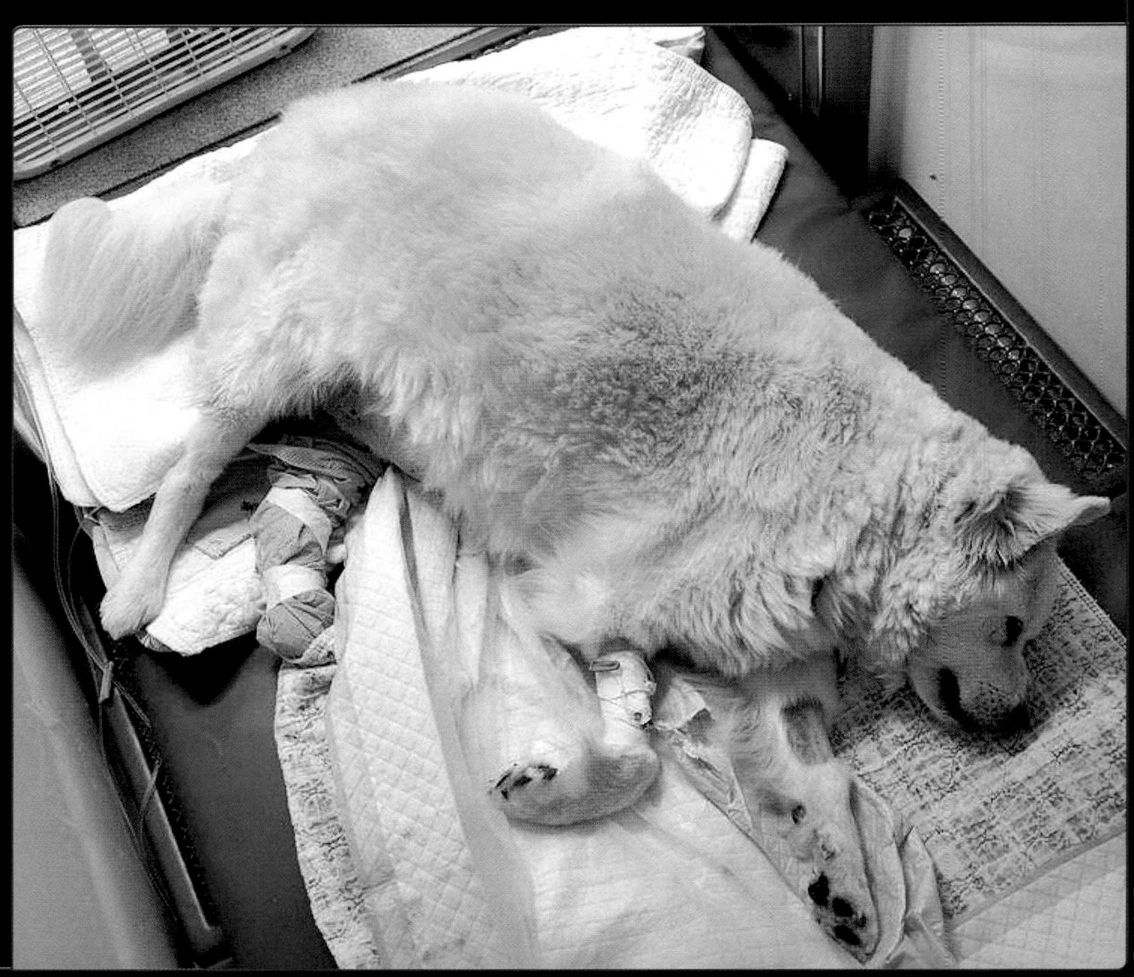

▲ This comatose Samoyed dog has hepatic encephalopathy.

10

Liver disorders

It was the famous French physiologist Claude Bernard (1838–1878) who established the liver in its rightful place as a vital organ, "a veritable laboratory of life" (Haubrich, 1997). In modern times, the liver is acknowledged as the largest solid organ in the body, totally supporting Bernard's teaching that the liver is essential to life. The liver has multiple vital functions including detoxification, glucose storage and release, lipid metabolism, bile formation to assist digestion, production of several proteins including clotting factors and immunoglobulins, hormone metabolism, hormone messenger production such as IGF1, and others. With all of these functions, it is not difficult to recognize the true importance of this organ.

Because of its functions as a 'toxic waste dump and clearing house' for toxins coming by way of the portal vein, it is no surprise to find that the liver is subject to various forms of pathology including fibrosis, parasite infection, sterile inflammation, septic inflammation, neoplasia, toxins, and infiltration by potentially injurious substances. Many of these pathologies can affect both young and old animals. Although there are many solitary forms of hepatopathy, inflammatory liver diseases can occur in conjunction with gallbladder disease, causing the syndrome of cholangiohepatitis with cholecystitis. This can pose potentially life-threatening situations to those afflicted with such maladies. Several of these disorders are illustrated in this section.

Haubrich WS (1997) *Medical Meanings: A Glossary of Word Origins*. American College of Physicians, Philadelphia.

10 Liver disorders

- Sepsis can cause cholangiostasis.
- Gas in the gallbladder is bad and is a surgical emergency.
- Bilirubinuria in cats signifies liver disease.
- Judicious J-tube or esophageal tube feeding can benefit the patient with acute pancreatitis.
- Anemic pallor plus icterus cause a yellow hue.
- Pink mucous membranes plus icterus cause a more orange color.

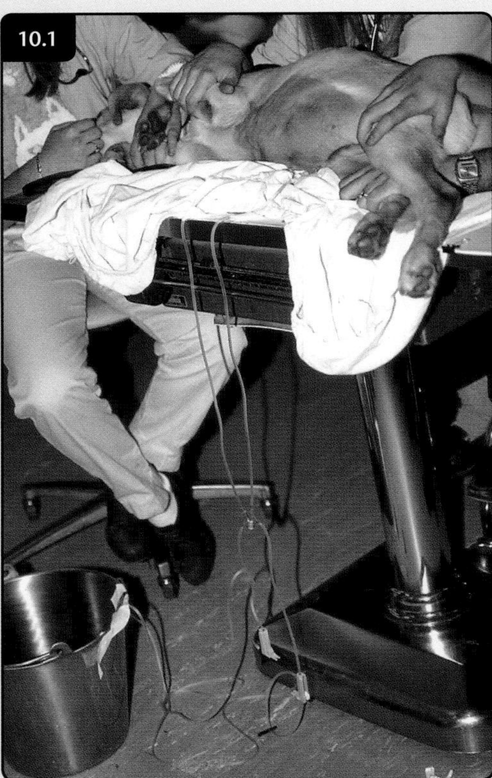

10.1. Rapid abdominocentesis. Ascites is a common complication of chronic liver disease. It occurs as a result of portal hypertension and co-existing hypoalbuminemia (causing less intravascular oncotic pressure). When 'tense' ascites occurs, relief for the diaphragm can be accomplished by abdominocentesis. This image shows the procedure being performed using either 18 gauge needles or polyethylene cannulas at the site of drainage. The fluid should drain passively by gravity. In order to avoid any possible adverse declines in blood pressure, some clinicians will simultaneously infuse crystalloid or colloid intravenously. The drain apparatus in this picture includes two 18 gauge needles, two intravenous tubing sets, one collecting container, and one table pad. Sedation is never necessary and the procedure generally takes 30–40 minutes.

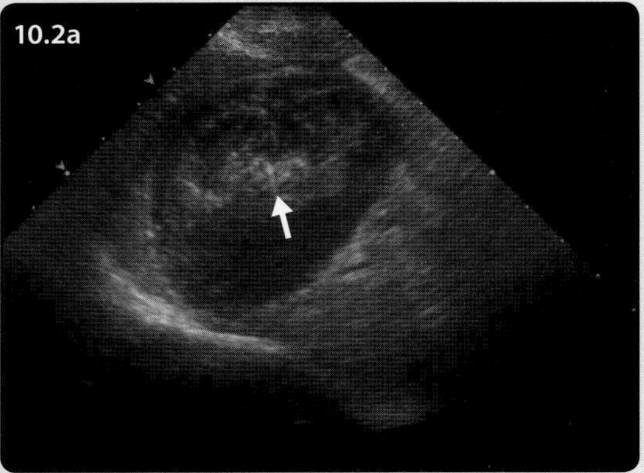

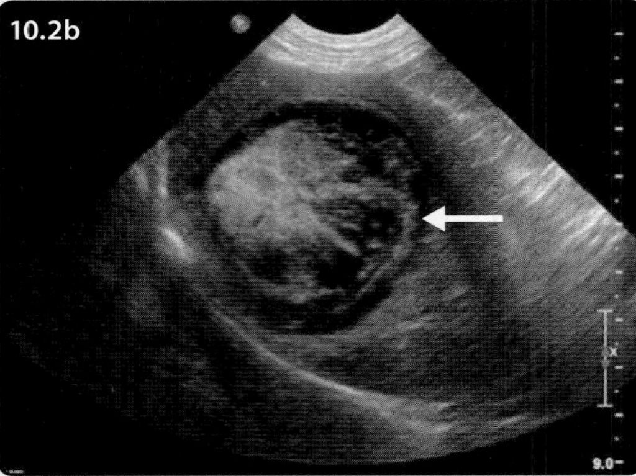

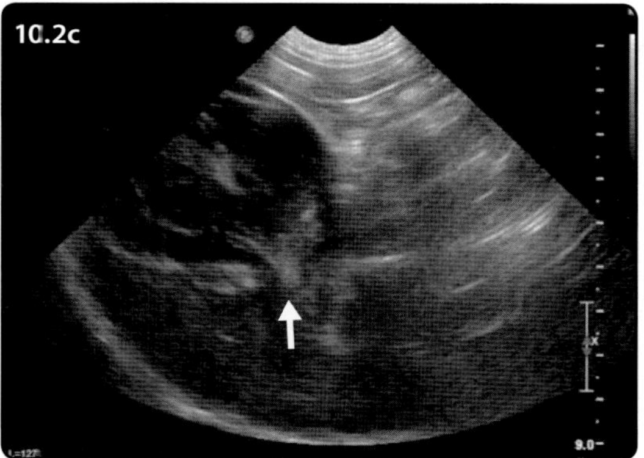

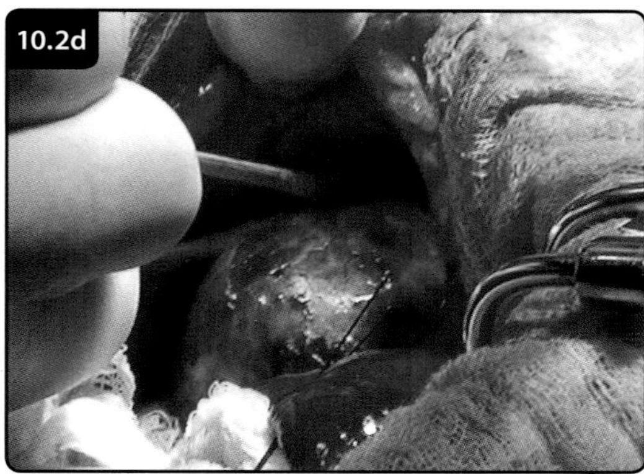

10.2a–d. Mucocele and cholecystitis in dogs. Figure 10.2a shows a gallbladder mucocele (arrow) identified on abdominal ultrasonography. Although some gallbladder mucoceles can be asymptomatic, many can be accompanied by cholecystitis, which is an indication for surgical cholecystectomy. Figures 10.2b, c show a gallbladder mucocele and an irregularity in the wall of the gallbladder (arrows) surrounded by an extraluminal fluid accumulation. This patient had a perforated gallbladder (Figure 10.2d) and a mucocele, and any delay in surgery could prove fatal.

10.3a, b. Cholecystitis on ultrasonography. Figure 10.3a shows a thickened cystic duct and sludge in the gallbladder. If surgery shows an inflamed gallbladder, it should not be opened and then sutured closed, because postoperative dehiscence is likely, as shown in Figure 10.3b where the dog returned to the hospital shortly after discharge because it developed bile peritonitis from the perforated gallbladder. The bile in the syringe was aspirated from the dog's abdominal cavity 3 days postoperatively. The dog was re-operated on for a cholecystectomy and died postoperatively from aspiration pneumonia.

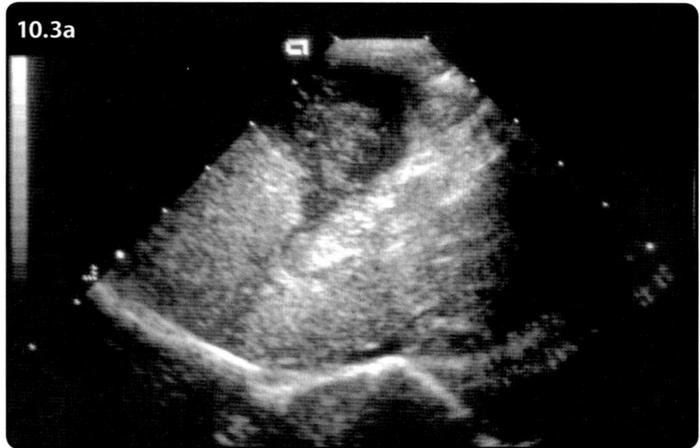

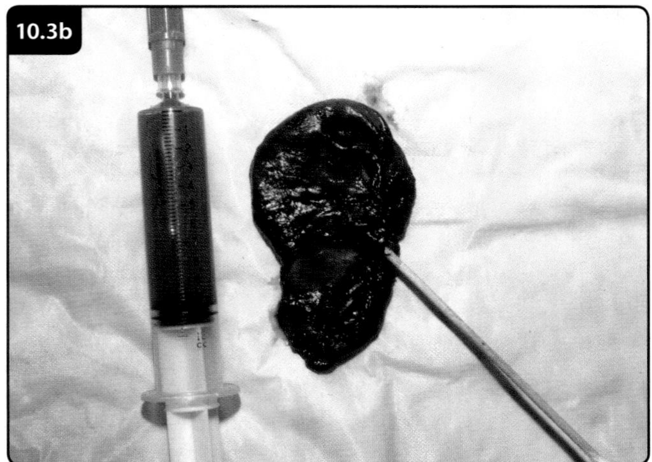

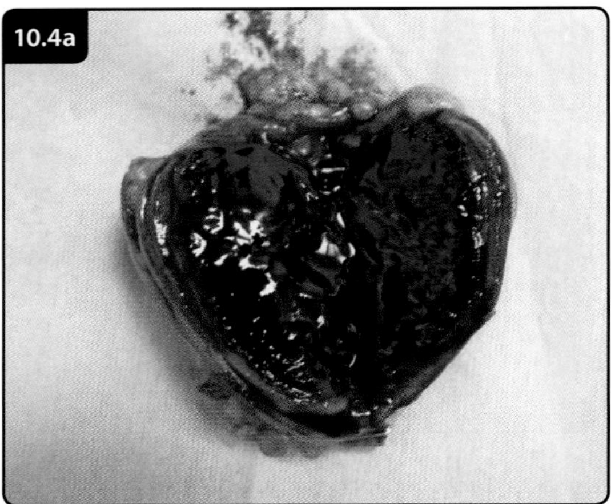

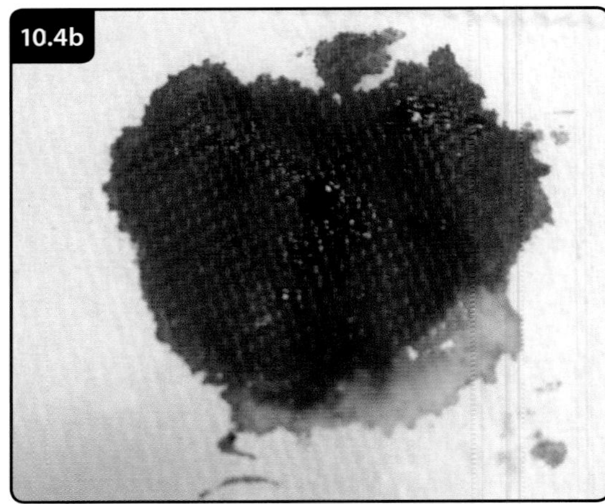

10.4a, b. Cholecystitis with hemobilia. These unusual images show blood in the lumen of the gallbladder. In humans, this is described as hemobilia and occurs as a result of a fistulous bleed from a blood vessel into the gallbladder. The typical gallbladder contents are either green or green–black (inspissated bile). The red imprint is from the blood contents seen in Figure 10.4a. Hemobilia can occur from gallstones, inflammation, vascular maldevelopment, tumors, coagulopathy, or liver biopsy. The cause in this dog was attributed to inflammation.

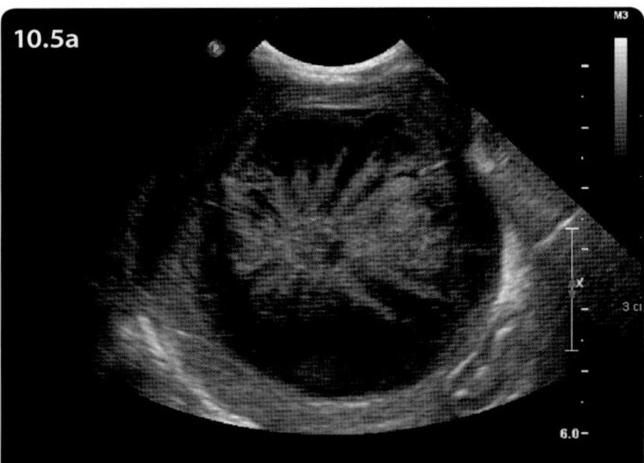

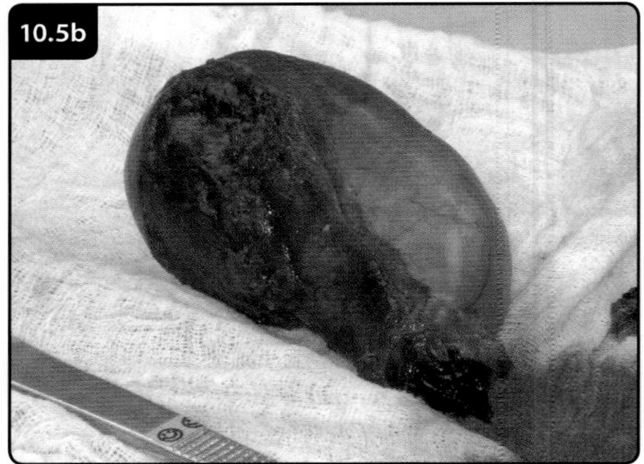

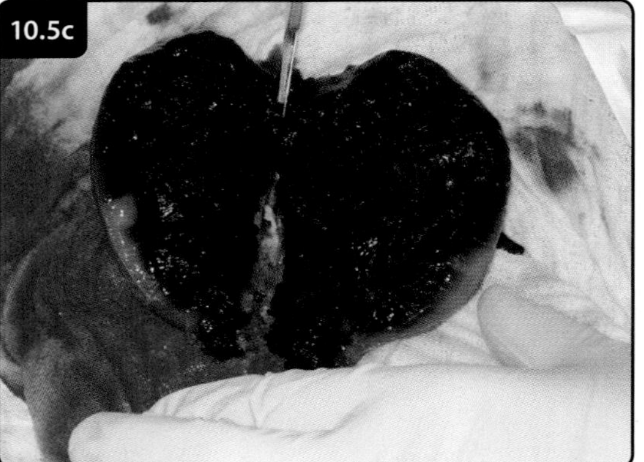

10.5a–c. Mucocele and inspissated bile in a dog. The ultrasound image shows a typical mucocele pattern (kiwi fruit pattern). Figure 10.5b shows the outer aspect of a cholecystitis gallbladder, while Figure 10.5c shows the gallbladder completely filled with inspissated bile. Dogs and cats affected with cholecystitis often have cholangiohepatitis, which requires a minimum of 6 weeks of antibiotic treatment.

10.6. Cholangiohepatitis, cholecystitis, and inspissated bile at necropsy. This specimen from a dog shows diffuse hepatobiliary disease. Gram-negative bacteria are frequently present, although gram-positive and anaerobic bacteria can occasionally be isolated.

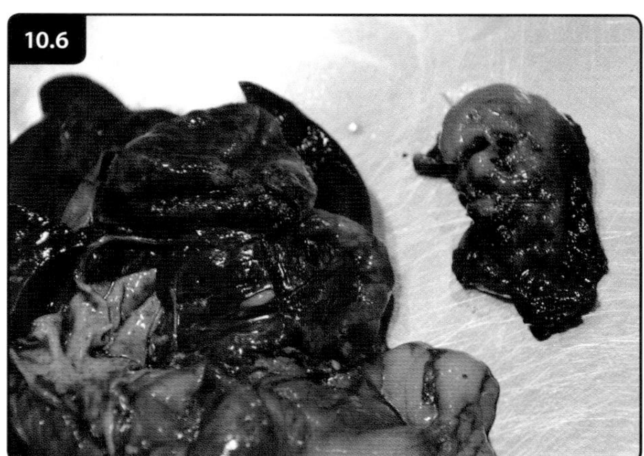

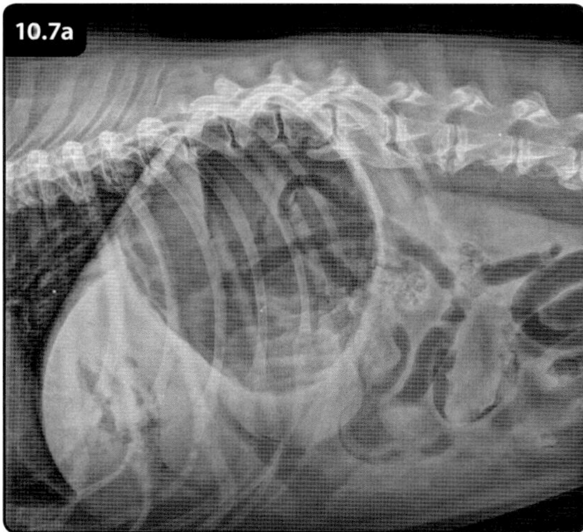

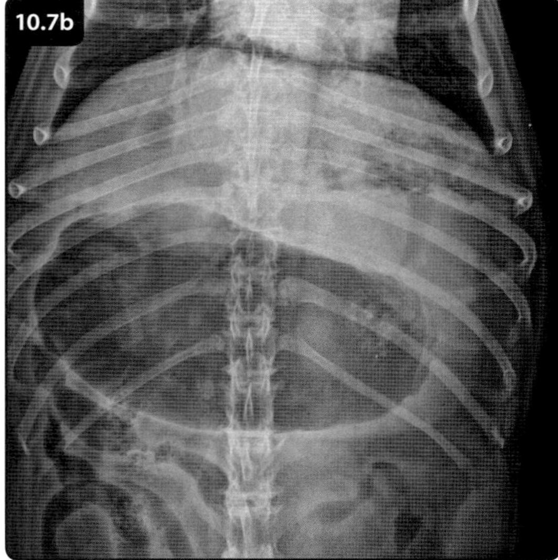

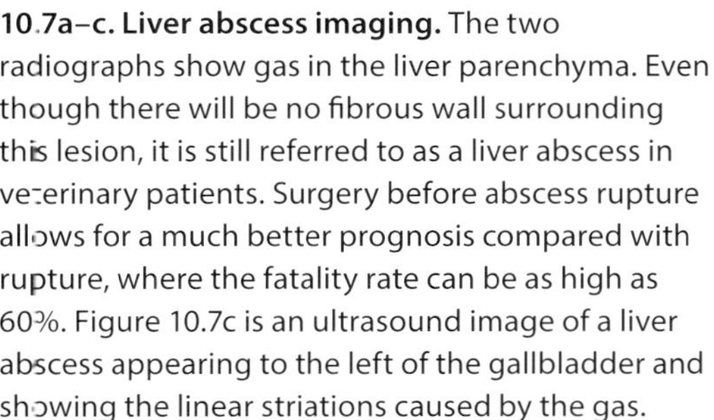

10.7a–c. Liver abscess imaging. The two radiographs show gas in the liver parenchyma. Even though there will be no fibrous wall surrounding this lesion, it is still referred to as a liver abscess in veterinary patients. Surgery before abscess rupture allows for a much better prognosis compared with rupture, where the fatality rate can be as high as 60%. Figure 10.7c is an ultrasound image of a liver abscess appearing to the left of the gallbladder and showing the linear striations caused by the gas.

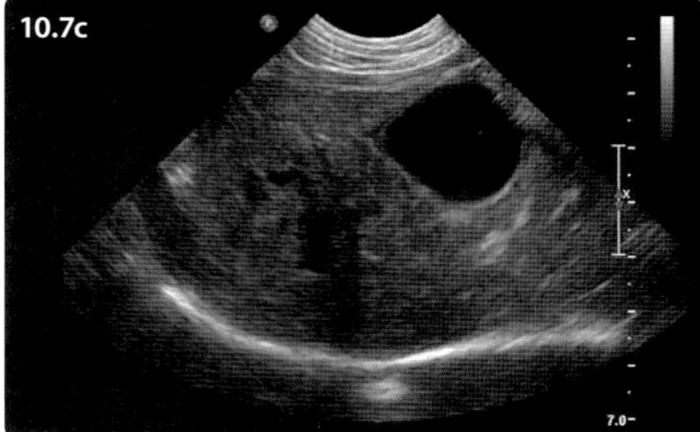

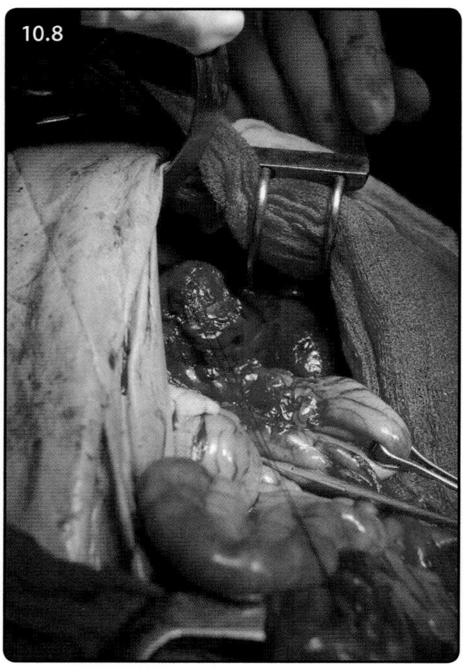

10.8. Liver abscess and cholecystitis in surgery. This intraoperative view shows the marked extent of the pathology in this dog. The procedure would entail cholecystectomy. Major involvement of a liver lobe would require a lobectomy as well. A localized abscess might fare well with drainage and an omental patch.

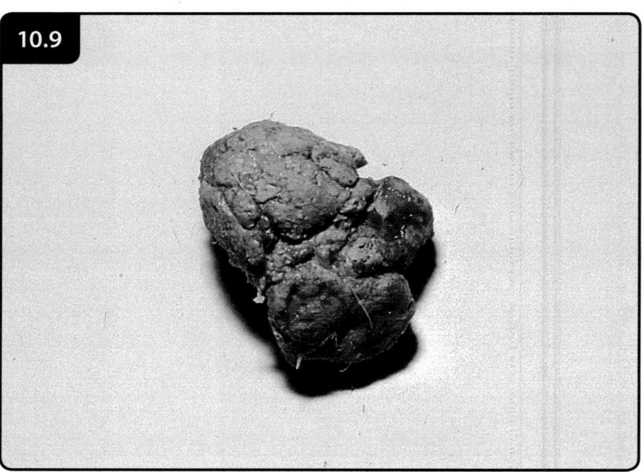

10.9. Acholic feces. This light colored stool specimen is the result of a complete extrahepatic bile duct obstruction preventing the passage of bile pigments through the GI tract. (See also Chapter 9, Case 9.6.) Stercobilin is a derivative of heme metabolism, a bile pigment derivative that is formed by air oxidation of stercobilinogen. It is a brown–orange–red pigmentation contributing to the color of feces and urine.

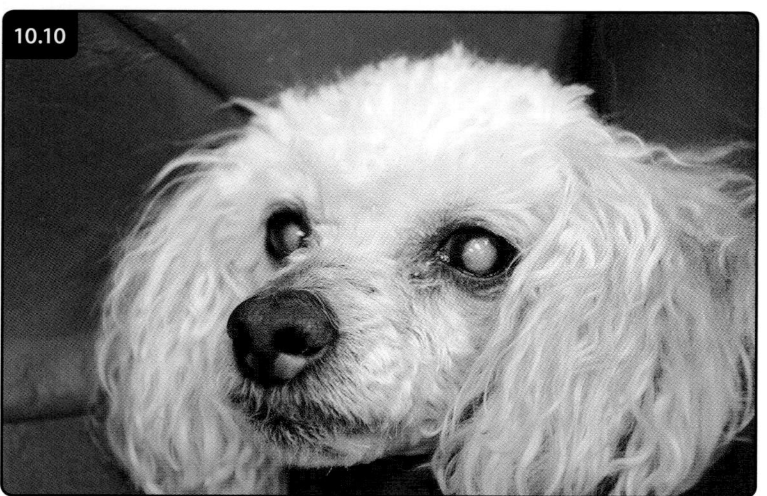

10.10. Bile stained cataract in a dog. Increased bilirubin blood levels will stain most tissues yellow. Rarely will hyperbilirubinemia stain a cataract yellow, as it did in this dog.

10.11. Bilirubinuria. There are several forms of natural pigmenturia including hematuria, hemoglobinuria, bilirubinuria, myoglobinuria, and chyluria. Hemoglobinuria and myoglobinuria cause renal tubule toxicity. Bilirubinuria appears as dark yellow pigment, but when hemoglobinuria is present simultaneously the color takes on a dark red tinge. The yellow tinge is visible on the white background of the paper container.

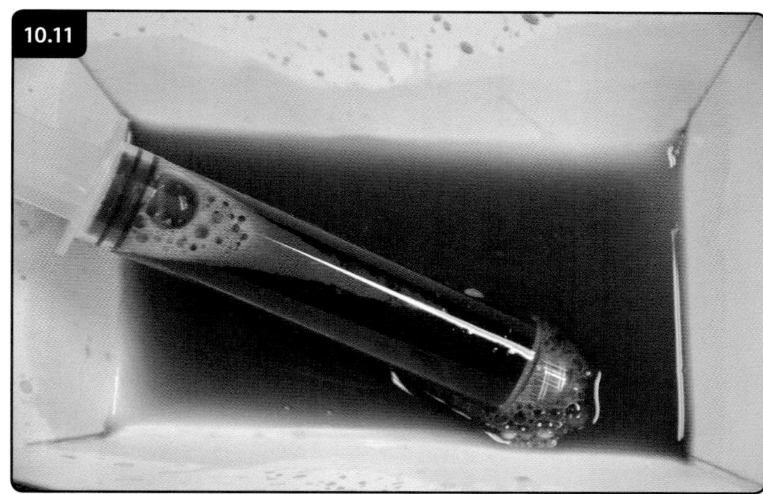

10.12. Fractured liver from cardiopulmonary resuscitation (CPR). This necropsy specimen shows that iatrogenic organ trauma can occur with CPR. The damage done to this patient might easily have contributed to its demise.

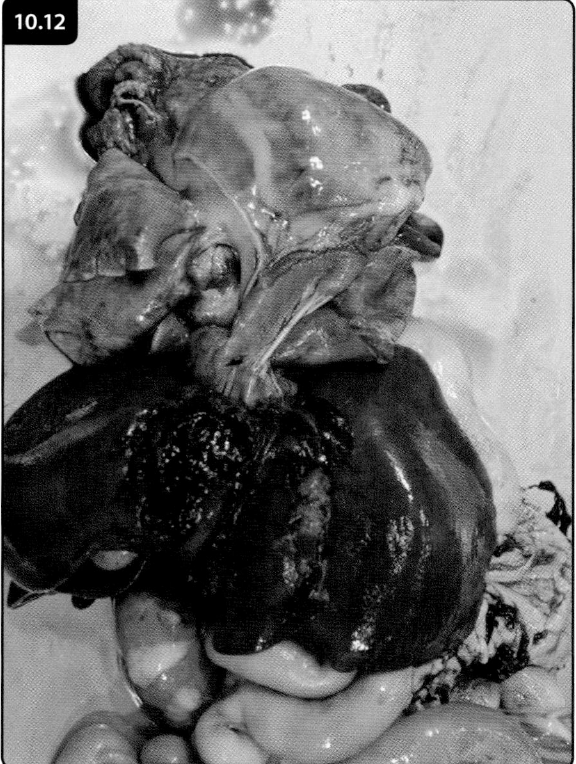

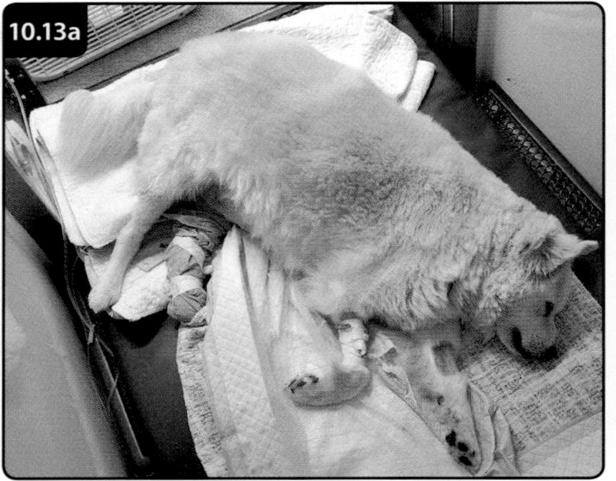

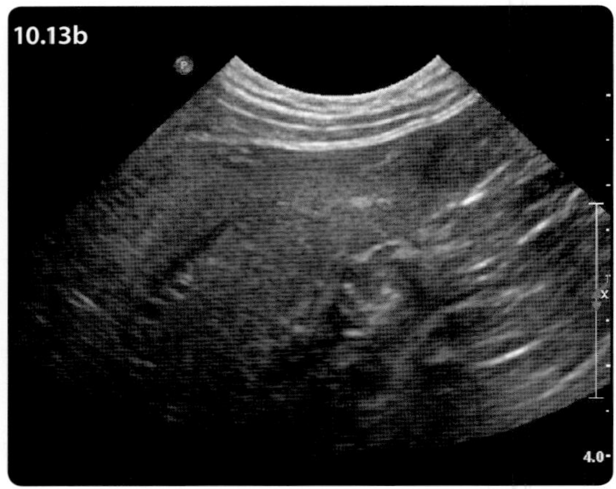

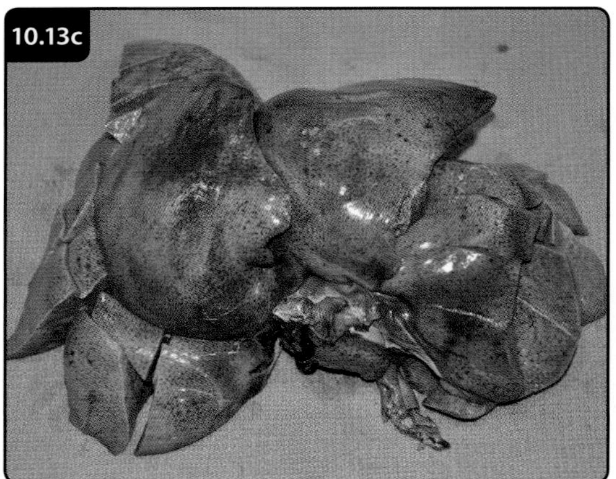

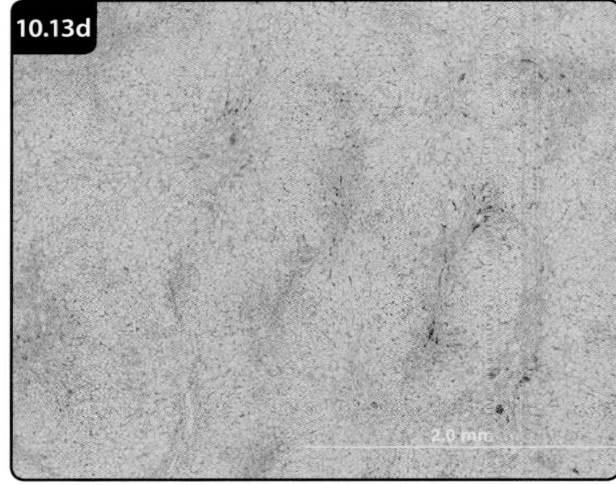

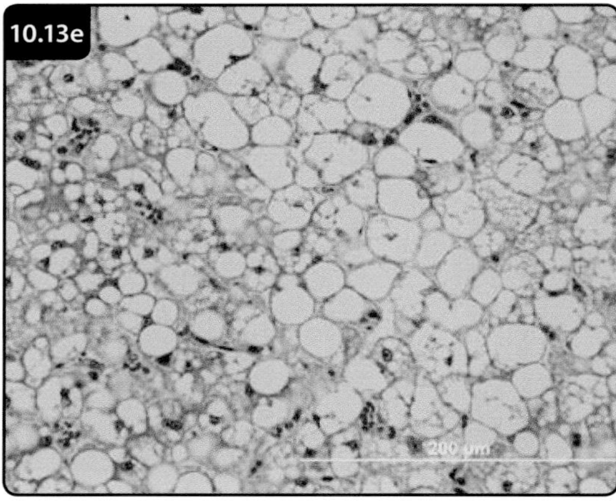

10.13a–e. Fatal hepatic lipidosis in a dog with diabetic ketoacidosis. This dog initially walked into the hospital, where it was diagnosed as having diabetes with ketoacidosis. Treatment followed established guidelines, but the dog lapsed into a stupor and then a coma by the third day in hospital despite improved diabetic laboratory parameters. The abdominal ultrasonogram shows a hyperechoic liver compatible with lipid infiltrate. At necropsy the liver was markedly enlarged and completely infiltrated with lipid. The low- and high-power histopathology images document the severity of this disease. The author has seen eight cases of fulminating hepatic lipidosis in dogs, all ending in death.

10.14. Macronodular cirrhosis in a dog. This progressive end-stage liver disease can occur in micronodular and macronodular forms. Cocker Spaniel dogs appear to have a higher incidence of the macronodular form compared with other breeds. Some of these cases present at a time when the liver enzymes are barely elevated because insufficient viable liver cells remain to release the enzymes into the blood stream. Icterus is not always present in these dogs despite the extensive pathology.

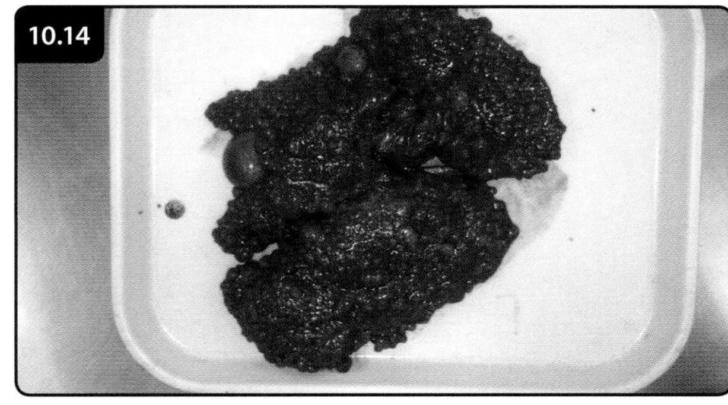

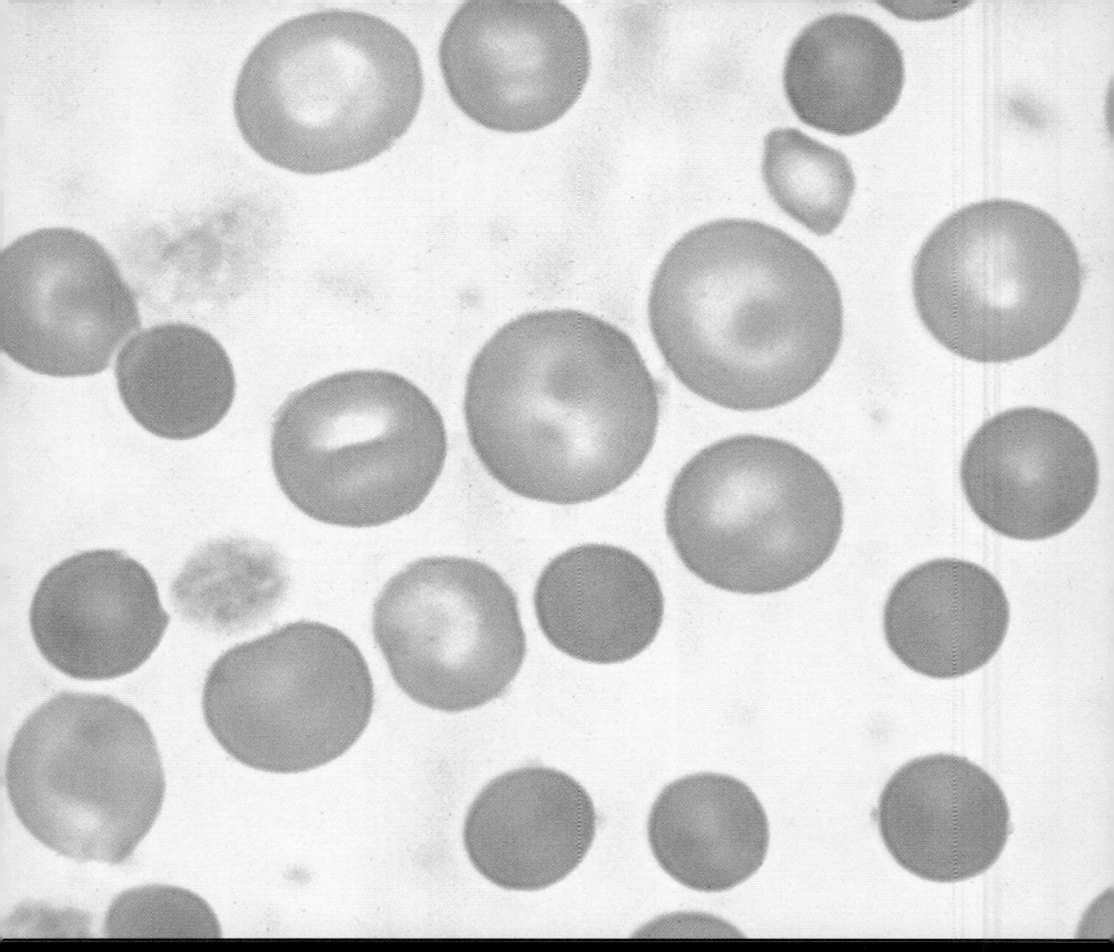

▲ This blood smear from a dog with immune-mediated hemolytic anemia shows very rounded red blood cel called spherocytes, which are typical of this disease.

11

Immune disorders

The word 'immunity' comes from the Latin *immunitas*, which to the Romans meant 'an exemption from taxes or from public military service' (Haubrich, 1997). In the late 19th century, when knowledge of toxins and infection evolved, the meaning was extended to refer to persons 'exempt from' or protected against the onslaught of foreign substances (Haubrich, 1997). This is accomplished by a very elaborate immunosurveillance system consisting of molecular and cellular networks involving B and T lymphocytes and immunoglobulins. When homeostasis is present the immune system is the great protector of its host, but when it functions inadequately, or should it turn against itself, the host will be met with various life-threatening insults.

In the case of autoimmunity, immunocytes fail to accept certain cells and tissues as their 'own self' and then proceed to destroy those cells, as seen with conditions such as immune-mediated hemolytic anemia, immune-mediated thrombocytopenia, rheumatoid arthritis, and systemic lupus erythematosus. In anaphylaxis, the exposure to a certain substance causes immunoglobulin E and complement to attach to mast cells and release their cellular contents, such as the interleukins, tissue necrosis factor, and many others. These then proceed to produce effects that cause hypersensitivity and/or systemic vasodilation and endothelial dysfunction, resulting in disorders ranging from mild conditions such as angioneurotic edema to serious conditions such as life-threatening vasocollapse, as seen with anaphylaxis or anaphylactoid reactions.

Haubrich WS (1997) *Medical Meanings: A Glossary of Word Origins*. American College of Physicians, Philadelphia.

11 Immune disorders

- Keep immune-mediated hemolytic anemia (IMHA) and immune-mediated thrombocytopenia patients on long-term every other day maintenance prednisone for 9–12 months after the initial loading and early maintenance periods (usually after 6 weeks) in order to avoid relapse.
- Observe for autoagglutination and spherocytes in IMHA.
- Fever and good appetite – think immune disease. Fever and anorexia – think infection.

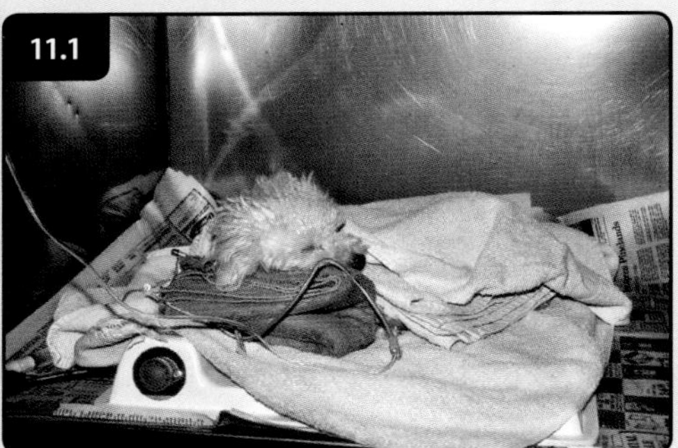

11.1. Anaphylaxis. This puppy was normal until 2 minutes after it received a vaccination, which caused it to go limp and become nearly unconscious. This was the 2nd vaccine of its series, so the sensitizing dose had been administered. Emergency treatment consisted of intravenous crystalloid, diphenhydramine, and intravenous glucocorticoids. The dog died 5 hours after it was admitted and treated. The omission of epinephrine in the treatment very likely could have contributed to the puppy's demise.

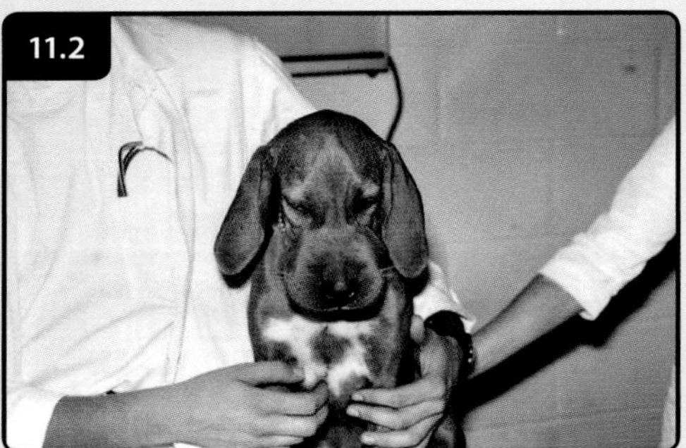

11.2. Angioedema. This puppy experienced facial pruritus and diffuse edema 30 minutes after it received its vaccination. It did not collapse and the vital signs were stable. Treatment in not-so-threatening type 1 hypersensitivity cases consists of antihistamines and glucocorticoids.

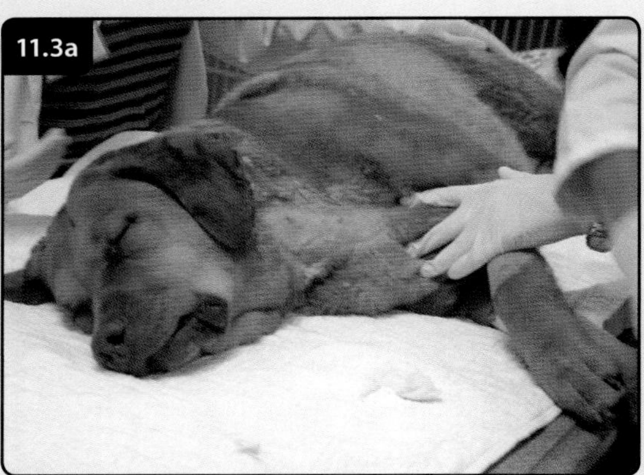

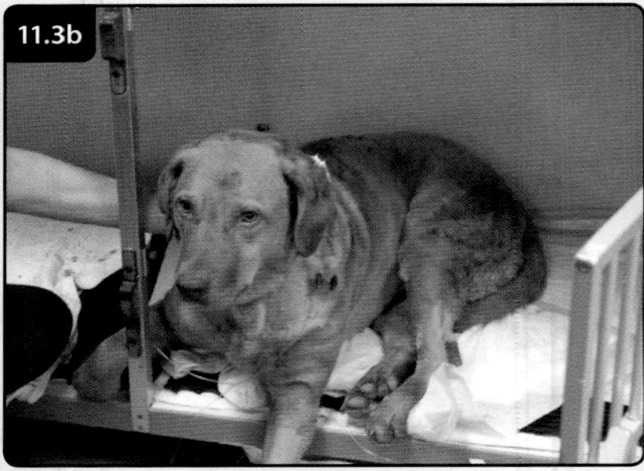

11.3a, b. Type 1 hypersensitivity. This dog (Figure 11.3a) presented in lateral recumbency with diffuse pitting edema and hypotension. A type 1 hypersensitivity was suspected and the dog responded well to epinephrine, intravenous crystalloid, diphenhydramine, and glucocorticoids (Figure 11.3b). The exact cause of this dog's hypersensitivity state was not determined.

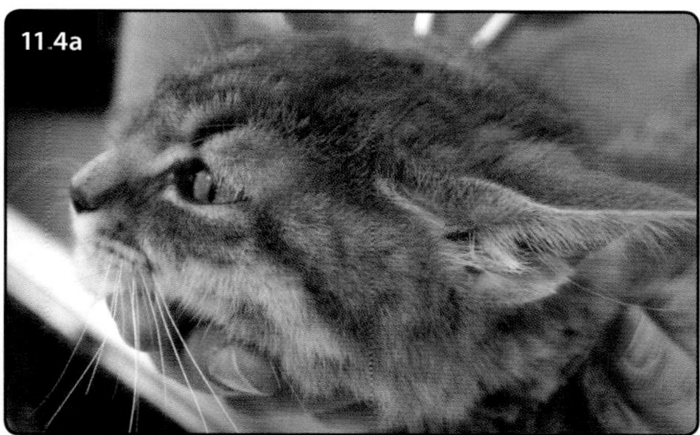

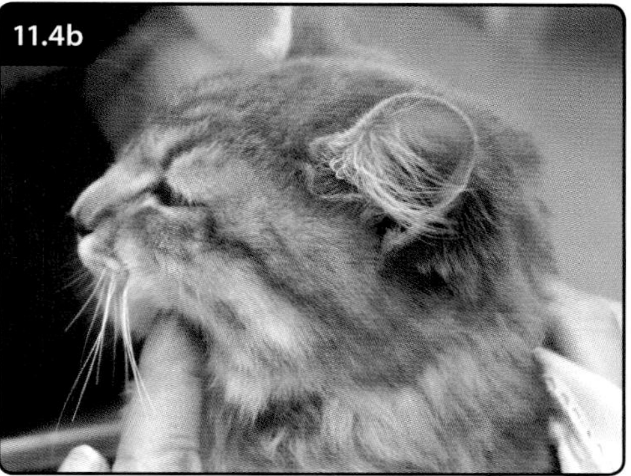

11.4a, b. Angioedema in a cat. This young cat presented with an acute-onset weakness and diffuse cool facial edema within 1 hour after it received a vaccination (Figure 11.4a). Anaphylaxis was diagnosed, which prompted immediate treatment with intravenous crystalloid, glucocorticoids, and an antihistamine. The cat was treated as an acute hypersensitivity, as described above, and it responded well within 24 hours (Figure 11.4b).

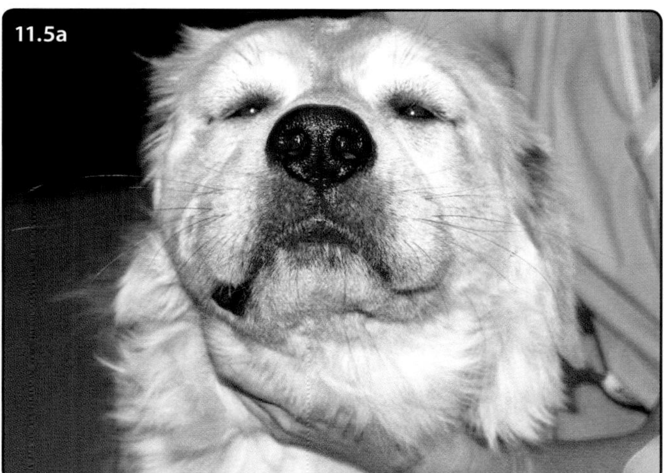

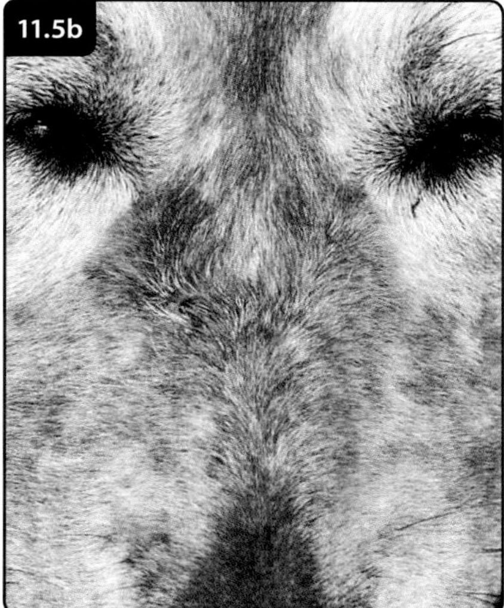

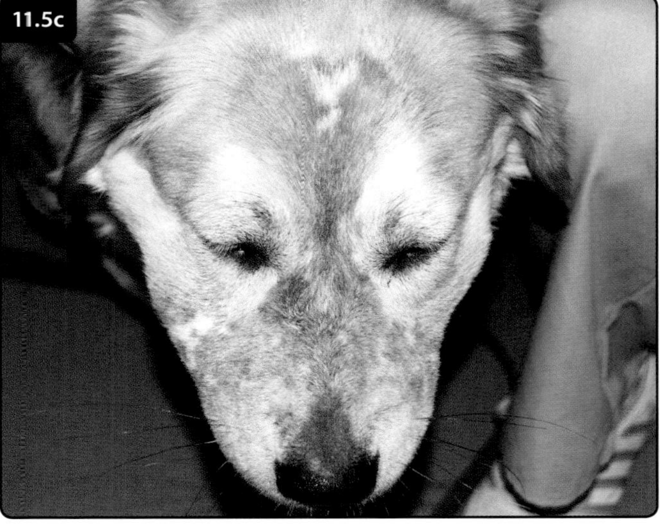

11.5a–c. Type 1 hypersensitivity to venomous hymenopteran. This dog was normal before it was let outside into its backyard. Minutes later it returned with facial erythema and pitting edema (Figure 11.5a). Figure 11.5b shows a small wound on the nasal bridge that probably represented contact with a stinging insect. The dog responded over hours to dexamethasone and diphenhydramine treatment (Figure 11.5c). Wasps, bees, and yellow jackets were all in the vicinity.

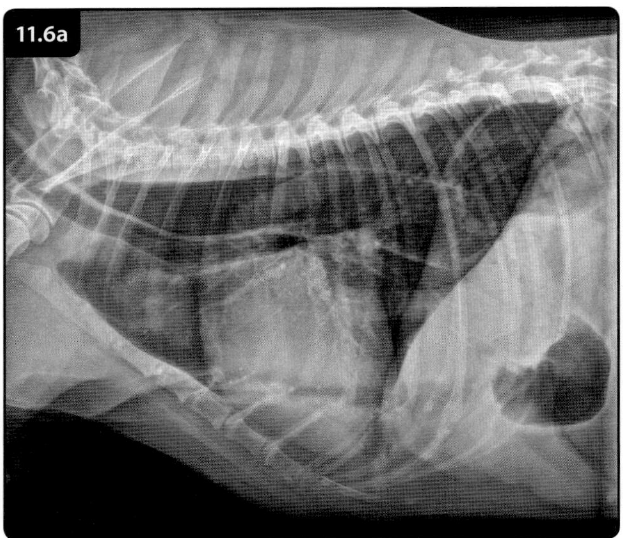

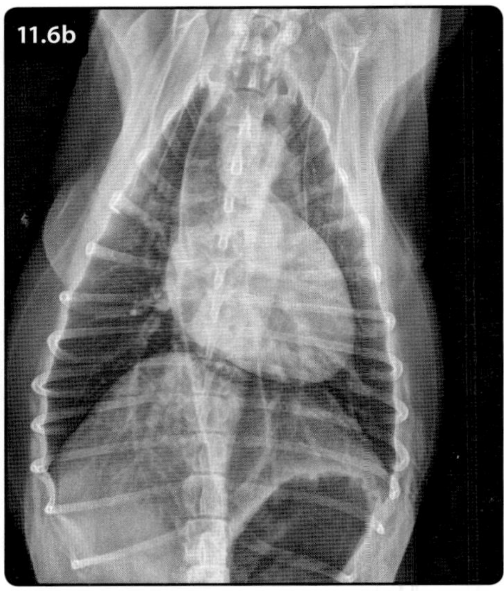

11.6a, b. Myasthenia gravis megaesophagus radiographs. These thoracic radiographs belong to a dog with periodic weakness that occurred with exercise, followed by spontaneous recovery until the next period of exertion. The dog was also regurgitating and megaesophagus was diagnosed, as seen on these radiographs. The diagnosis of myasthenia gravis was confirmed with the acetylcholine esterase antibody test and the dog responded to pyridostigmine treatment. Aspiration pneumonia is a long-term threat to dogs affected with this disorder.

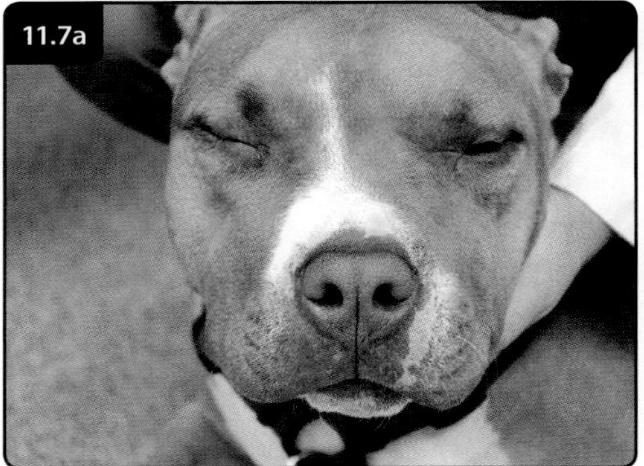

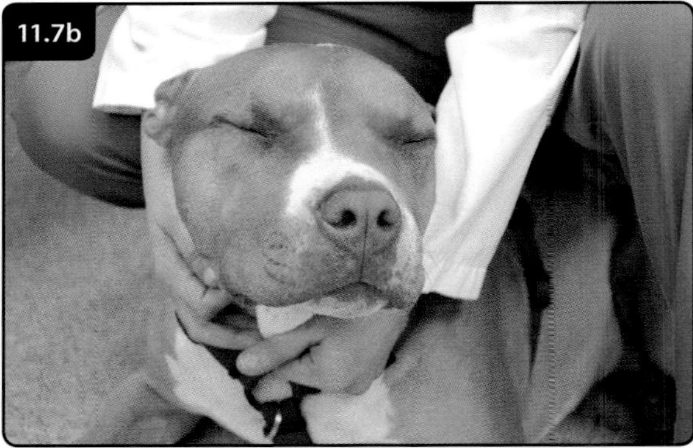

11.7a, b. Angioneurotic edema. This condition is an acute type 1 hypersensitivity response either to something ingested or perhaps the result of being stung by a venomous hymenopteran. The initial edema differs from hemorrhagic lymphedema caused by pit viper venom in that the latter is dark red and nonpruritic. The dog in this figure responded well to treatment for type 1 hypersensitivity using antihistamine and glucocorticoid drugs.

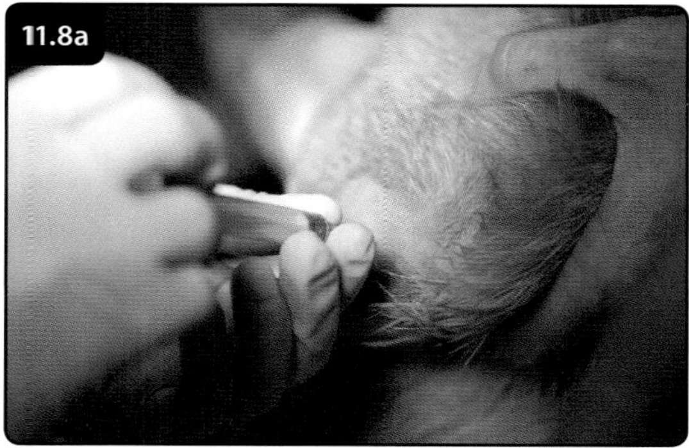

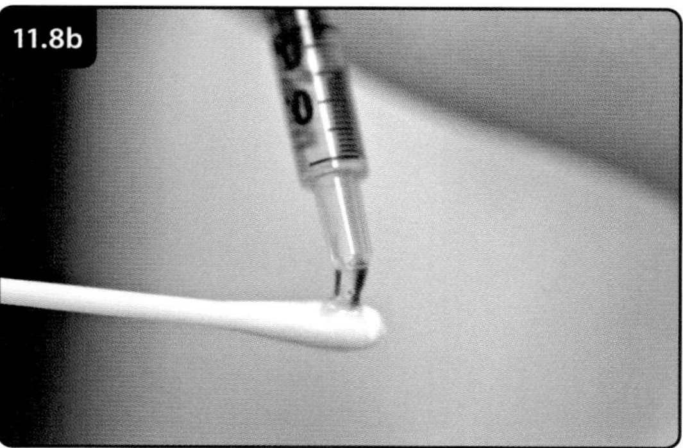

11.8a, b. Immune-mediated polyarthropathy joint fluid. Immune-mediated polyarthropathy in dogs is characterized by multiple joint swelling, lameness, and fever. The diagnosis is based on the clinical signs and the cytology of a joint fluid aspirate. The joint aspiration procedure is done with the dog under sedation, with the site of sampling depending on the joint involved. A complete sterile technique using a drape is recommended. Inflamed joint fluid loses its viscus quality and becomes more watery. The cytology shows many neutrophils, which can number >50,000/µl without any evidence of bacteria. This condition is very responsive to glucocorticoid treatment, which usually has to be administered at maintenance doses for months to avoid relapse. Some cases relapse despite optimal immunosuppression.

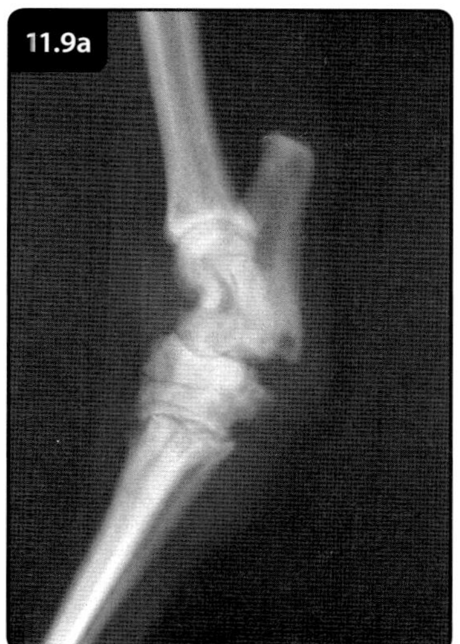

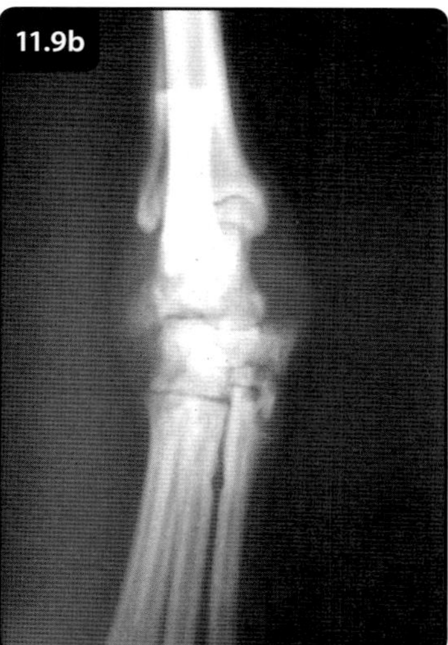

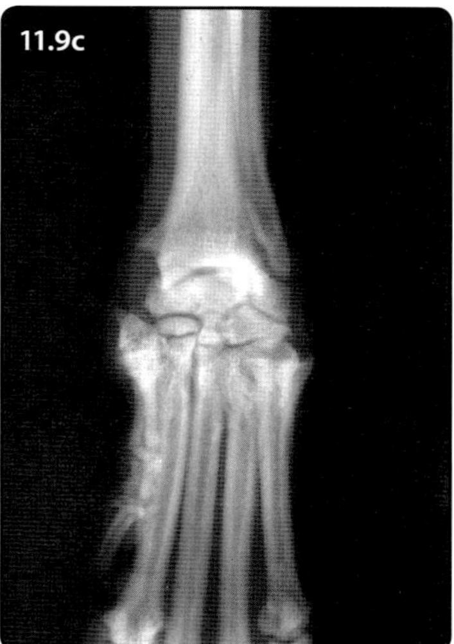

11.9a–c. Immune-mediated polyarthropathy radiographs. These radiographs of a dog's tarsus show signs of erosive immune-mediated joint disease similar to rheumatoid arthritis. The images show periarticular soft tissue swelling, bone erosion and bone proliferation, and some collapse of the interarticular spaces. There is some subluxation as well. Figure 11.9c is from a less advanced case and shows some bone proliferation medially and soft tissue swelling. A joint fluid analysis would typically have a watery texture and increased white blood cell numbers without evidence of bacteria.

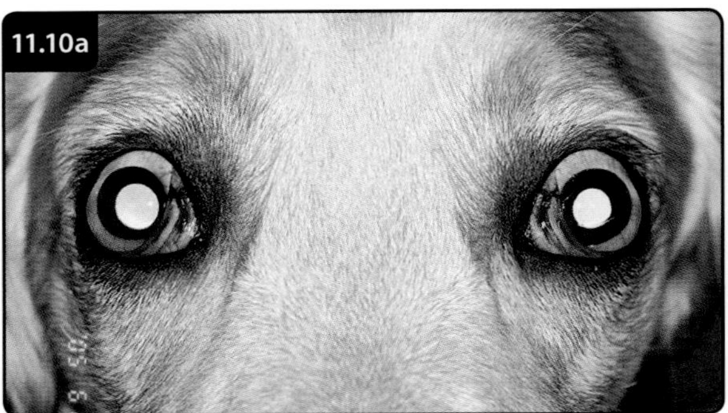

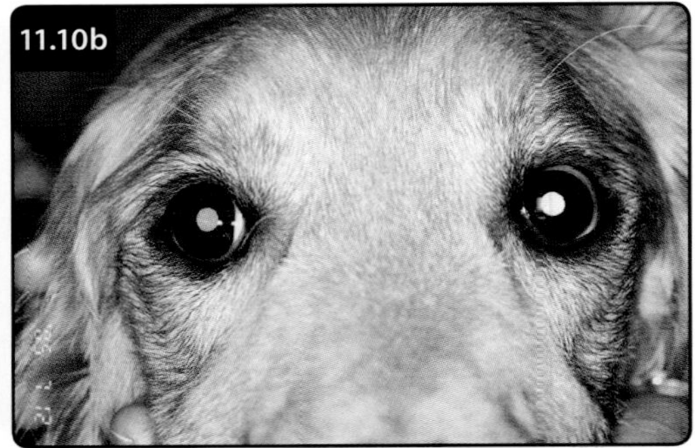

11.10a, b. Immune-mediated myositis. The exophthalmos in Figure 11.10a is typical of a dog with immune-mediated myositis with extraocular muscle involvement. The masticatory muscles are commonly involved and a masticatory muscle antibody test is available to help confirm the diagnosis. This disease is usually rapidly responsive to glucocorticoid treatment (Figure 11.10b), which must be administered at maintenance doses for several months in order to prevent relapse. After several months, the masticatory muscles might atrophy because of chronic inflammatory disease or from the effects of long-term steroid use. No functional impairment occurs unless the resulting fibrosis fuses the muscles involved with the temporomandibular joint, causing the dog to be unable to open its mouth (trismus). (Courtesy Ophthalmology Service, University of Florida)

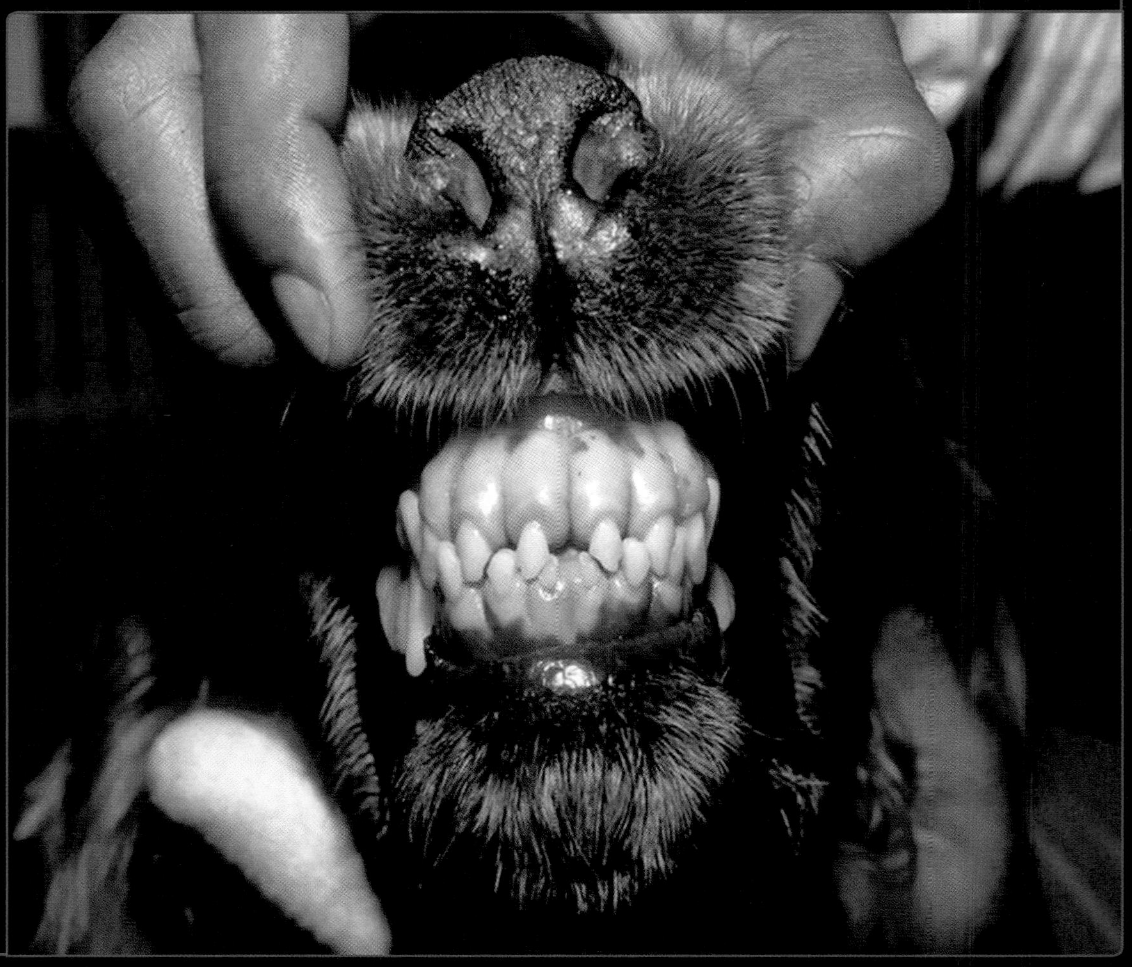

▲ This Irish Setter dog has gingival hyperplasia and widened spaces between dentition typical of acromegaly.

12

Endocrine disorders

ENDOCRINOLOGY is derived from the Greek word *endon*, meaning within, and *krin*, meaning to separate. Disorders of this medical discipline include several interesting syndromes, a number of which involve metabolism, including fluid and electrolyte disorders. Endocrinopathies can involve different organ systems throughout the body, thereby requiring the clinician to have a broad knowledge base in order to fully understand the pathophysiology, which might be very complex. Routine diagnostic tests are used to assess a patient with an endocrine disorder, but special tests are required in order to fully evaluate the endocrine disorders.

The images in this section illustrate the highlights of several endocrinopathies and should prove useful to the practicing clinician.

12 Endocrine disorders

- Hypercholesterolemia plus elevated creatine kinase – rule out hypothyroidism; hypocholesterolemia – rule out Addison's disease.
- Do not forget K+ when treating diabetic ketoacidosis.
- Oliguric diabetics have marked hyperglycemia.
- Marked hyperglycemia with minimal glycosuria – consider oliguria/anuria.
- Morning marked glycosuria and afternoon diminished glycosuria – typifies transient insulin response (need split dose).
- Blood glucose meters are not very accurate at the high and low ends of the scale.
- When fludrocortisone (Florinef®) does not work well, use desoxycorticosterone pivalate and prednisone. Keep an eye out for the atypical addisonian.
- If you have a diabetic dog with Cushing's disease that is receiving both insulin and o,p′-DDD (mitotane), and the dog becomes weak and depressed, remember this:
  - If the dog is o,p′-DDD toxic, its appetite will have been absent that day and vomiting may or may not have occurred.
  - If the dog is insulin overdosed, it very likely will have eaten that morning. Coma and seizures can be present.
  - If the dog has both hypoglycemia and o,p′-DDD toxicity, any combination of all of the above can occur. This is where 'treat for the treatable' comes in if laboratory tests are unavailable, where treatment would call for both dextrose and glucocorticoid.

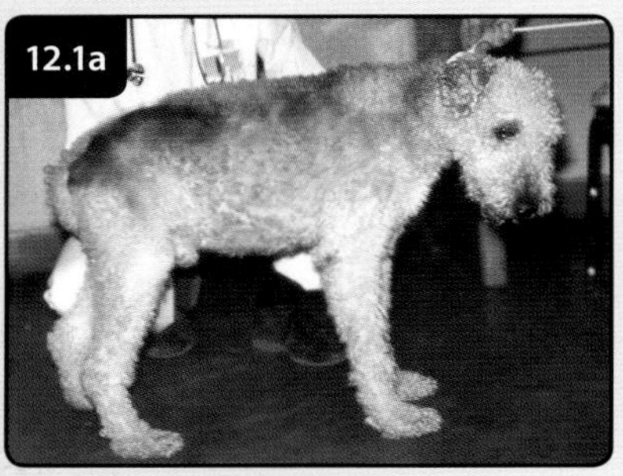

12.1a–c. Cushing's disease dog. This Airedale was diagnosed with pituitary Cushing's disease. Figure 12.1a shows the dog before beginning o,p′-DDD (mitotane) treatment, and the following figures show the dog's progressive improvement. Hair regrowth can begin as early as 6 weeks after beginning treatment with either mitotane or trilostane; however, in some dogs hair growth might take longer than 1 year. This Airedale shows a remarkable response over a 6-month period. Note that in most dogs the new hair color will be considerably darker than the original hair.

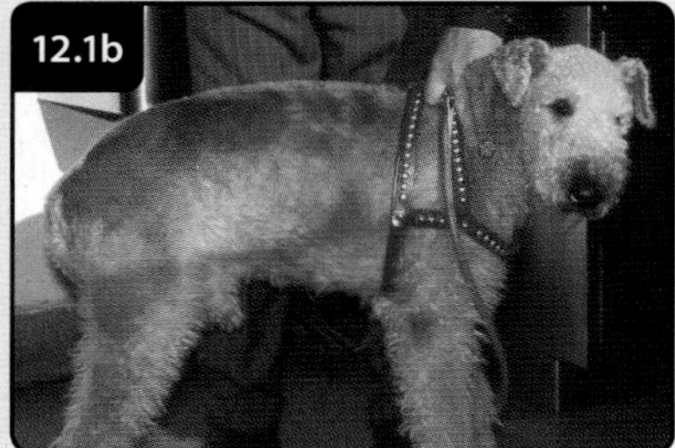

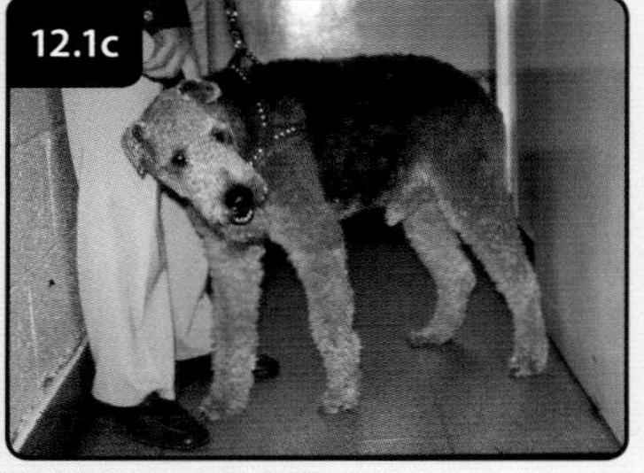

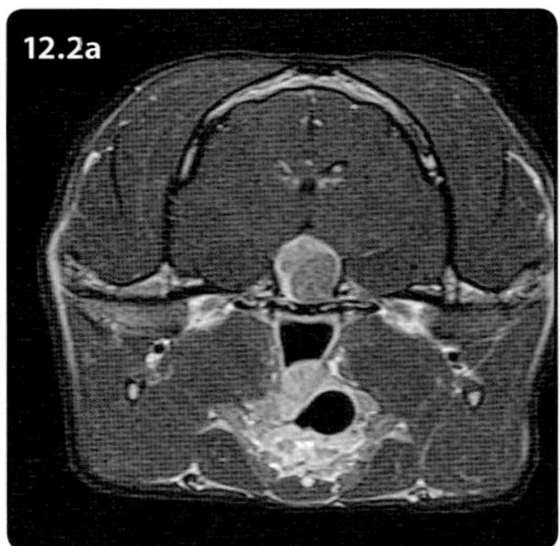
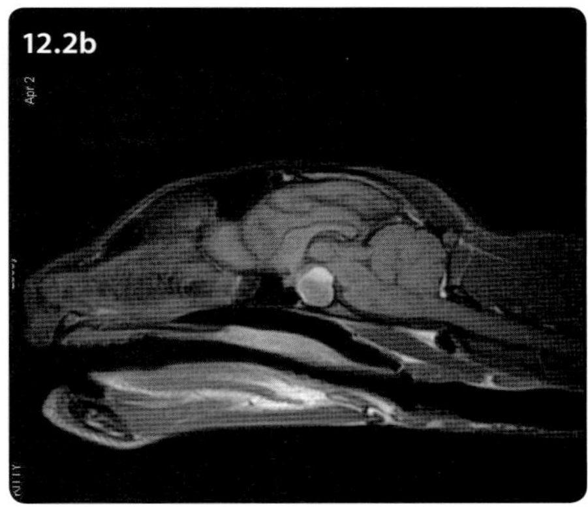

12.2a, b. Feline acromegaly. Shown is an MR image of a cat with acromegaly which, unlike the dog (see Case 12.3), has a pituitary tumor as the primary underlying cause. These frontal and sagittal images clearly show the pituitary macroadenoma. Almost all cats with acromegaly are also diabetic at the time of diagnosis because of peripheral insulin resistance caused by the growth hormone. The insulin-like growth factor-1 test is a surrogate diagnostic test when plasma growth hormone assays are unavailable. Fractional radiation is the current treatment until surgery becomes more commonplace.

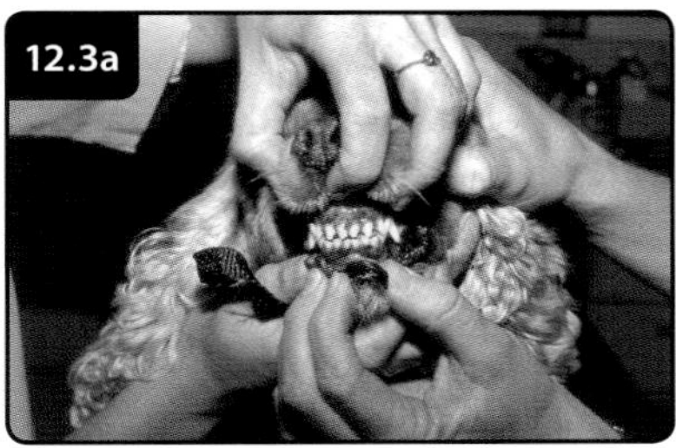
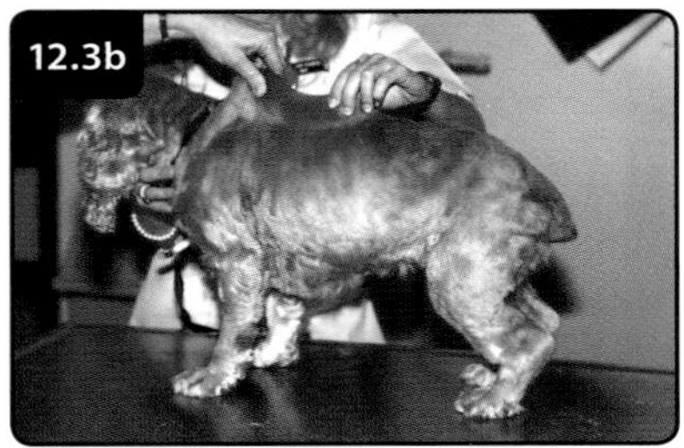

12.3a, b. Acromegaly in the dog. In most dogs, acromegaly occurs as a result of increased progesterone levels. In this Cocker Spaniel it resulted from previous medroxyprogesterone injections that were given for behavior modification. The widened interdental spaces (resulting from maxillary spreading) (Figure 12.3a) are typical of this syndrome in both dogs and cats, along with other signs such as redundant skin folds (Figure 12.3b), pharyngeal hyperplasia, and enlargement of the distal extremities. The condition is reversible following the return to normal progesterone blood levels.

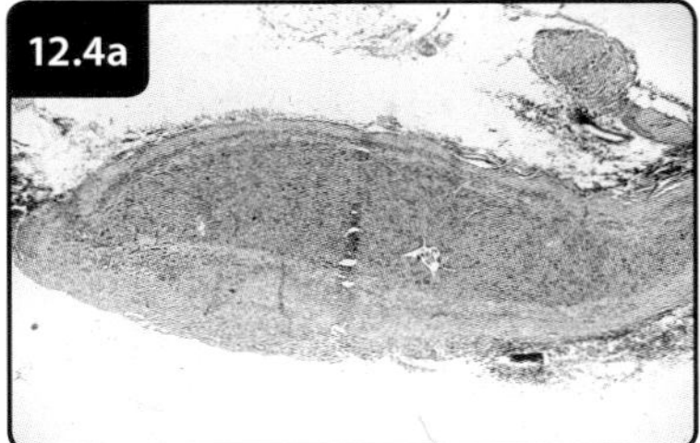
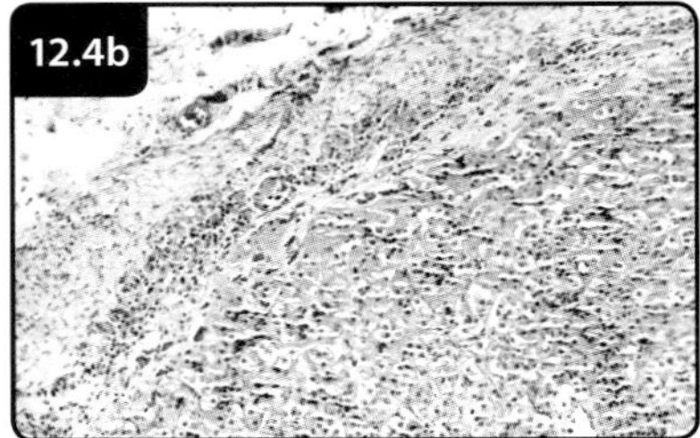
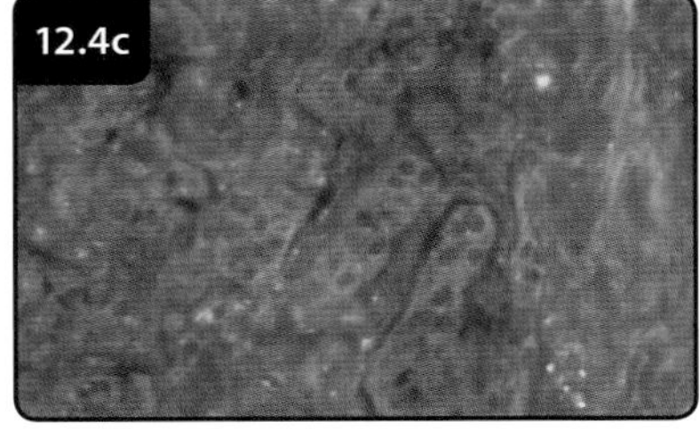

12.4a–c. Autoimmune adrenalitis in the dog. These three images are histopathologic specimens from a dog with Addison's disease. Figure 12.4a shows a markedly diminished adrenal cortex while Figure 12.4b shows lymphocyte infiltrates in the cortex amongst a collapsed and diminished adrenal cortex, suggesting immune-mediated destruction. Figure 12.4c shows positive indirect immunofluorescent staining (yellow highlights) on a normal adrenal tissue template documenting autoimmune adrenalitis in the dog. This same type of lesion has been described in dogs with co-existing autoimmune thyroiditis, allowing for the diagnosis of autoimmune endocrinopathy.

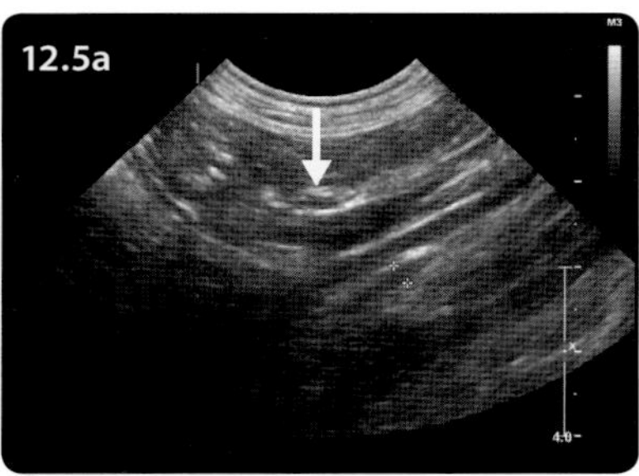
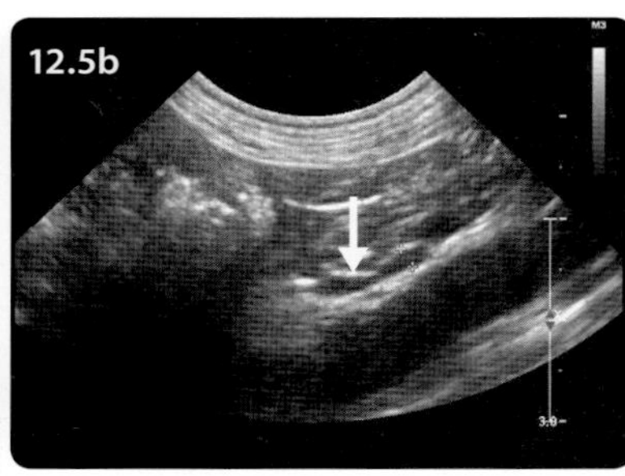

12.5a, b. Ultrasonographic appearance of Addison's disease in the dog. Shown are the right and left adrenal glands (arrows) of an addisonian dog showing diminished size bilaterally. The normal adrenal width is 7 mm. This finding is not demonstrable in every case, but it does support the diagnosis along with blood cortisol concentrations that are <1.0 μg/dl (<27.59 nmol/l).

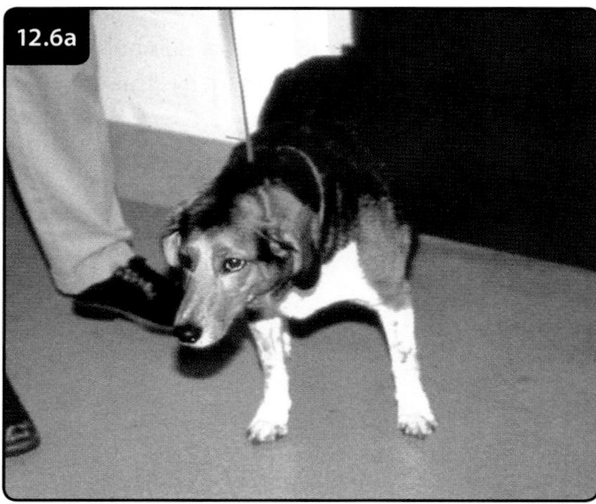
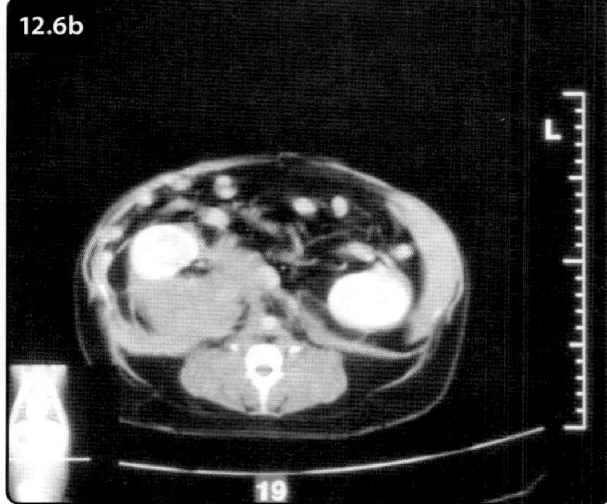
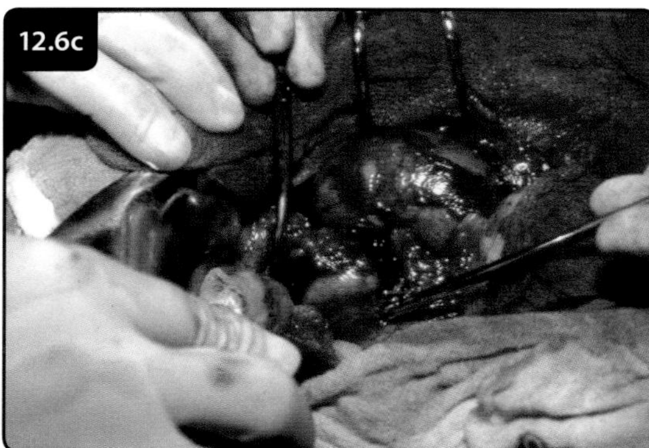
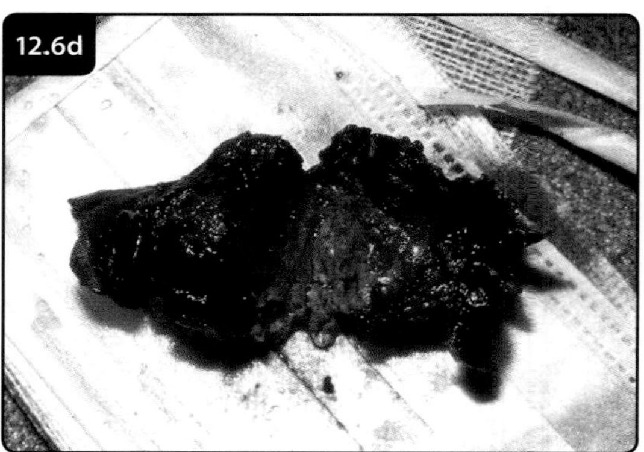

12.6a–d. Periadrenal cortical carcinoma hemorrhage. This 9-year-old neutered male Beagle (Figure 12.6a) was evaluated for polydipsia and polyuria. The blood test results were compatible with Cushing's syndrome. Initial abdominal ultrasound imaging noted an adrenal mass. Thoracic radiographs were normal. The dog became acutely hypotensive that same evening before the next day's scheduled surgical exploratory. Overnight intravenous fluids stabilized the dog. A preoperative CT study (Figure 12.6b) showed fluid surrounding a right-sided adrenal mass, which turned out to be acute hemorrhage in the periadrenal region, as evident at surgery (Figures 12.c, d). The bleeding could have been consequent to accidental blunt abdominal trauma or it could have occurred spontaneously. The histopathologic diagnosis was adrenocortical carcinoma.

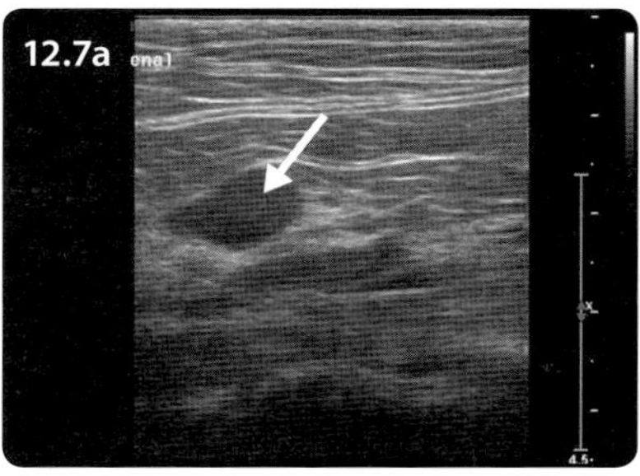

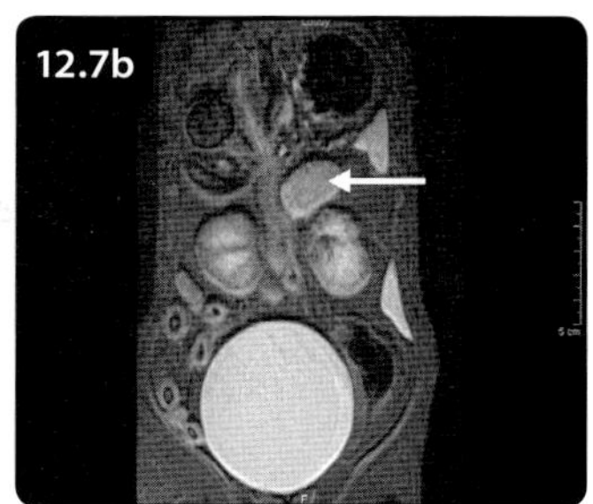

12.7a–c. Aldosteronoma in a cat. This tumor originates from the zona glomerulosa of the adrenal cortex. The clinical effects are associated with hypokalemia and an increase in total body sodium while the serum sodium concentration can be normal. The clinical effects include muscular weakness from the hypokalemia and hypertension caused by the increased total body sodium. Shown is an abdominal ultrasound image of an adrenal tumor that was further imaged with MRI to clarify the presence of any metastasis or caudal vena cava involvement. Figure 12.7c shows the neoplastic adrenal gland at surgery. Care must be taken to avoid accidental incising of the caudal vena cava and any extra-adrenal blood vessels. Some of these patients can have adrenocortical insufficiency postoperatively if the tumor was producing both aldosterone and cortisol.

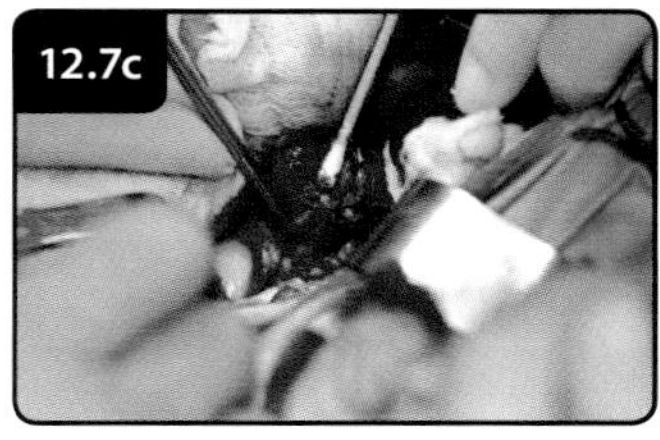

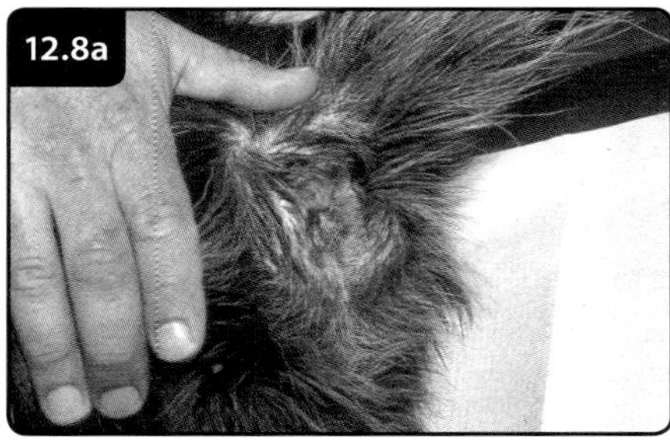

12.8b Hoag – 11-yr-old K9 Mix

WBC × 10^3	9.0	Phos	5.7
PCV	50.9	Cl^-	120
BUN	132	Amylase	9130
Creat.	5.6	S. G. (urine)	1.008
Calcium	16.0	RBC	10-12
		Cast	Occa. Hyaline granular

12.8a, b. Hypercalcemia of malignancy. This condition is the most common cause of hypercalcemia in the dog. Lymphoma and anal sac carcinoma (Figure 12.8a) are the most common tumors associated with this paraneoplastic syndrome. The parathyroid hormone level is low in these cases because of negative feedback inhibition, while some dogs will show a positive parathyroid hormone-related peptide test. The azotemia and isosthenuria in this dog's work up (Figure 12.8b) reflect nephrocalcinosis, which can result from sustained hypercalcemia. Treatment entails controlling the hypercalcemia and any renal dysfunction, and treating the primary neoplasm.

12.9. Immune thyroiditis. This histopathologic image illustrates autoimmune thyroiditis in a dog, as evident by the lymphocytic infiltrate. Some of these dogs might also have autoimmune adrenalitis, as described in Case 12.4 (Figures 12.4a–c). Most dogs will not show signs during the lymphocytic infiltrative stage of the disease until the majority of the thyroid gland is involved. Many of these dogs will be positive for antithyroid antibodies, but treatment with thyroid replacement will not be indicated until the serum thyroxine concentration is below normal.

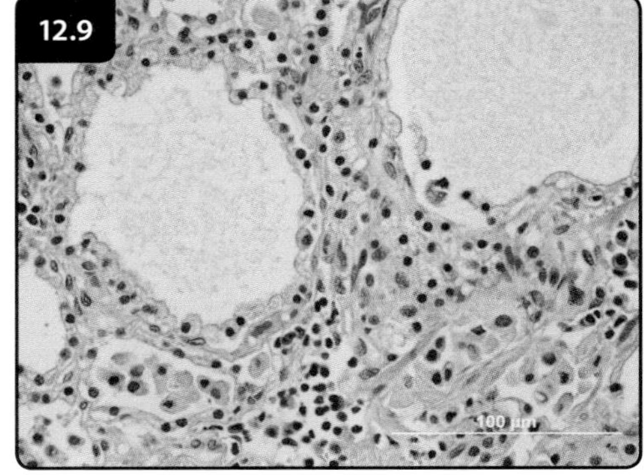

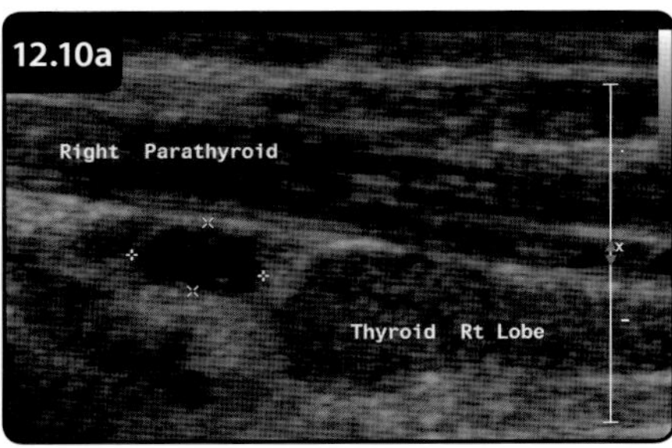

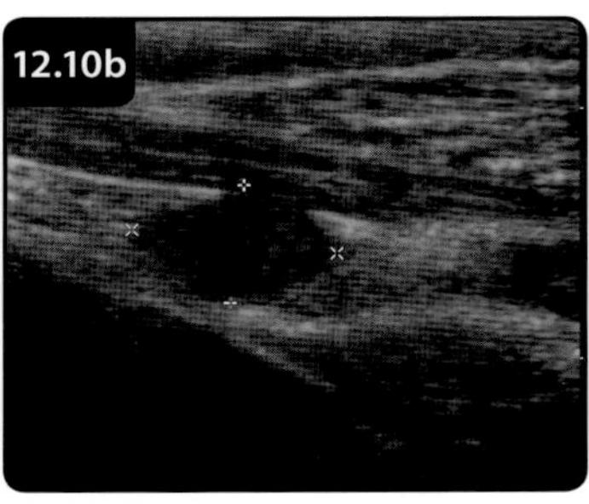

12.10a, b. Bilateral parathyroid adenomas in a dog. This dog had hypercalcemia and hypophosphatemia in addition to an elevated parathyroid serum level, which is diagnostic for primary hyperparathyroidism. The dog was sent to surgery and two enlarged parathyroid glands were removed. Histopathology confirmed the diagnosis of bilateral parathyroid adenomas. Postoperative management entails monitoring for hypocalcemia, which should then be treated with calcium and/or vitamin D supplementation. This complication occurs as a result of negative feedback inhibition of parathyroid hormone from the remaining parathyroid glands, which have become atrophic. This atrophy will reverse over days or weeks.

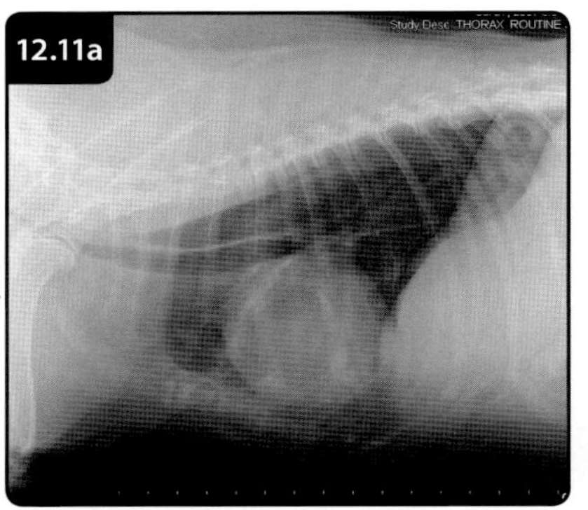

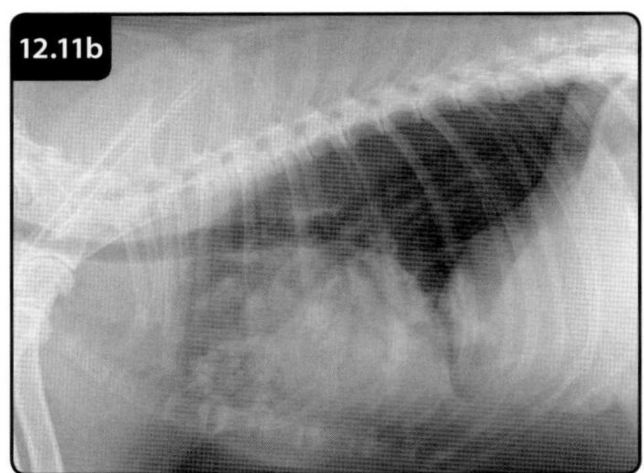

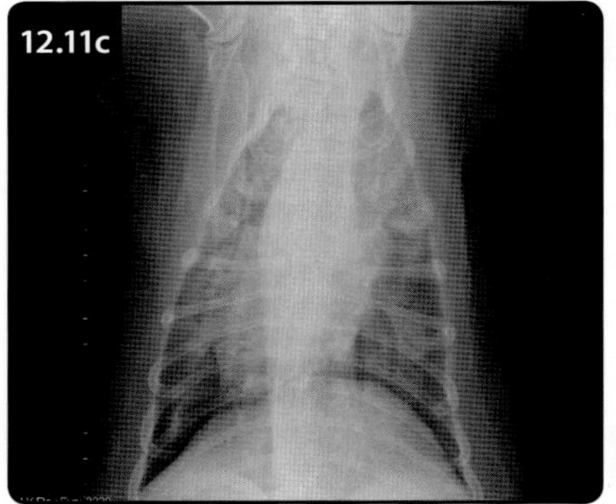

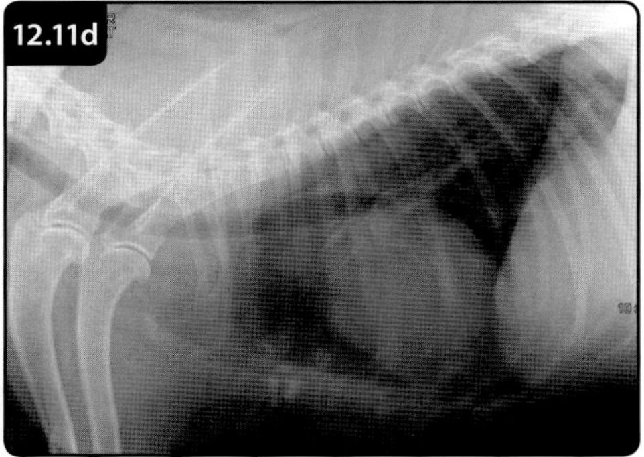

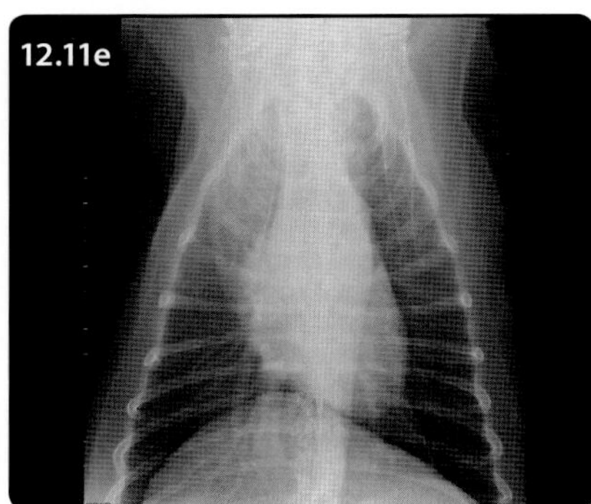

12.11a–e. Hypothyroidism and megaesophagus. Figure 12.11a show a megaesophagus in a dog that was recently diagnosed with hypothyroidism. There was no aspiration at first, but this did occur a week later (Figures 12.b, c). The dog was treated with antibiotics and L-thyroxine (levothyroxine) and responded well to treatment. Figures 12.11d, e, taken about 3 weeks later, found that the megaesophagus had disappeared, as had the pneumonia. Megaesophagus has been associated with hypothyroidism, but several authors have challenged this association. The dog shown in this sequence of radiographs provides evidence that perhaps the association is real in some cases.

12.12. Severe inflammatory calcinosis cutis. This young dog was diagnosed with primary hypoparathyroidism based on his clinical signs of neuromuscular irritability, muscular weakness, and generalized seizures. It had hypocalcemia, hyperphosphatemia, and a low parathyroid hormone serum concentration. The dog was treated with diluted calcium gluconate subcutaneously as per recommendations in the veterinary literature, and this caused the formation of severe inflammatory calcinosis cutis, which led to the dog's demise. Shown is the markedly inflamed trunkal skin of this dog. Although many dogs do not show this type of reaction, there have been some cases reported in the literature that should cause us to use this therapeutic modality with caution.

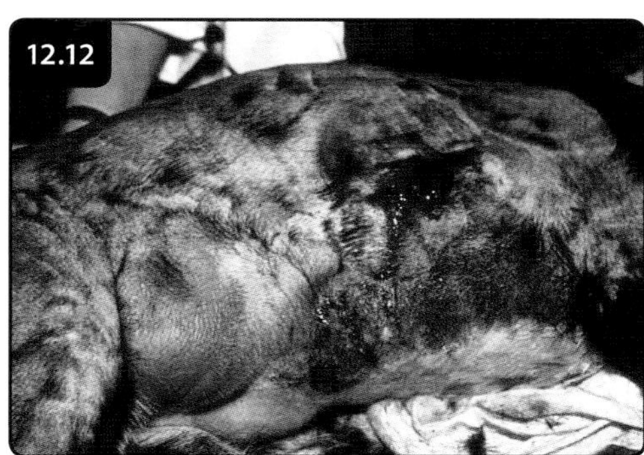

12.13a–d. Acromegaly and pituitary Cushing's disease in a diabetic cat. This diabetic cat (Figure 12.13a) had progressive insulin resistance. Its insulin glargine dose exceeded 18 units twice daily. The medical work up diagnosed this cat as having a pituitary tumor that was causing bilateral adrenocortical hyperplasia. An elevated response with ACTH stimulation confirmed pituitary Cushing's disease, which led to an additional presumptive diagnosis of acromegaly of pituitary origin. She also had a markedly elevated insulin-like growth factor-1 concentration, which led to an additional presumptive diagnosis of acromegaly. The cat did not show any gross physical changes compatible with either acromegaly or Cushing's disease, perhaps because of the early diagnosis before morphologic signs occurred. The abdominal ultrasound images (Figures 12.13b, c) show bilateral adrenal gland enlargements, and the CT scan (Figure 12.13d) shows a pituitary tumor. Treatment consisted of insulin glargine, trilostane, and pituitary irradiation. The cat had a minimal response to fractional radiation treatments and was euthanized 2 months later.

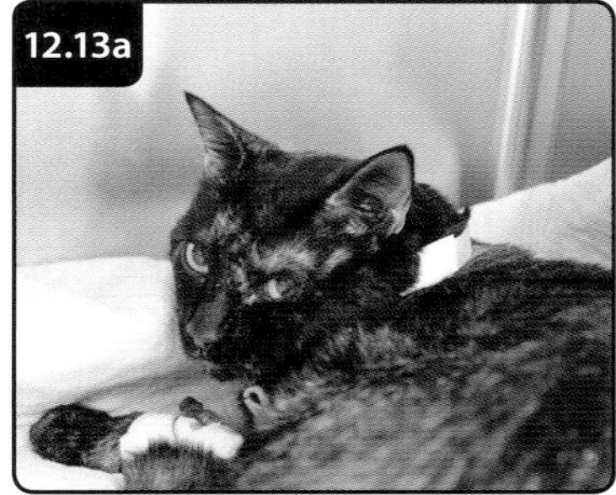

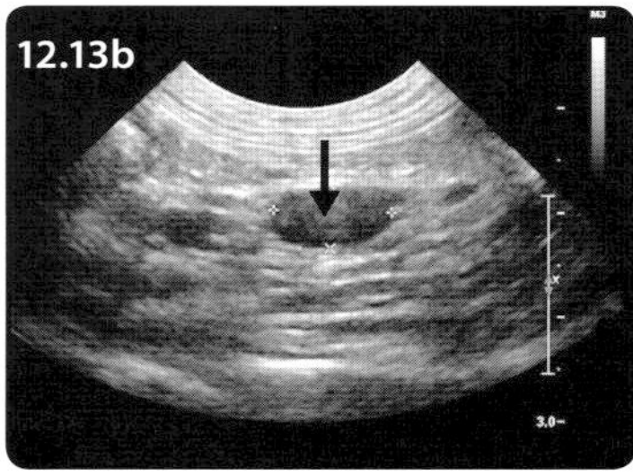

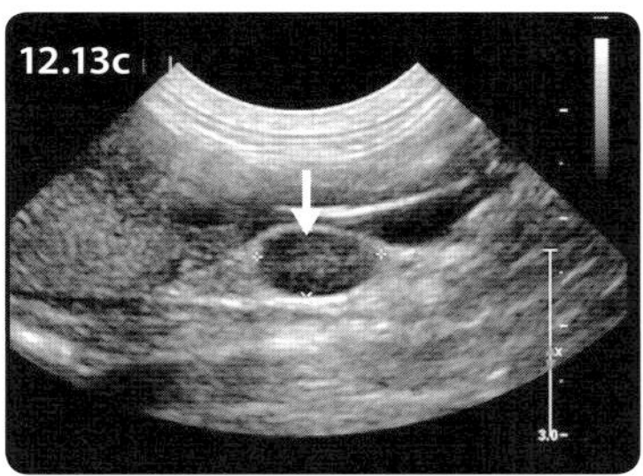

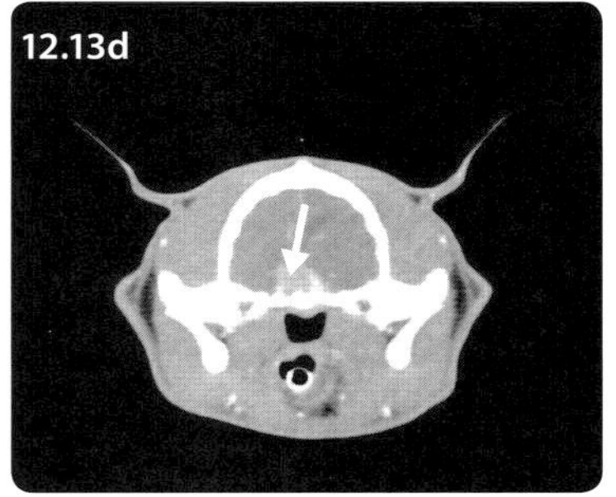

12.14. Metastatic insulinoma. This abdominal CT scan was obtained from a dog showing neurologic signs associated with hypoglycemia (neuroglycopenia). The pancreas is seen as a white structure between the liver lobes (arrowhead). The contrast media highlights the pancreas, which contained a beta cell carcinoma, and the small round areas on the liver representing metastatic lesions (arrow), showing that the liver is the most common site for metastasis with this neoplasm. Surgical debulking, along with the use of certain medications such as prednisone and diazoxide, is palliative and might prolong the period of euglycemia postoperatively.

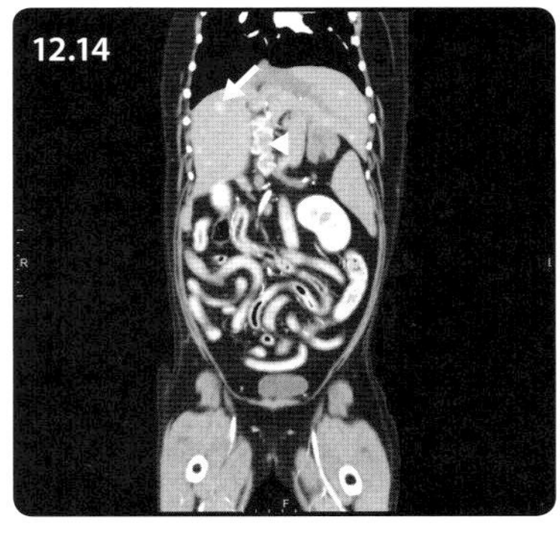

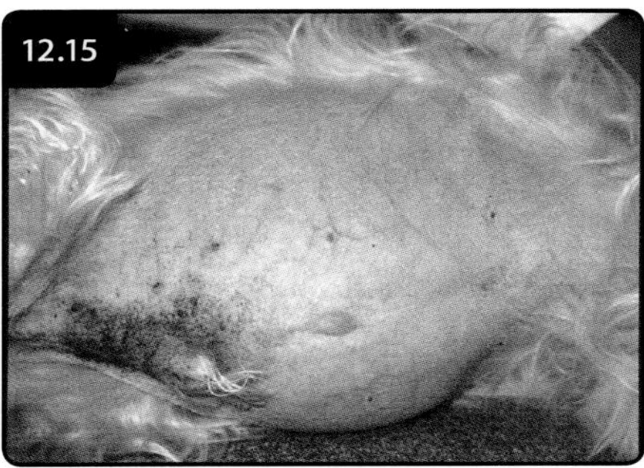

12.15. Cushing's disease in the dog. The Maltese dog in this image shows typical cushingoid abdominal distension, thin skin, small whitish skin deposits representing calcinosis cutis, and hyperpigmentation. The umbilical hernia was likely associated with the stretching of the abdominal wall. This dog was also a poorly controlled diabetic because of the co-existing hypercortisolism. He was treated with o,p'-DDD (mitotane) and the diabetic condition stabilized, accompanied by an overall improvement in the dog's condition.

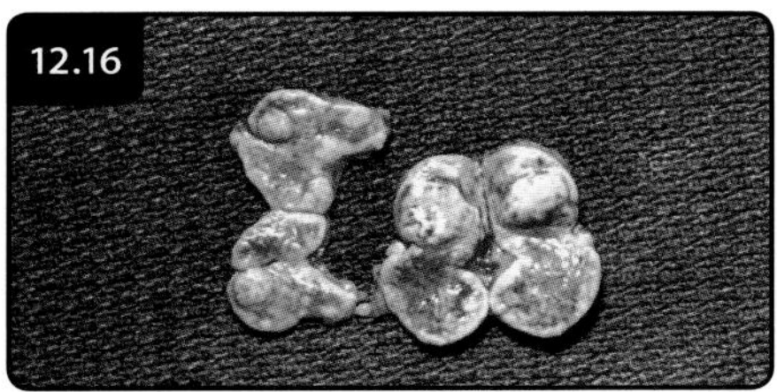

12.16. Adrenal nodular hyperplasia. These adrenal glands came from a dog with pituitary-dependent adrenocortical hyperplasia. On ultrasound examination this lesion is virtually impossible to distinguish from neoplasia unless the nodules remain static over a period of months without showing a malignant tendency for invasive growth. Dogs with this lesion show typical signs and diagnostic test results as other dogs with pituitary-dependent hyperadrenocorticism, and they usually respond well to treatment. Some dogs might show a tendency for repeated escape from therapeutic control, thus requiring repeated loading doses of their oral medication, as was the case in this dog.

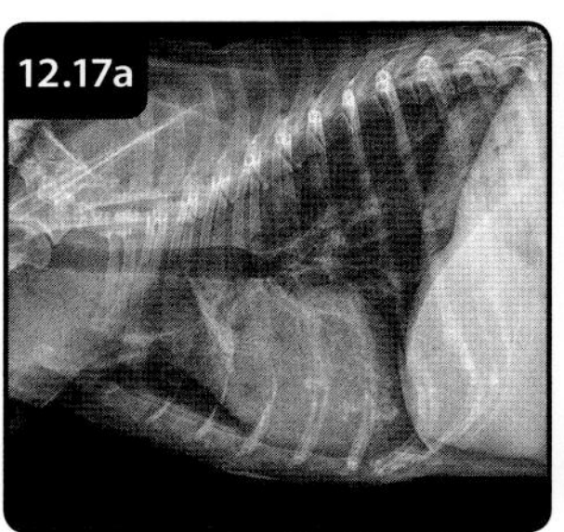

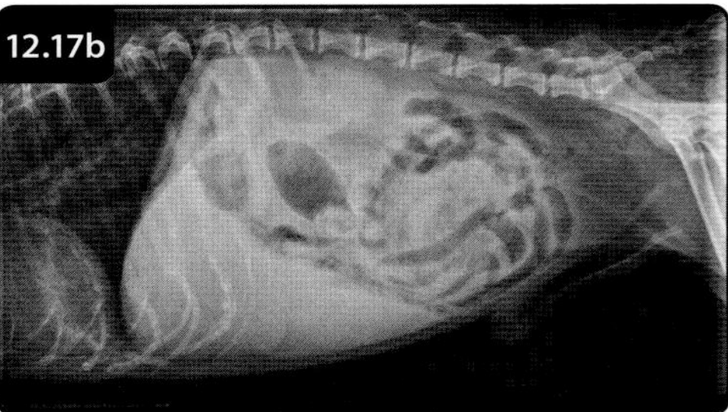

12.17a, b. Calcinosis cutis and pulmonary parenchymal mineralization. These thoracic radiographs of a Cushing's disease dog show diffuse pulmonary parenchymal mineralization and subtle areas of subcutaneous mineral deposits in the sternum representing dystrophic pulmonary calcification and calcinosis cutis, respectively. The lateral abdominal radiograph shows the typical pot belly and hepatomegaly of the same Cushing's dog. The hepatomegaly occurs from glycogen deposition in the liver, and this accounts for the increased liver transaminase enzymes and serum alkaline phosphatase enzyme.

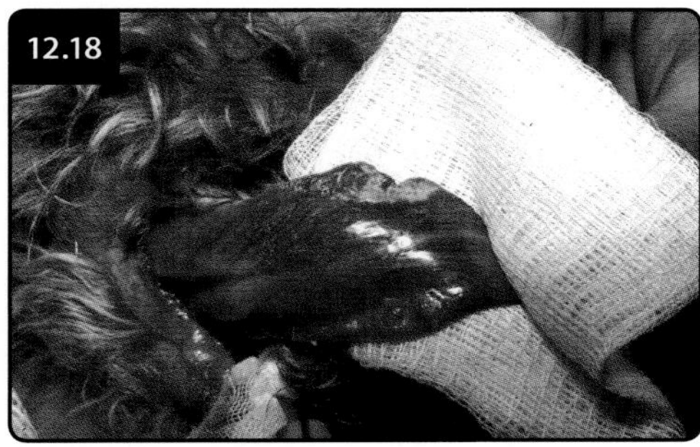

12.18. Lingual calcinosis cutis. This is the tongue of a dog with Cushing's disease. The calcium deposits in the soft tissues of a Cushing's dog are a dystrophic tissue change that occurs from chronic hypercortisolemia. Calcinosis cutis has various patterns and different tissue involvements. These lesions might eventually disappear after the patient is successfully treated and serum cortisol levels return to normal.

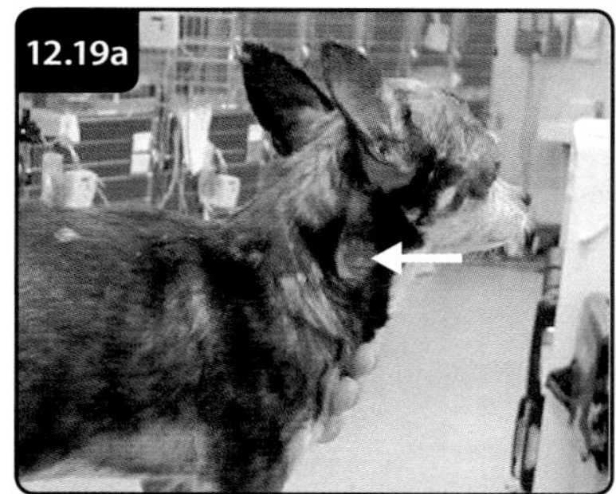

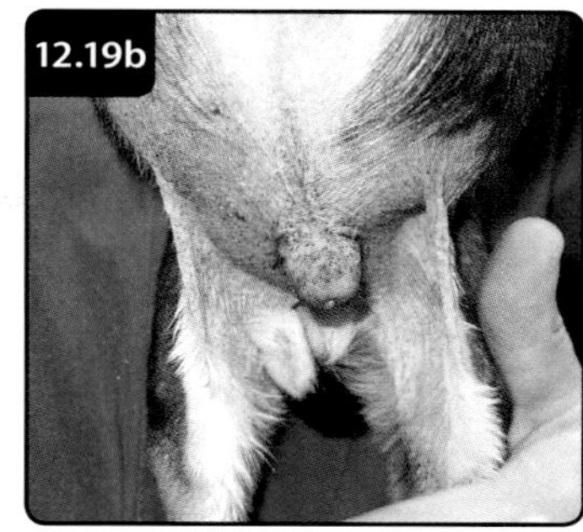

12.19a, b. Skin changes from Cushing's disease. This Terrier shows the typical skin pathology of the Cushing's disease dog. Note the areas of alopecia, thin skin, hyperpigmentation, a plaque of calcinosis cutis on his neck (arrow), epidermal atrophy, and abdominal distension. All of these changes will resolve over weeks to months with successful treatment of the underlying disease.

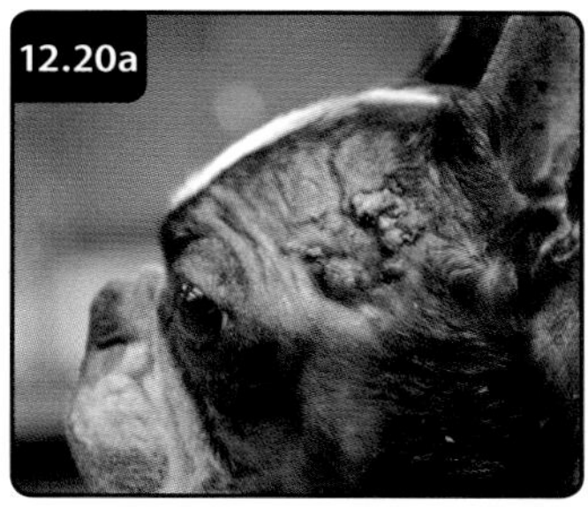

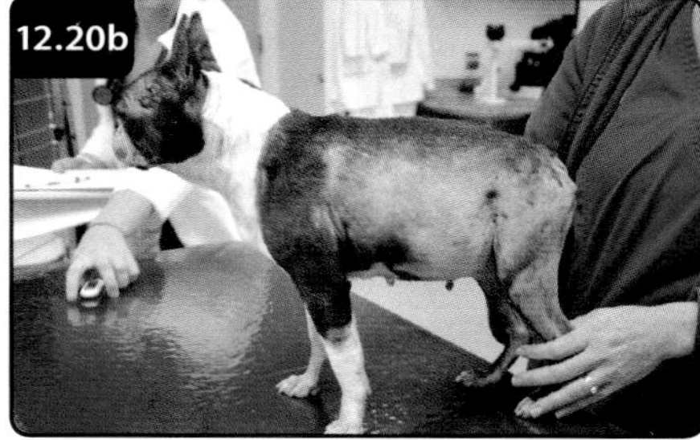

12.20a, b. Cushing's skin changes. This Boston Bulldog has pituitary-dependent Cushing's disease. She shows obvious trunkal alopecia, thin skin, and facial calcinosis cutis. These lesions will predictably improve with restoration of normal serum cortisol concentrations. The calcinosis cutis lesions might require months before they resolve. There is no explanation why calcinosis cutis appears in some dogs while avoiding others. There is no topical treatment for this condition other than time and the return to normal blood cortisol levels.

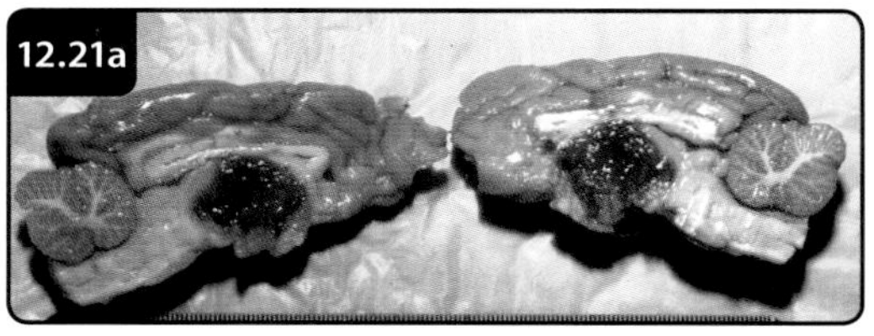

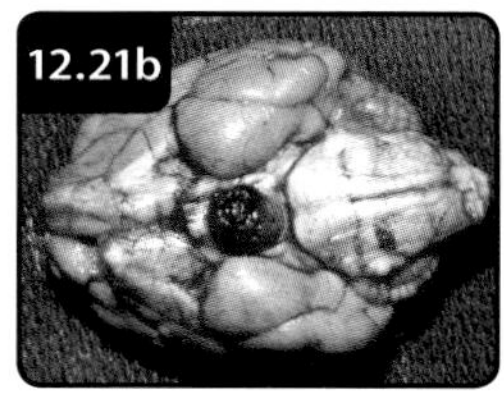

12.21 a, b. Pituitary apoplexy in the dog. A minority of dogs (10–20%) with pituitary-dependent Cushing's disease will experience growth of their pituitary tumor, where it will change from a microadenoma to a macroadenoma. Some of those with macroadenoma will be victim to pituitary apoplexy when the tumor causes an acute hemorrhage in the diencephalon and causes the dog to become demented and show other neurologic signs, such as head pressing or circling, or lapse into a semistuporous state and become recumbent. The term pituitary apoplexy refers to a hemorrhagic stroke, as first described in humans in the late 19th century. The condition is usually fatal in the dog because there is no treatment other than to wait and monitor the neurologic course. Most pet owners will elect euthanasia because of the significant degree of neurologic impairment and the continued growth of the macroadenoma. The large amount of tissue involvement makes surgical treatment unfeasible. Shown is a sagittal section of the brain at postmortem examination showing the degree of extension involving the diencephalon (Figure 12.21a). The other brain specimen (Figure 12.21b) is uncut and shows only the superficial aspects of a macroadenoma that also hemorrhaged.

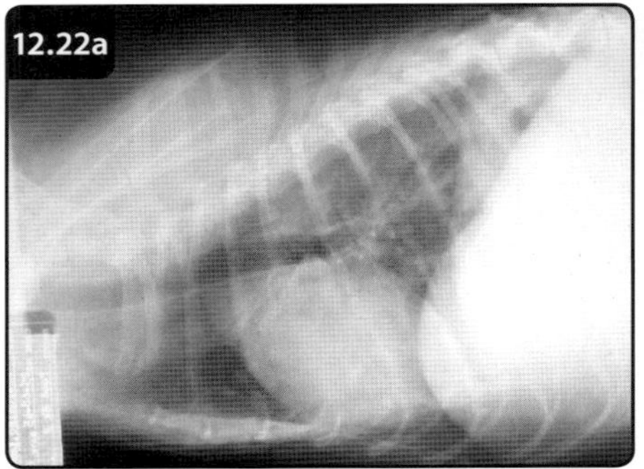

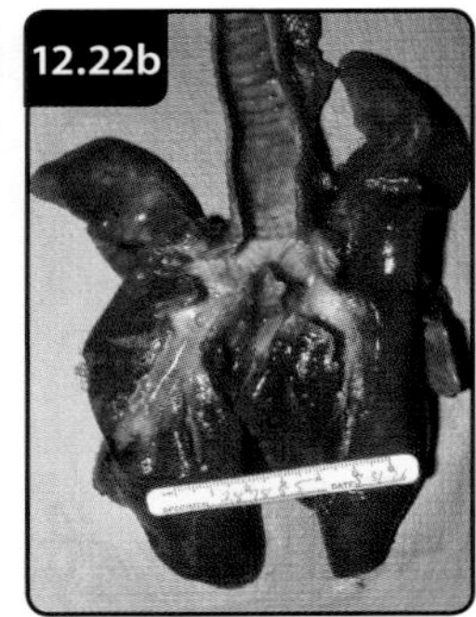

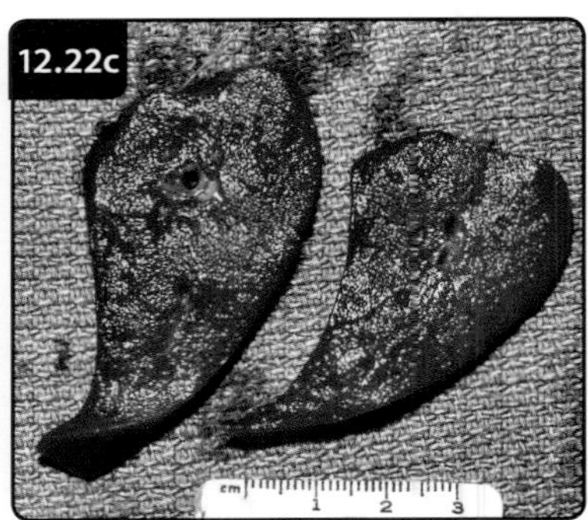

12.22a–c. Cushing's disease-induced pulmonary lung mineralization. Certain dystrophic tissue changes can occur because of hypercortisolism. The lungs can become mineralized and dogs with this problem will have signs of chronic lung disease, as shown with exercise intolerance and shortness of breath. This change is untreatable and irreversible despite treatment of the Cushing's disease. The lung disease has an insidious onset. On chest auscultation, there will be accentuated dry lung sounds and radiographs will show diffuse pulmonary interstitial mineralization (Figure 12.22a). At necropsy the lungs appear hyperemic (Figure 12.22b), and on incising the lungs, they feel gritty (Figure 12.22c).

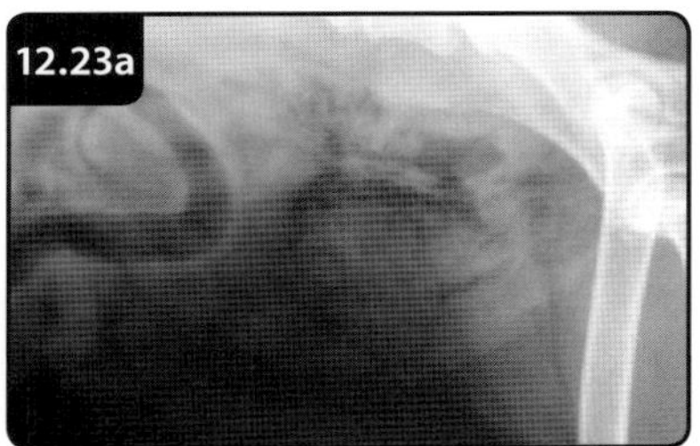

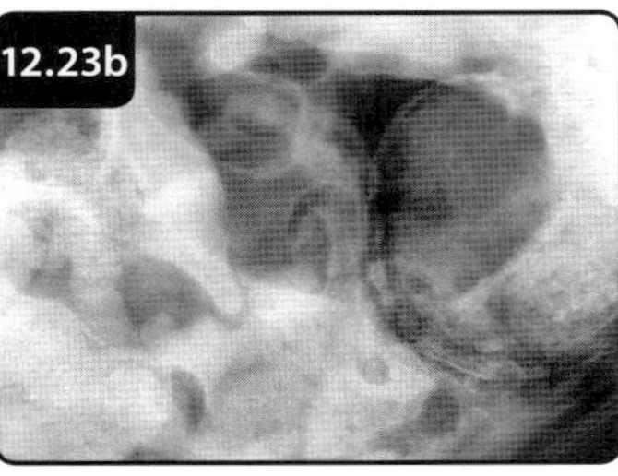

12.23a, b. Emphysematous cystitis in diabetic dogs. These two lateral abdominal radiographs are taken from two different dogs, both of them showing emphysematous cystitis. The pathogenesis of this condition involves a bacterial cystitis in the presence of glycosuria. The urine glucose undergoes fermentation by the bacteria and the resultant gas formation accumulates in the bladder submucosa and sometimes the surrounding bladder wall, as shown in Figures 12.23a and 12.23b, respectively.

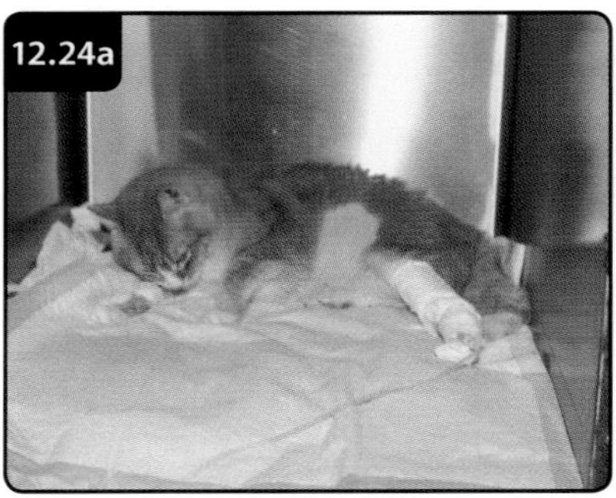

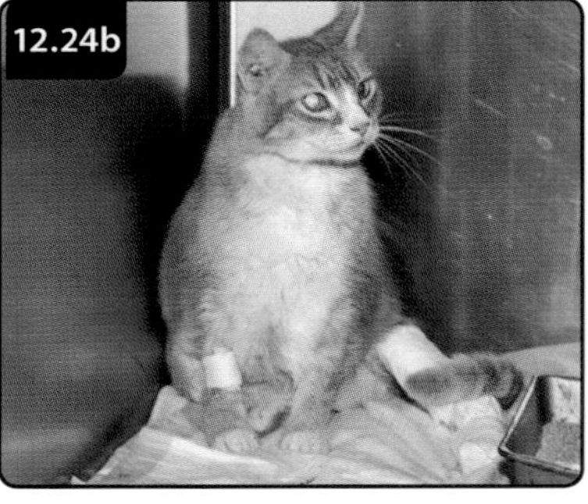

12.24a, b. Diabetic hypokalemic myopathy. This condition occurs in both dogs and cats, with muscular weakness being the main clinical sign. The cat in Figure 12.24a shows typical cervical flexion, which is due to the marked muscular weakness that is often present when the serum potassium decreases below 3.0 mmol/l (mEq/l). The lower the potassium declines the more progressive the weakness becomes, which can worsen to the point of respiratory failure because of weak muscles of respiration and, perhaps, the diaphragm. The ventral cervical flexion occurs because dogs and cats do not have a ligamentum nuchae, which would help keep the head extended despite the weak cervical muscles. Treatment involves administering potassium chloride, which is diluted in the intravenous fluids. In most cases, the muscular strength returns within 24 hours (Figure 12.24b).

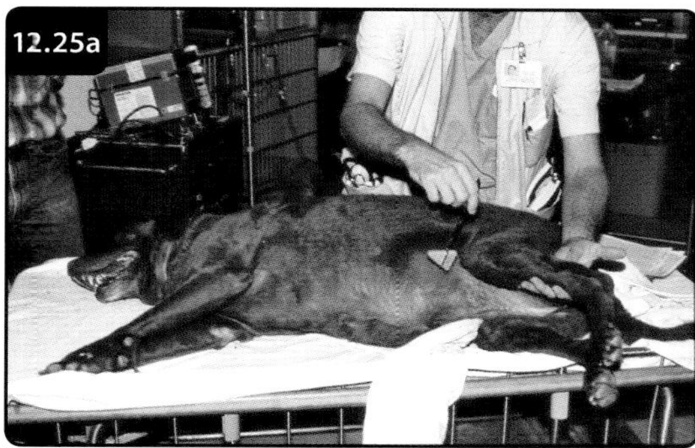

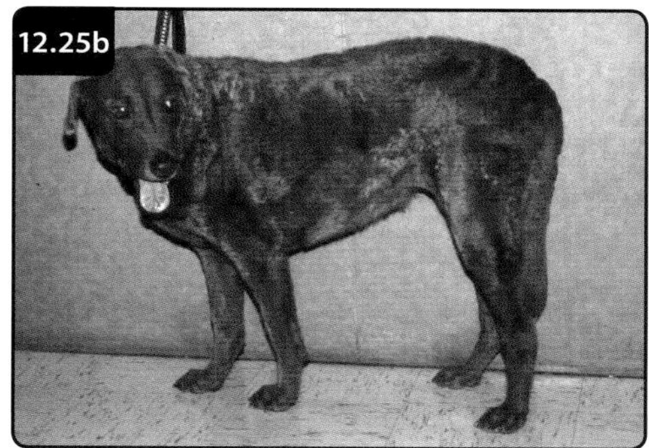

12.25 a, b. Diabetic neuropathy. This complication can occur in the dog and in the cat. In the latter, the typical appearance is plantar posturing. In the dog, the neuropathy appears as a lumbar cord myelopathy where the patient has bilateral hindlimb weakness that can range in severity from paraparesis to paraplegia. The pathology involves a demyelination of the spinal cord, which results from a combination of factors such as oxygen radical generation, capillary basement thickening, and certain biochemical derangements such as the sorbitol–polyol pathway. The condition is reversible, as shown. The rehabilitation in this dog took several months and involved diabetic regulation, weight loss, and physical therapy. Much of the latter was done using the owner's swimming pool. The dog returned to normal neurologic function.

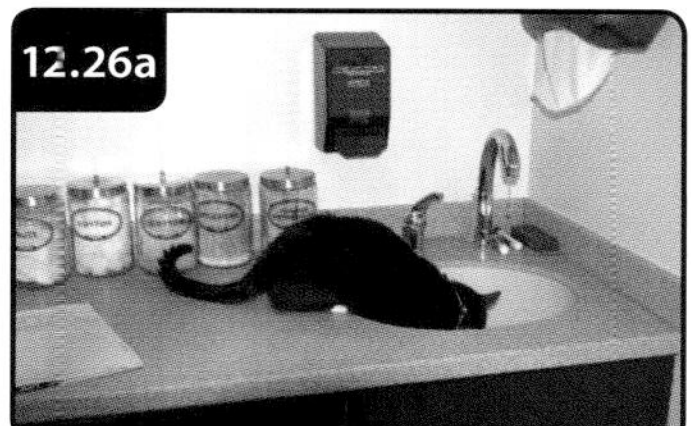

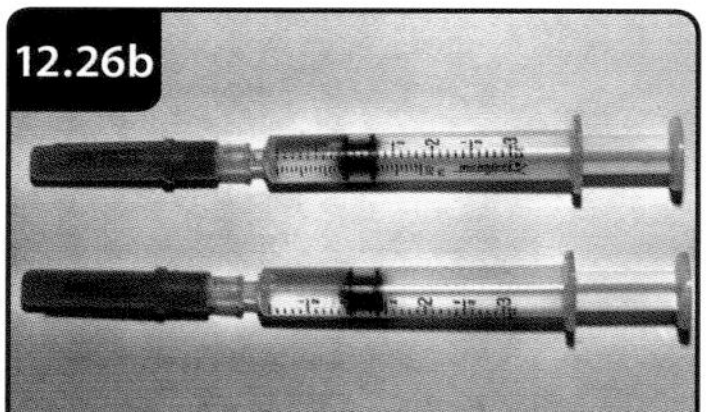

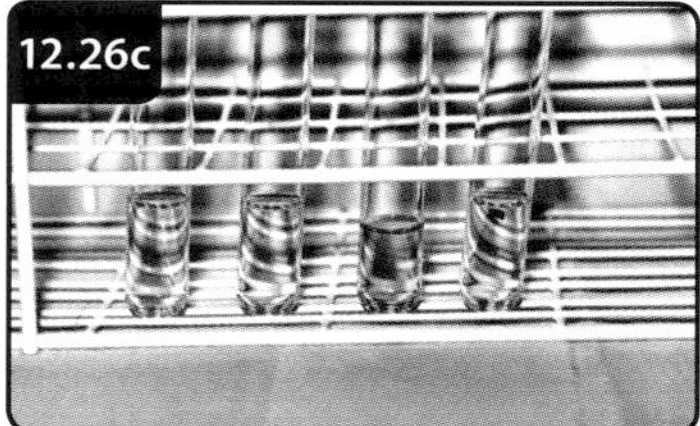

12.26a–c. Diabetes insipidus (DI). This condition is due to an antidiuretic hormone (ADH) deficiency (pituitary DI) or to resistance of the distal nephron to the actions of ADH. Extreme polydipsia (Figure 12.26a) and polyuria (PD-PU) are the hallmark clinical signs, which are due to a water diuresis state because of the absence or ineffectiveness of ADH. The polydipsia will exceed 100 ml/kg/day. The medical work up will rule out the majority of the causes of PD and PU. The water deprivation test distinguishes DI from psychogenic PD (PPD); the patient with PPD will show an ability to concentrate its urine after several hours of water deprivation. Figure 12.26b shows the baseline urine sample and the one taken after water deprivation, showing the dilute urine on the bottom at baseline and the more concentrated sample on top after the water deprivation test compatible with PPD. The dog with DI will be unable to concentrate its urine with water deprivation. The ADH challenge test will differentiate pituitary DI from nephrogenic DI where the pituitary patient will be able to concentrate its urine within 1–2 hours after it receives ADH, as shown in the successive urine samples in Figure 12.26c, whereas the nephrogenic patient will not show such a response. Sometimes, a gradual water withdrawal over 12–24 hours is necessary to help restore the renal counter-current multiplier mechanism in order to allow for urine concentrating ability.

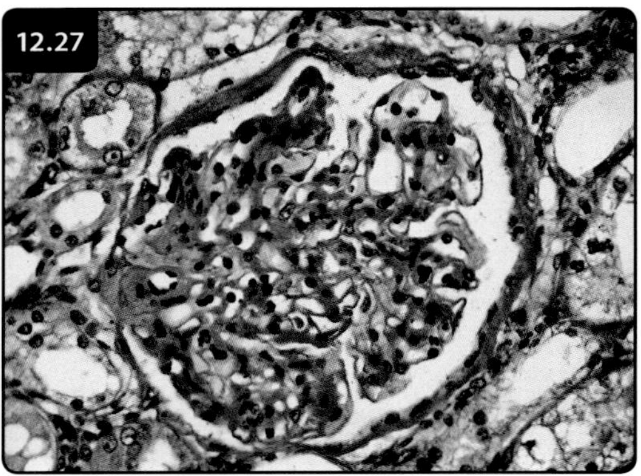

12.27. Diabetic glomerulopathy. Although dogs and cats do not suffer from as many diabetic '-opathies' as humans, they do acquire some of them. Glomerulopathy is one such disorder that can have progressive and devastating effects on the animal if it progresses to advanced kidney injury. One form of diabetic kidney disease is glomerulosclerosis, which is shown in Figure 12.27. Such a lesion would clinically appear as one characterized by albuminuria, proteinuria, systemic and glomerular hypertension, and eventually tubular dysfunction. The prognosis is guarded to grave with advanced disease.

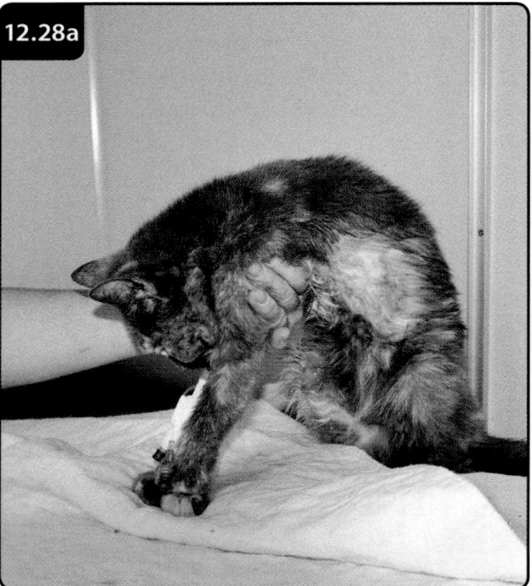

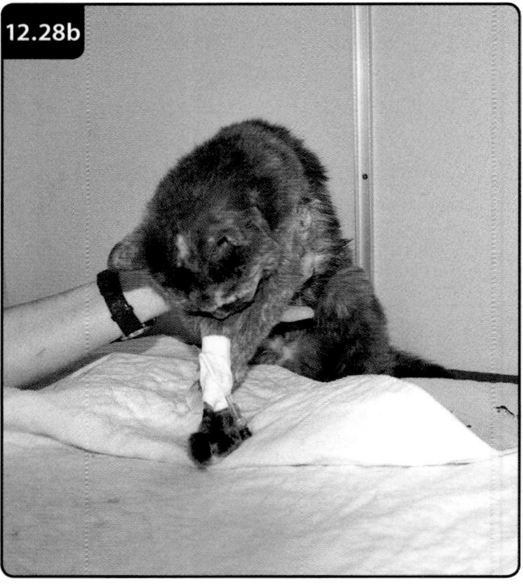

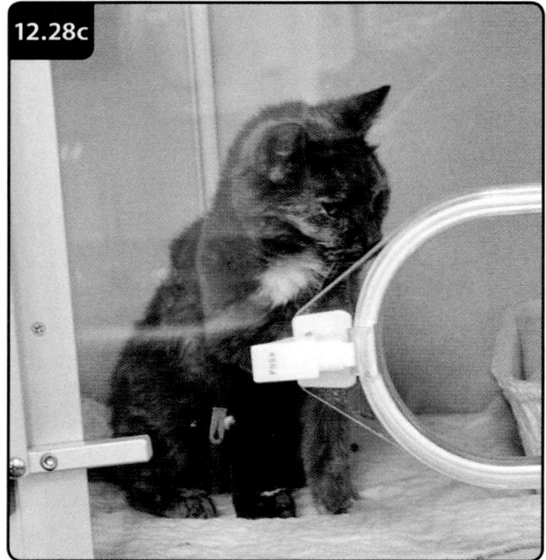

12.28a–c. Hypokalemia with hyperthyroidism in a cat. Although hypokalemia in the cat is commonly seen in diabetes, hyperaldosteronism, and chronic kidney disease, it might also occur in other debilitating diseases characterized by polydipsia and polyuria, as was shown in this hyperthyroid cat. Treatment with potassium chloride administered over a 24-hour period brought about improved muscular function, as seen in the three images. The cat continued to improve after euthyroid function was restored.

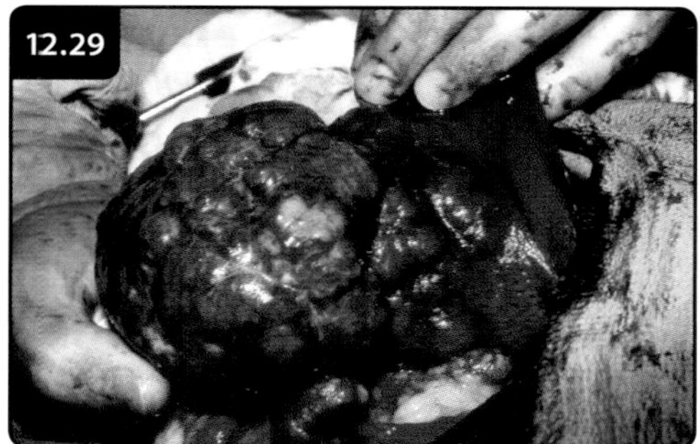

12.29. Paraneoplastic hypoglycemia. Hypoglycemia in the adult dog can be caused by several different disorders including insulinoma, septic shock, adrenocortical insufficiency, xylitol intoxication, chronic liver disease, and paraneoplastic disease. The hepatoma in Figure 12.29 was the sole cause of the dog's hypoglycemia, which was as low as 34 mg/dl (1.89 mmol/l). The hypoglycemia disappeared after tumor resection. Several other tumors can do the same because of the production of insulin-like growth factor-2.

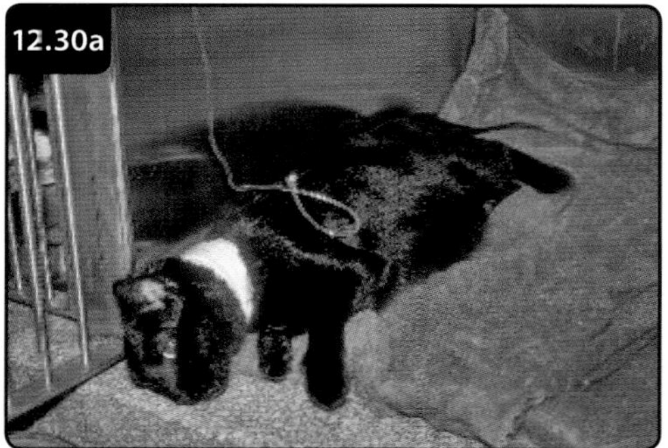

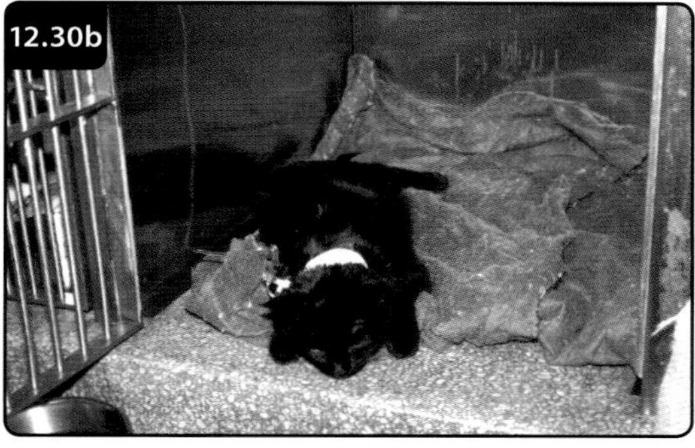

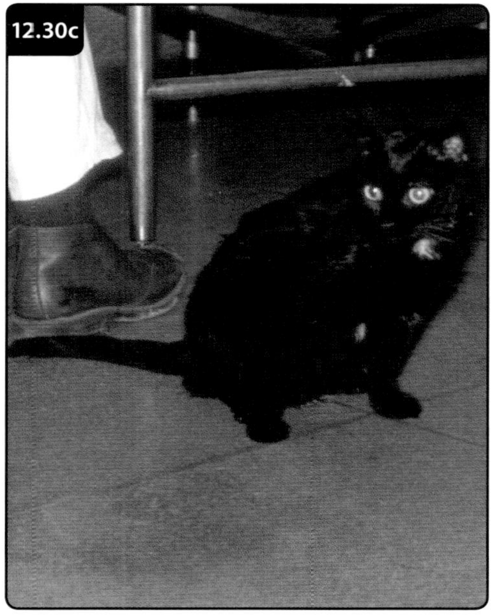

12.30a–c. Diabetic hyperosmolar nonketotic syndrome. This is one of the emergency presentations of the decompensated diabetic dog and cat. The condition results from a diminished amount of insulin necessary for glucose transport in the peripheral tissues, but enough insulin to enter the portal vein and be transported to the liver, where it will deter ketogenesis. The extreme hyperglycemia results from poor utilization, marked dehydration, and impaired glycosuria associated with renal dysfunction, thus allowing the blood glucose level to exceed 700 mg/dl (38.9 mmol/l). The resulting plasma hyperosmolality will cause osmotic disequilibrium in the brain and various neurologic signs, especially stupor and coma. Treatment calls for a gradual lowering of the blood glucose concentration, which should not exceed a rate of decline of 75–100 mg/dl [4.16–5.55 mmol/l]/hour. Figures 12.30a, b illustrate the comatose state this cat had at the time of admission, and Figure 12.30c shows the return to normal neurologic function by day 3 of hospitalization.

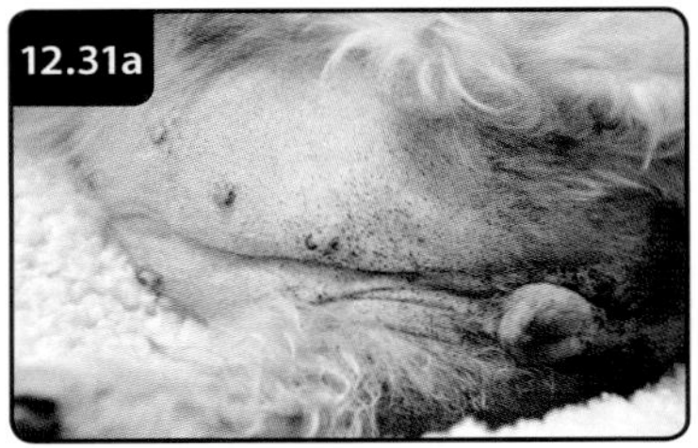
12.31a

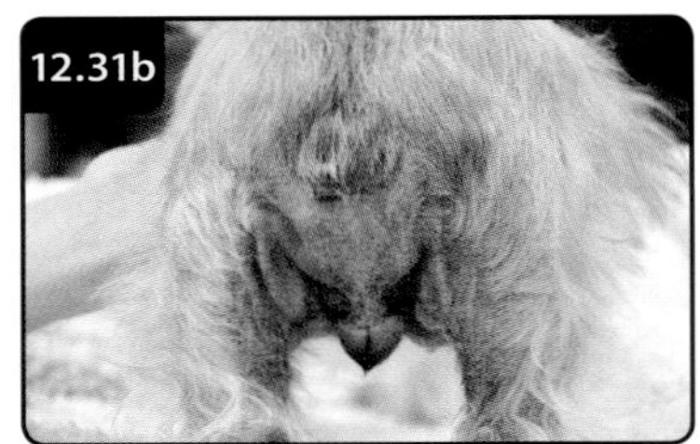
12.31b

12.31a, b. Hyperestrinism in a dog. This condition is commonly caused by cystic ovaries, but it is also caused by ovarian granulosa cell tumors in the female and testicular tumors in the male. It can also occur through contact with the owner's estrogen cream or prescribed estrogens. The clinical features are clearly shown in Figures 12.31a, b, including vulvar edema, skin hyperpigmentation, caudal and ventral abdominal alopecia, and slight nipple enlargement. Successful treatment depends on removing the source of estrogens.

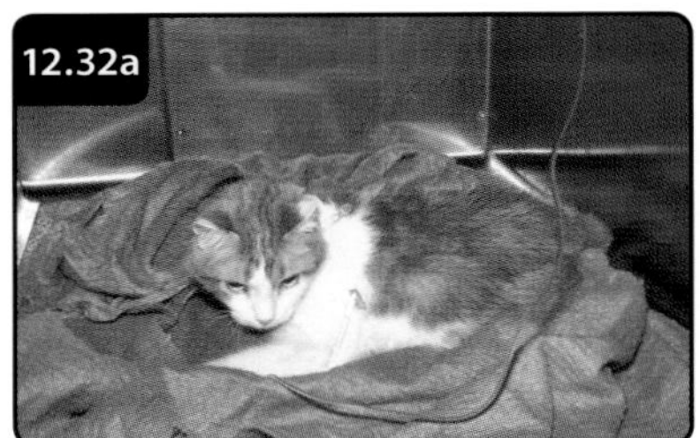
12.32a

12.32a–c. Insulin-induced hypoglycemic seizure. Hypoglycemic episodes usually have two components. This first is dominated by stimulation of the sympathetic nervous system and is characterized as excitatory, vocalization, and sometimes random scurrying. The epinephrine response is the body's attempt to counteract the hypoglycemia by attempting to raise the blood glucose level via glycogenolysis and gluconeogenesis. The second component is encephalopathic and is characterized with dementia progressing to overt seizure activity. The images show a diabetic cat experiencing a hypoglycemic seizure. Figure 12.32a shows the cat in a preictal phase of seizure, with a startled facial expression that is immediately followed by a grand mal component (Figures 12.32b, c) and then the motionless postictal phase of its epileptic seizure (not shown). The hypoglycemia was treated with an intravenous bolus of 50% dextrose at 1.0 ml/kg body weight, and the insulin dose was subsequently decreased.

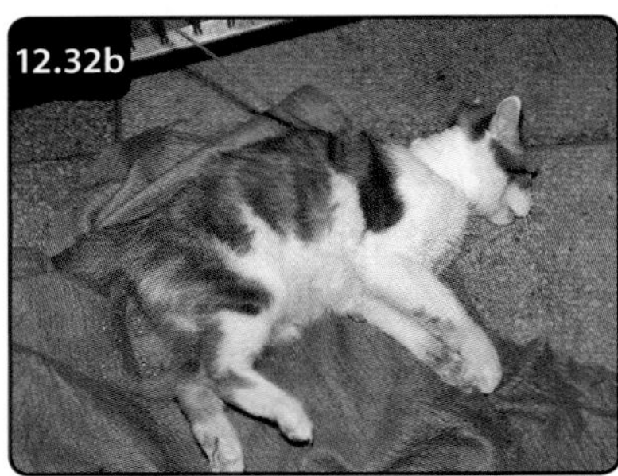
12.32b

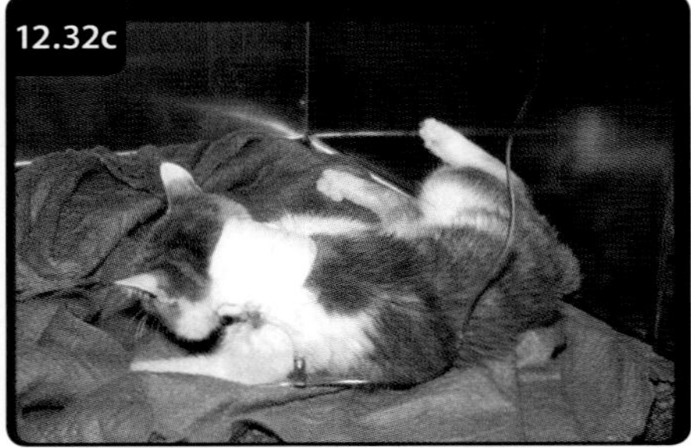
12.32c

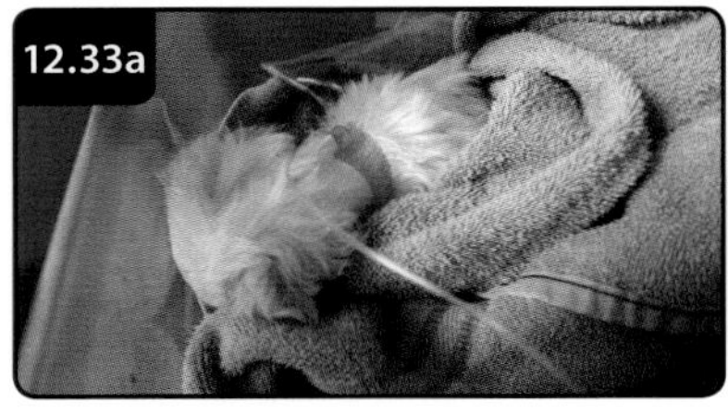
12.33a

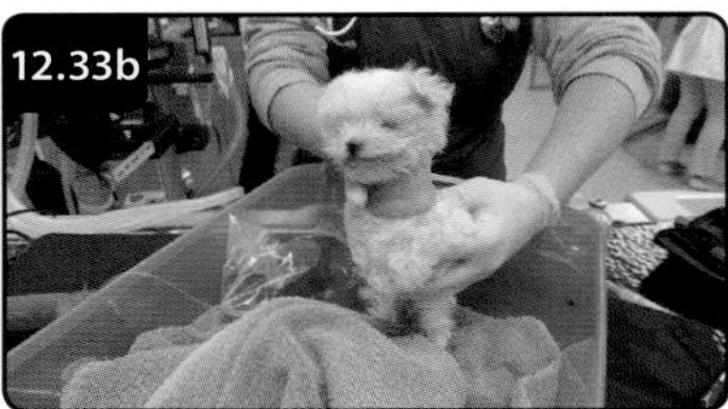
12.33b

12.33a, b. Pediatric hypoglycemia. This Maltese puppy presented with hypoglycemic stupor (Figure 12.33a). The puppy had not eaten in 24 hours and it had a hookworm infestation. Very young animals are particularly predisposed to hypoglycemia because of their limited ability to counteract it through adequate glycogenolysis and gluconeogenesis. Treatment entails providing glucose and treating any underlying condition that has predisposed the patient to hypoglycemia, as was done in this puppy (Figure 12.33b).

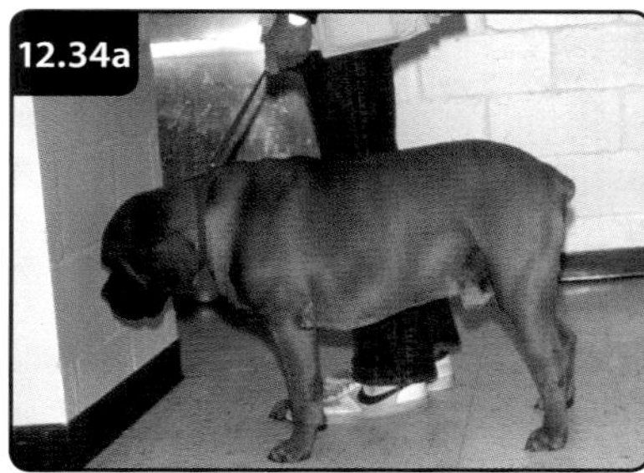
12.34a

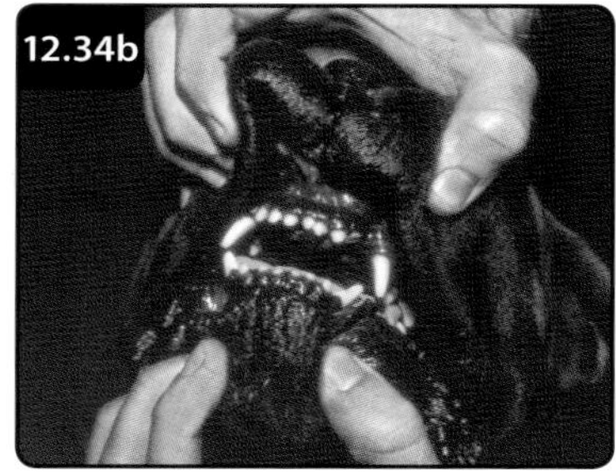
12.34b

12.34a, b. Hypothyroidism and acromegaly in a Boxer dog. These images show a Boxer dog that was diagnosed as having hypothyroidism. Its physical features were found to be similar to those of a Bull Mastiff. The widened interdental spaces were further suggestive of acromegaly (Figure 12.34b). The insulin-like growth factor-1 serum level was subsequently found to be elevated, thus adding further evidence to its acromegalic-like condition. The increased growth hormone (GH) release in hypothyroid dogs may be the result of the absence of a response element for thyroid hormone within the canine pituitary GH gene and alterations in suprapituitary regulation.

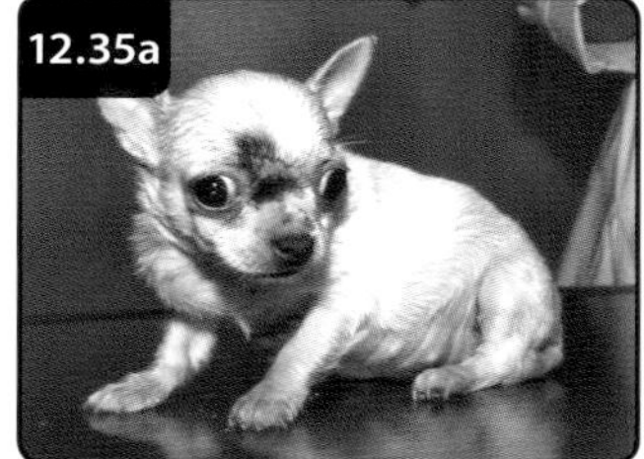
12.35a

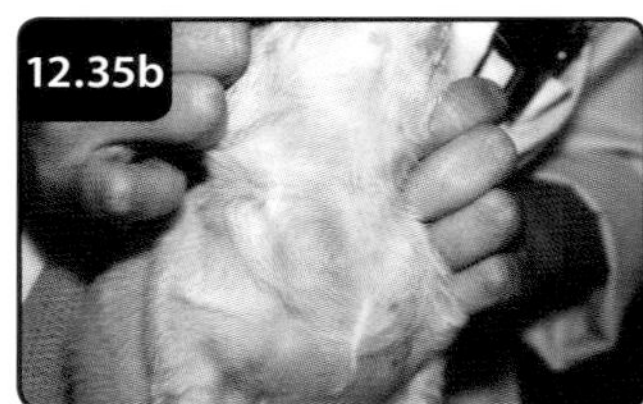
12.35b

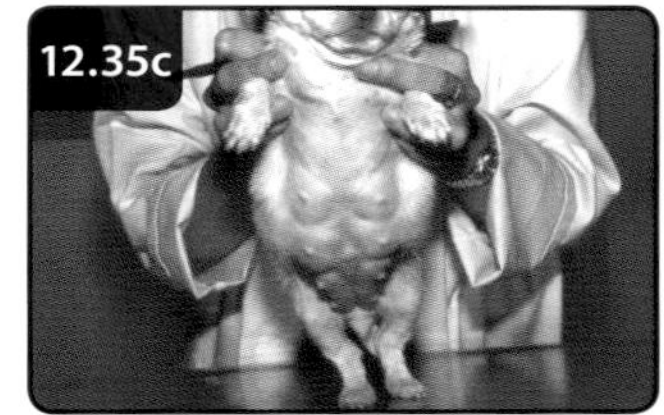
12.35c

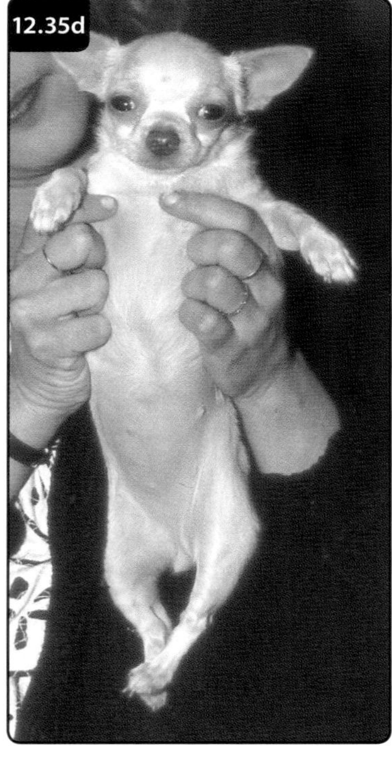
12.35d

12.35a–d. Hypothyroidism from dietary iodine deficiency. This young Chihuahua was referred for lethargy, stunted development, and noticeable gynecomastia. The owner had been giving the dog a home-cooked diet that was subsequently evaluated and found to be deficient in iodine. The owner had been applying gentian violet to the dog's head following some kind of self-imposed home treatment. The physical examination findings showed a mentally dull dog (Figure 12.35a) and a pathetic facial expression typical of severe hypothyroidism. In addition, she had stunted growth and palpable bilateral cervical masses that were actually large goiters (Figure 12.35b), and gynecomastia (Figure 12.35c). The goiters resulted from the thyroid gland's inability to produce and secrete thyroxine and the hormone deficiency stimulated the pituitary to secrete excess thyroid-stimulating hormone (TSH). This in turn resulted in excess thyroid colloid accumulation and distended follicles, which causes the glandular enlargement. The gynecomastia results from excess prolactin secretion as a result of the hypothyroid condition. Treatment consisted of providing a balanced canine diet. Figure 12.35d shows the dog markedly improved and acting normal at home. Iodine deficiency is rarely seen in western diets because most foods are supplemented with iodized salt. Seafood is also a common source of iodine. This dog showed similar signs to those that people from iodine deficient goiter belt areas of the USA used to show. The hypothyroid condition in toddlers leads to the development of cretinism and its attendant mental retardation. Perhaps the dog's mental dullness represented this change but actual retardation was impossible to assess; however, treatment with iodine was curative.

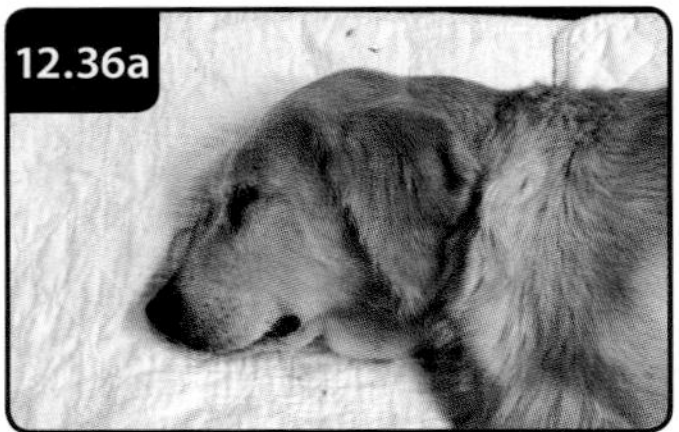

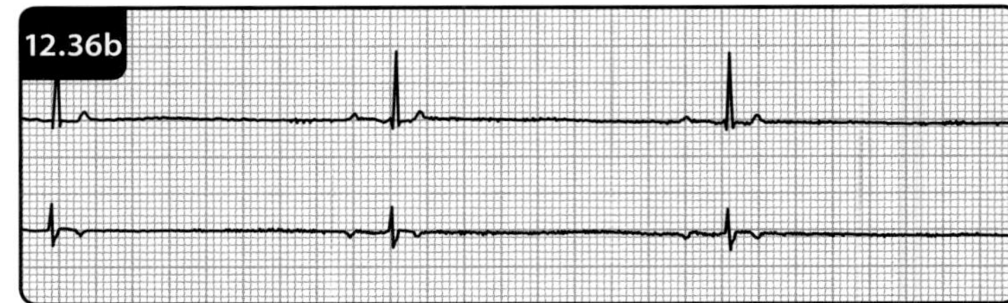

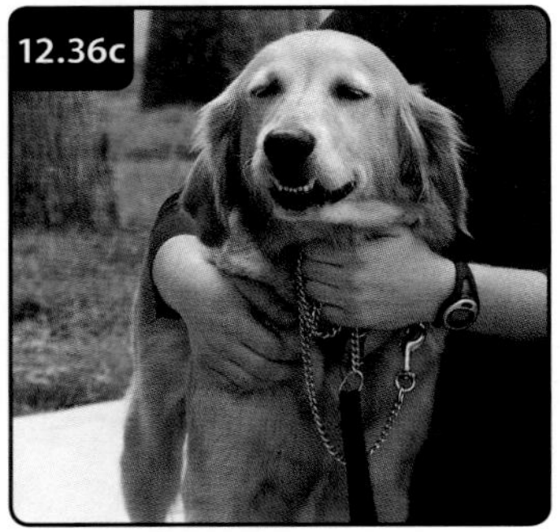

12.36a–c. Hypothyroid myxedema crisis in a dog with pyometra. This 5-year-old female Golden Retriever underwent surgery for a pyometra. Postoperatively, the dog would not regain consciousness from anesthesia, and she became very hypothermic at 98°F (36.7°C) (Figure 12.36a). Her heart rate decreased to 40 beats per minute and her ECG R wave complexes were noted to be abnormally short, measuring 0.5 mv (Figure 12.36b). Preoperatively, the dog's history had no major signs of hypothyroidism other than a vague sluggishness that the owners failed to have evaluated. Preoperative blood work showed a mild anemia (PCV = 38% [0.38 l/l]) and mild hypercholesterolemia (381 mg/dl [9.87 mmol/l]). Serum T4 was 0.34 ng/dl (4.38 pmol/l) (reference interval 1.45–3.5 [18.7–45.0]). Serum cortisol was normal at 4.0 µg/dl (110.5 nmol/l). L-thyroxine (levothyroxine) (0.02 mg/kg) was added to the postoperative treatment plan and the dog was remarkably improved by the next day (Figure 12.36c).

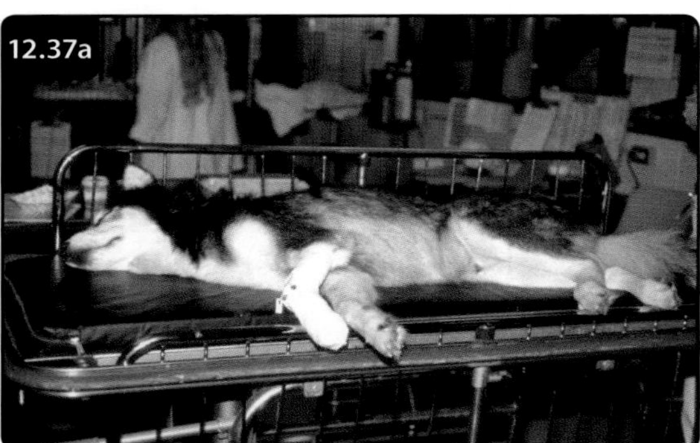

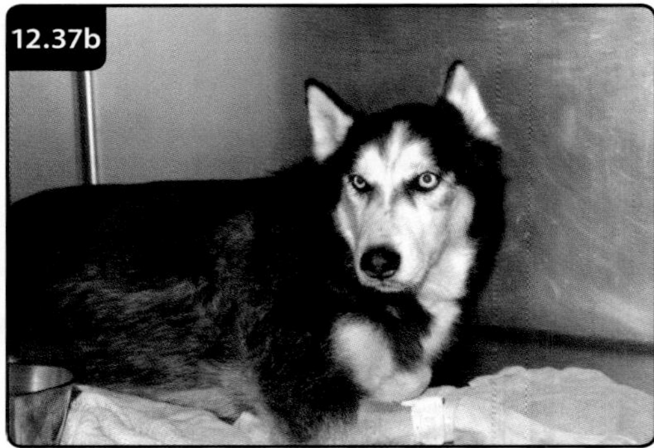

12.37a, b. Hypothyroid myxedema and hypothyroid neuropathy. This young male Malamute was referred to the neurology service for the primary complaint of progressive generalized weakness of 1 month's duration. Preanesthetic blood test results showed a mild anemia with the PCV at 32% (0.32 l/l) and an elevated serum cholesterol at 550 mg/dl (14.25 mmol/l). Spinal radiographs and cerebrospinal fluid evaluations were normal. The dog became hypothermic under anesthesia and would not recover despite discontinuation of the anesthetic (Figure 12.37a). The ECG R waves were of short amplitude. Hypothyroid myxedema was tentatively diagnosed and blood for a thyroid-stimulating hormone stimulation test was sent to the laboratory. In the meantime, the dog responded well to treatment consisting of L-thyroxine (levothyroxine), prednisolone, and slow warming over the next 18 hours. He recovered by the next day (12.37b) and his neurologic disorder disappeared over the next month with thyroid hormone replacement. The total thyroxine test results for both pre-and post-TSH stimulation were 0.5 µg/dl; reference low <1.0 (6.44 nmol/l; reference low <6.44).

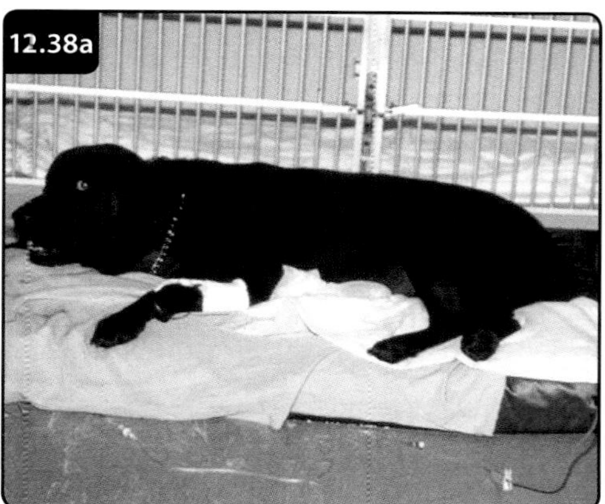

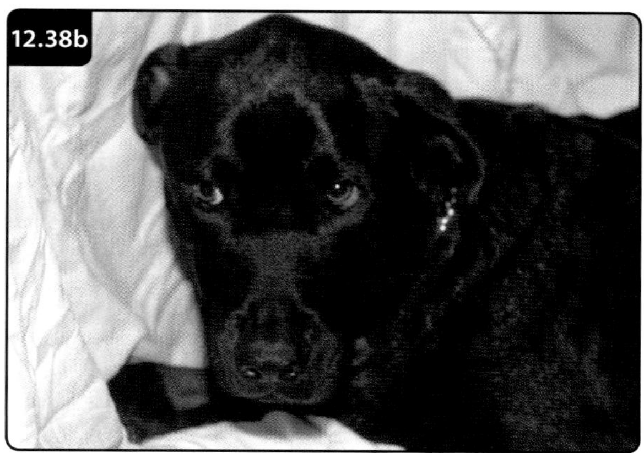

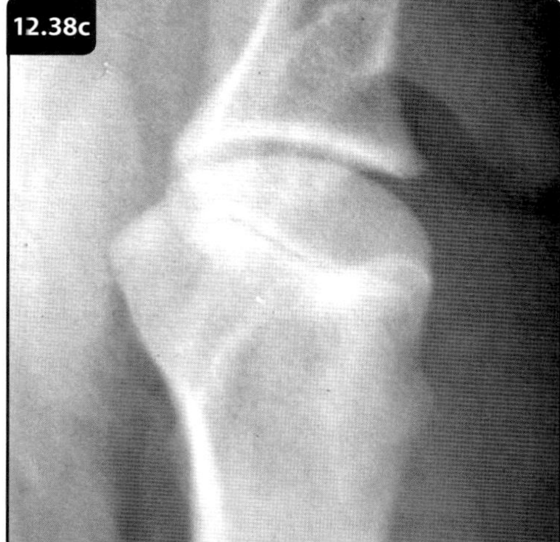

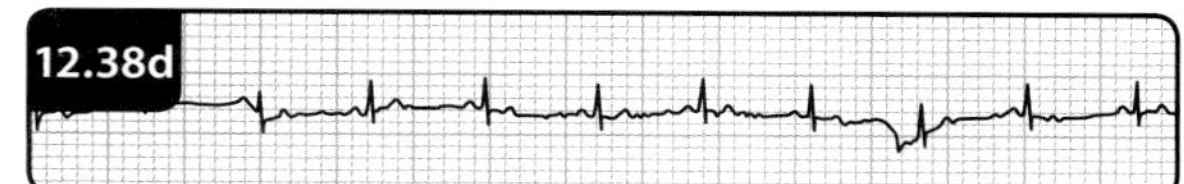

12.38a–d. Hypothyroid neuropathy in a dog. This 18-month-old Labrador Retriever was seen by the neurology clinic for the complaint of diffuse weakness and abnormal cranial nerve function (Figure 12.38a). He had nonlocalizing weakness and dysconjugate eye movements (Figure 12.38b). His signs were compatible with a diffuse neuropathy. Radiographs of his chest and shoulder showed unfused growth plates (Figure 12.38c) while his ECG showed small amplitude R waves (Figure 12.38d). The serum thyroxine concentration was abnormally low (exact value unavailable). The dog became normal after receiving thyroxine treatment.

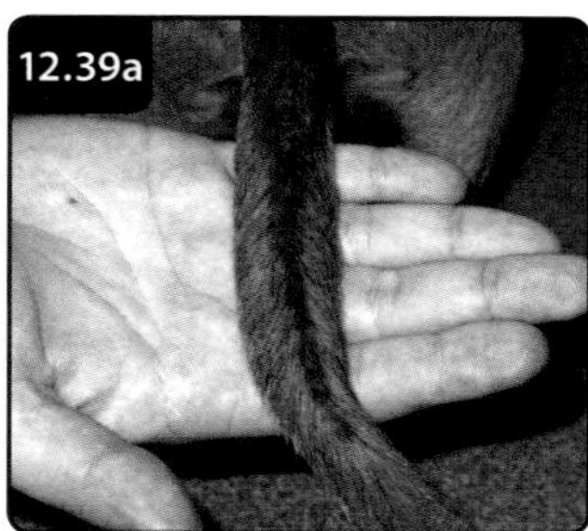

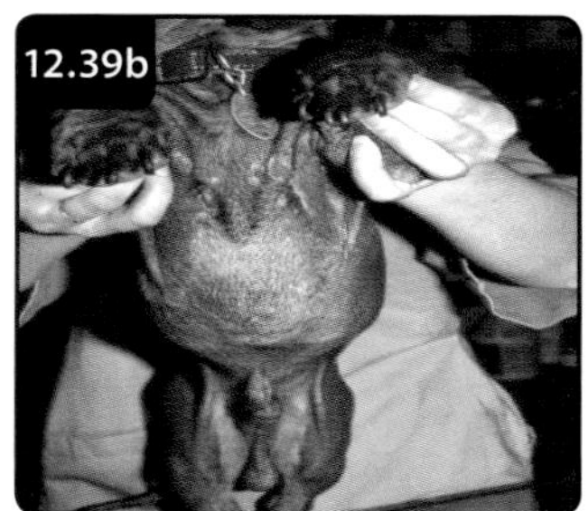

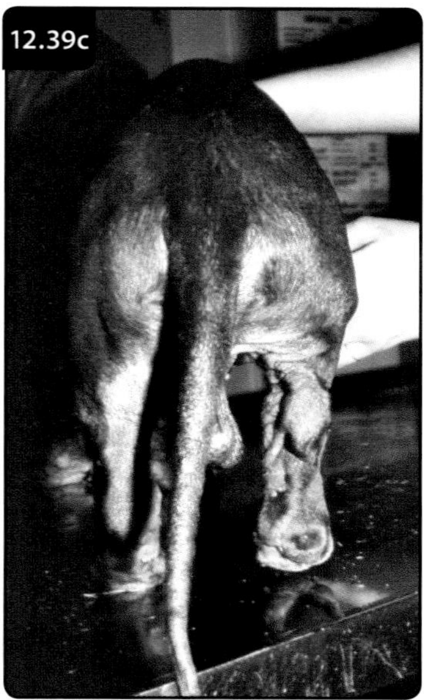

12.39a–c. Hypothyroidism dermatologic changes. There are several dermatologic abnormalities caused by hypothyroidism. This dog (Figure 12.39a) shows early alopecia and hyperpigmentation of its tail (rat tail). The dog in Figures 12.39b, c shows axillary 'acanthosis nigricans' and a more advanced 'rat tail' lesion. These changes do not affect every hypothyroid dog; however, they are reversible with thyroid replacement hormone treatment.

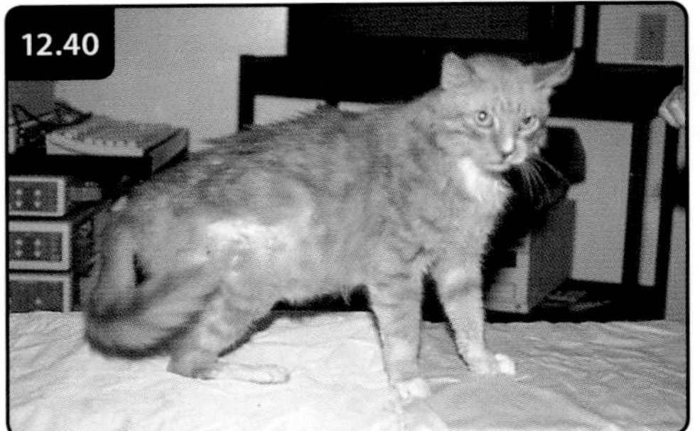

12.40. Diabetes mellitus and Cushing's syndrome in a cat. This cat is showing the plantar posture typical of diabetes mellitus, and alopecia and a distended abdomen caused by hypercortisolism. The diabetes was caused by the Cushing's disorder, which in turn was caused by long-term injectable glucocorticoid treatment. The latter was documented with the history and an unresponsive ACTH stimulation test. The diabetes required insulin treatment for several weeks, but it and the Cushing's features eventually disappeared after the effects of the glucocorticoid drug dissipated, which required about 6 weeks.

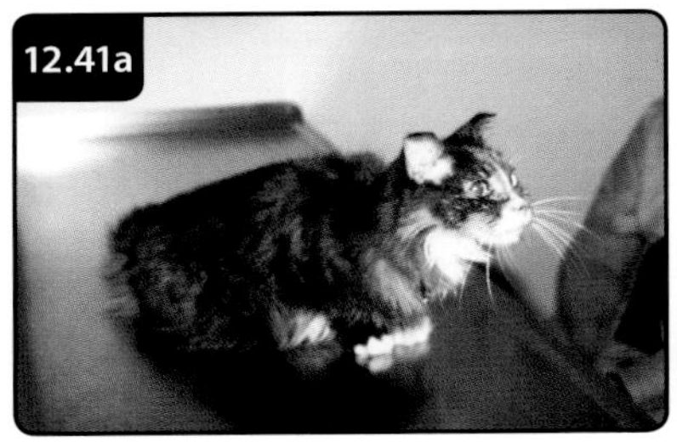

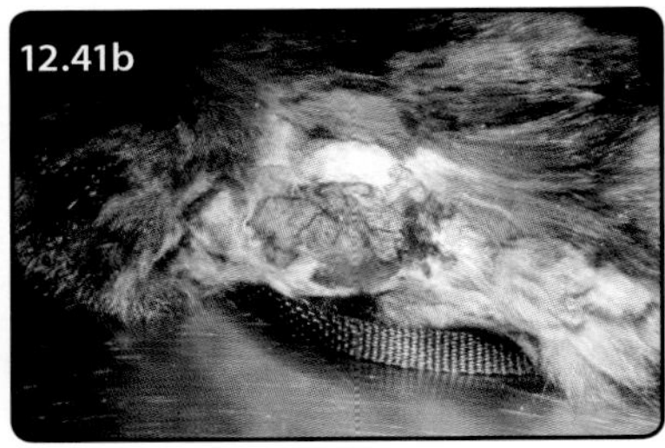

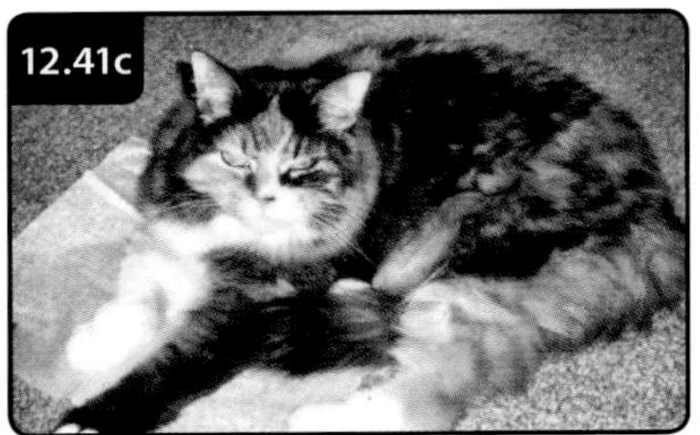

12.41a–c. Iatrogenic Cushing's disease in a cat. This domestic longhair cat became overtly cushingoid after it received a large dose of triamcinolone. Her examination showed hair coat thinning, very friable skin, ear tip folding, and palpable hepatomegaly (Figures 12.41a, b). Liver enzymes were elevated and fine needle aspiration biopsy of the liver showed diffuse vacuolization that stained positive for glycogen, similar to the Cushing's dog. The cat was hyperglycemic but not a clinical diabetic. The cat improved as the effects of the glucocorticoid dissipated, and she returned to normal after several months (Figure 12.41c).

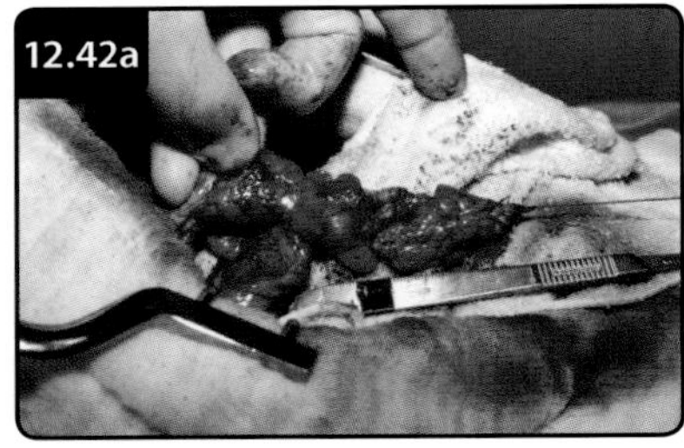

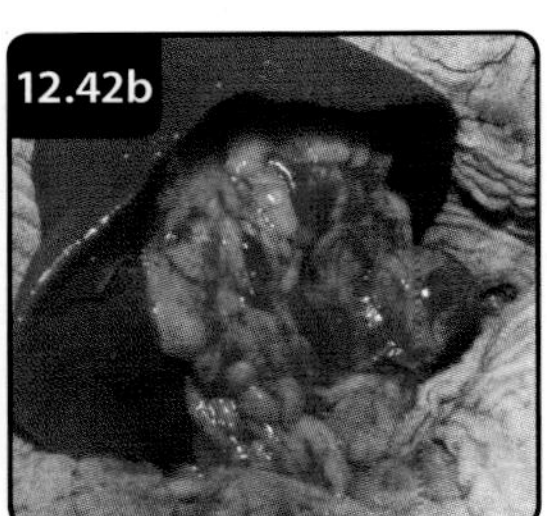

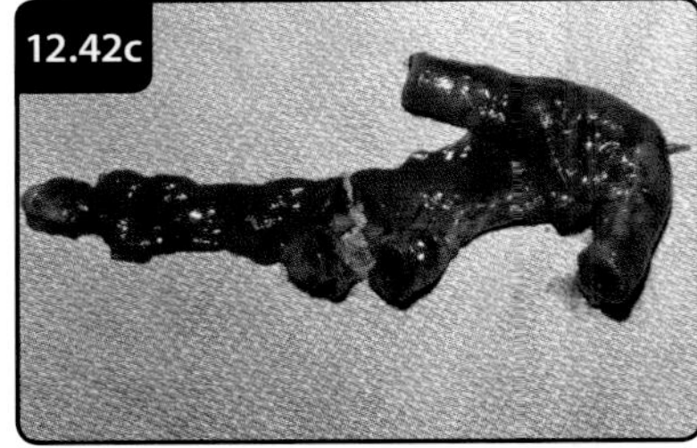

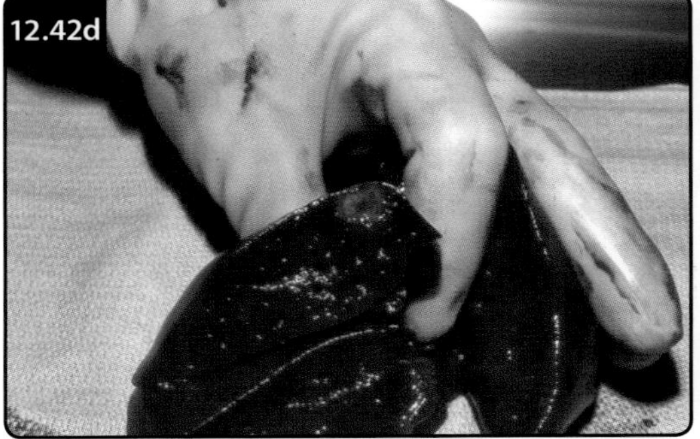

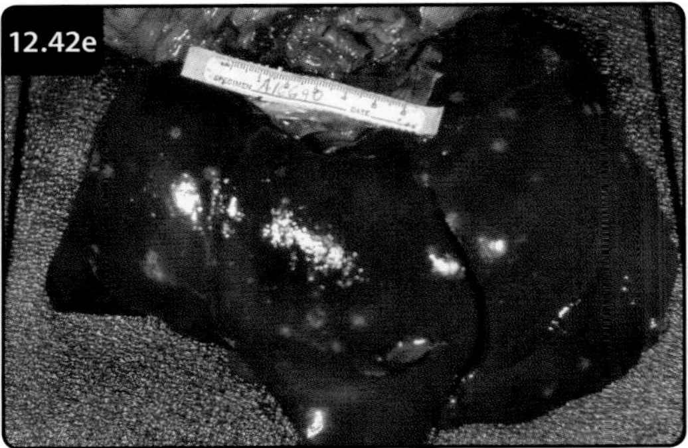

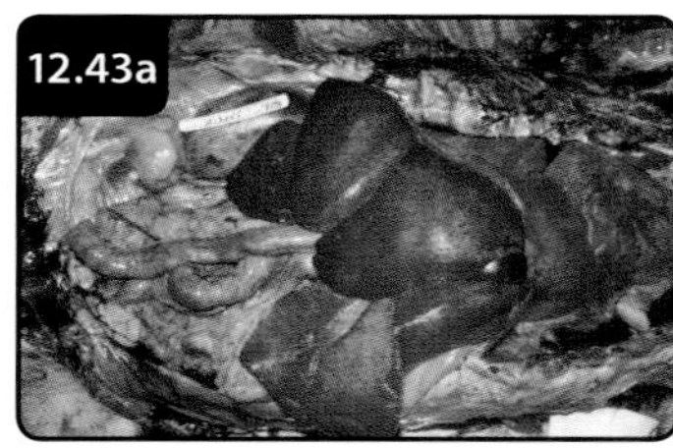

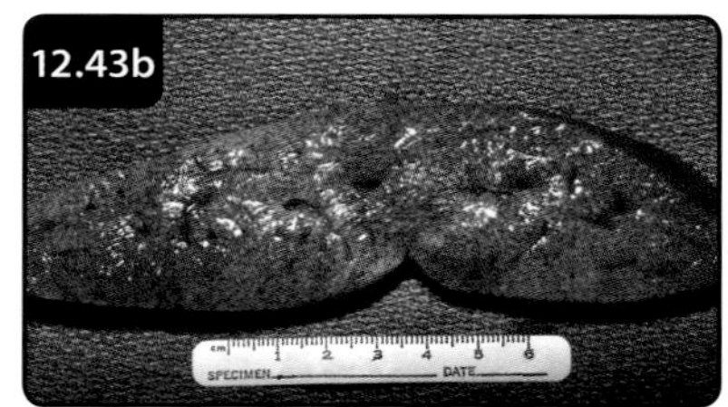

12.43a, b. Fatal hepatic lipidosis in the diabetic dog. Most cases of hepatic lipidosis in the diabetic dog are taken rather nonchalantly because of the reversibility of this condition with treatment for the primary disease. In rare cases, and for unknown reasons, the lipidosis becomes progressive and overwhelming and causes the dog to go into liver failure. The necropsy of this dog was the end result of an intact female dog that went into diestrus, which caused marked insulin resistance and extreme hepatic lipidosis. The blood glucose and ketoacidosis eventually came under control, but the liver disease progressed to acute hepatic failure. Figures 12.43a, b show gross hepatomegaly and the diffuse fatty infiltrate. Other examples of this condition are discussed in Chapter 10 (Liver disorders).

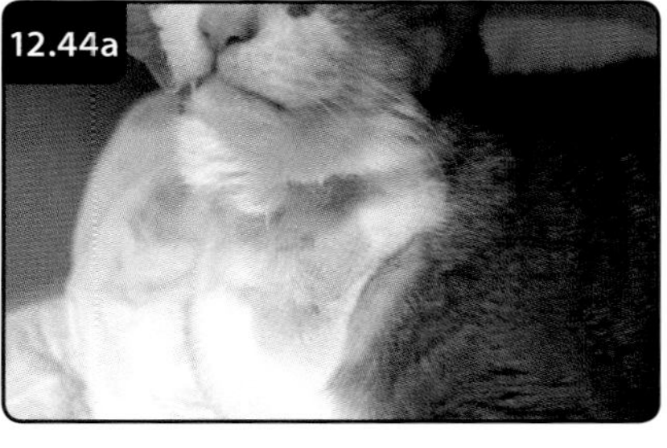

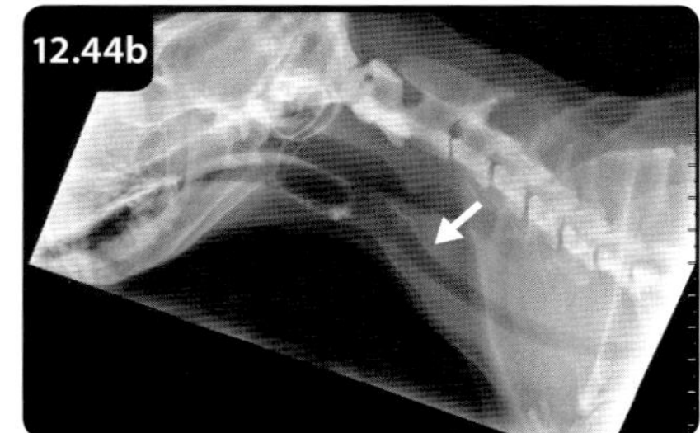

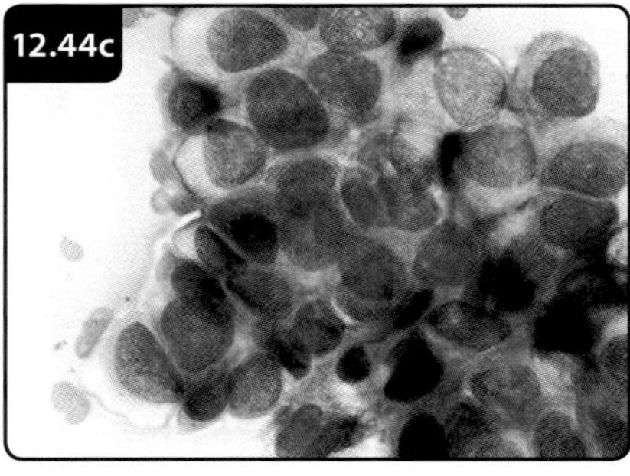

12.44a–c. Malignant hyperthyroidism in a cat. Most cases of hyperthyroidism in the cat (98%) are due to adenomatous hyperplasia and there is a favorable prognosis with treatment in most cases. The cat shown in Figure 12.44a had mild clinical hyperthyroidism and a readily palpable mass in its neck that felt more extensive than the typical goiter. The lateral radiograph (Figure 12.44b) shows a space-occupying mass effect in the area caudal to the larynx (arrow), and the cytology sample (Figure 12.44c), taken by fine needle aspiration of the enlarged thyroid gland, shows cells with atypia compatible with features of a carcinoma. Radioisotope treatment can be used to treat this condition, but isolation of the patient would be very long because of the large dose of radiation required. Palliative treatment with methimazole was done in this patient.

12.42a–e. Insulinoma in the dog. Beta cell carcinoma (insulinoma) most commonly occurs in middle-aged to older dogs. The clinical signs are related to the neurologic signs of hypoglycemia (neuroglycopenia). Most of these tumors are located in the pancreas (Figure 12.42a) but some can occur in the parapancreatic region, as shown in Figure 12.42b, with the tumor lying in the mesentery beside the pancreas. These tumors have a high rate of metastasis, with the liver being the primary site of malignant spread. Figure 12.42c shows regrowth of the insulinoma in a dog that had a beta cell tumor resected from its pancreas 1 year previously. This time the dog again had neuroglycopenia, which proved to be refractory to medical treatment using mainly diazoxide and prednisone. At necropsy the dog had focal metastasis to the liver (Figure 12.42d). The infiltration of the tumor is seen on cut section. The liver specimen in Figure 12.42e is from a dog that had been diagnosed with insulinoma approximately 6 months previously. Multiple metastases are present as white deposits throughout the liver.

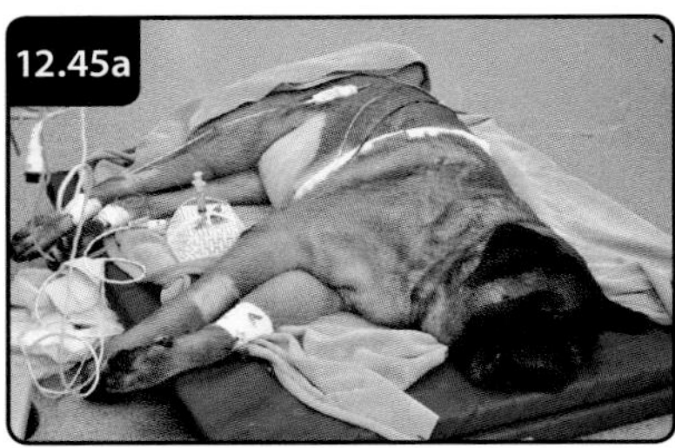

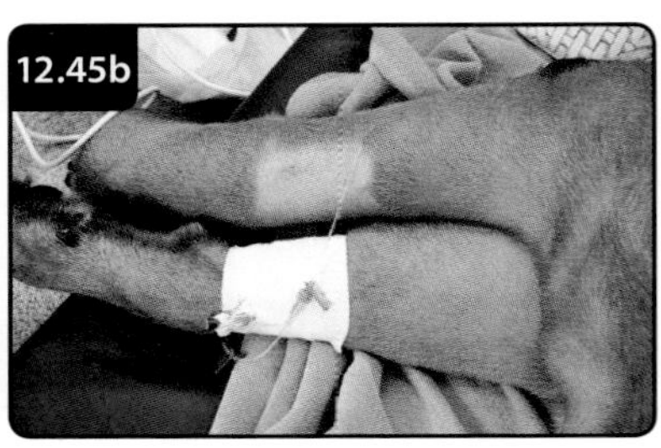

12.45a, b. Intravenous fluid intolerance in a hypothyroid myxedema dog. This dog's swollen forelimbs occurred because of its fluid intolerance during a myxedema crisis. Clinically, the dog's skin had a water-soaked sponge texture. Patients with this condition are characteristically in a water excess state from the myxedema and they rapidly show signs of overload during treatment. The water excess condition can also cause hyponatremia. Treatment at this point calls for water restriction while the dog continues to receive its thyroxine replacement.

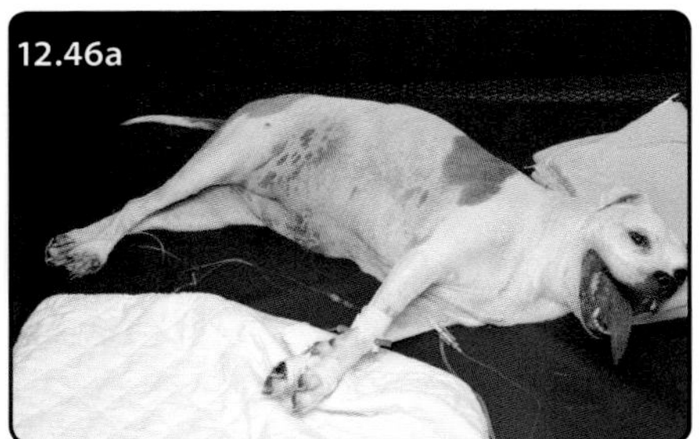

12.46a–c. Invasive pheochromocytoma. This Labrador Retriever is laterally recumbent because of lumbar spinal cord spread of a malignant pheochromocytoma. Approximately 50% of these tumors are malignant and they can invade nearby structures such as the posterior vena cava and the spinal cord. This is why an abdominal ultrasound examination is sometimes requested as part of the neurologic work up. Figure 12.46a shows a dog with spinal invasion, which is further elaborated on the MR images, which show actual spinal cord infiltration by the tumor (Figures 12.46b, c, arrows). The prognosis is grave because this disorder is not amenable to surgical correction.

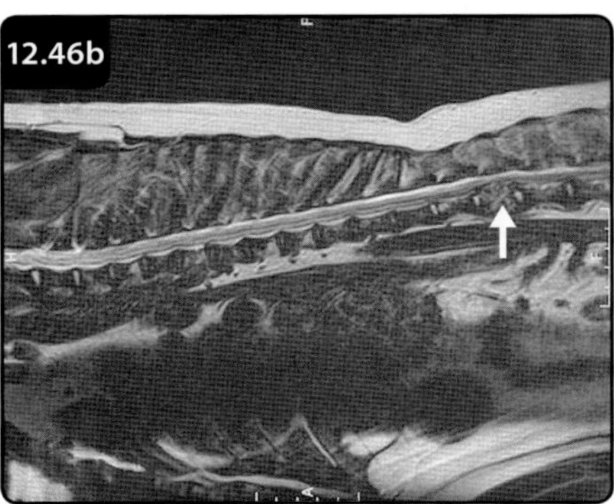

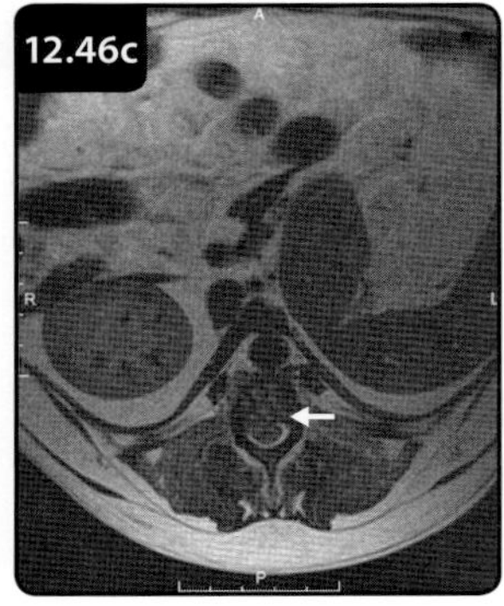

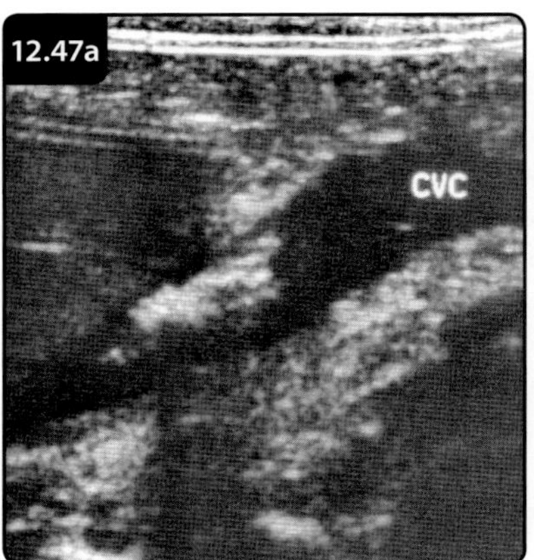

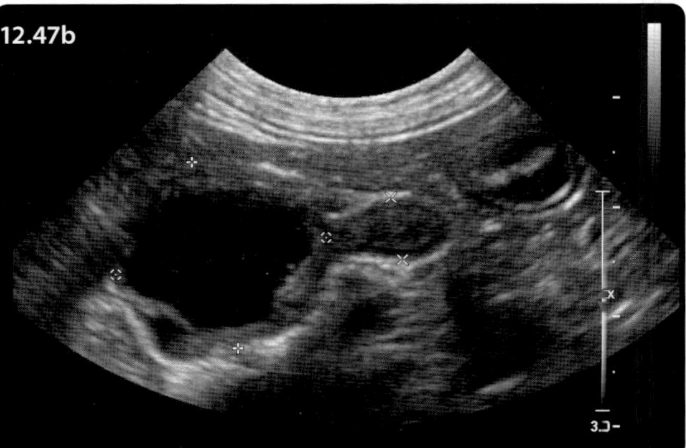

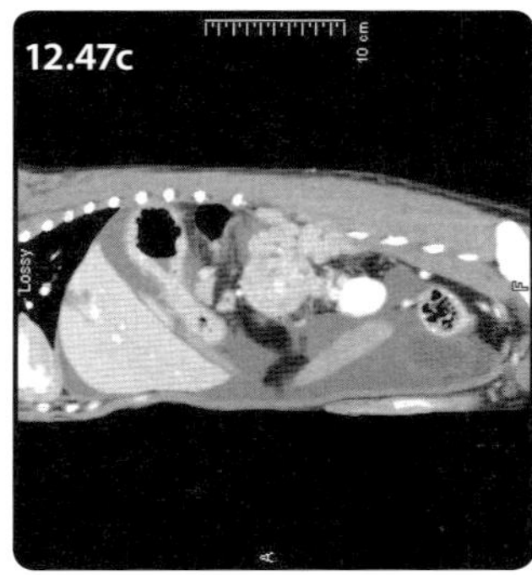

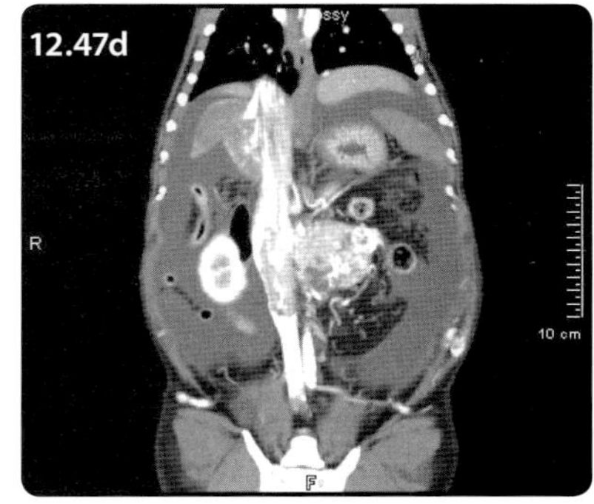

12.47a–d. Adrenal tumor imaging. Figure 12.47a is an abdominal ultrasonographic view of a malignant adrenal tumor invading the caudal vena cava. Figure 12.47b depicts a marked polar expansion of an adrenal gland tumor. There is no way to distinguish the various types of adrenal tumors on ultrasound or abdominal CT evaluation. The two abdominal CT scans are of a different dog (Figures 12.47c, d) and show an adrenal tumor displacing the caudal vena cava. There is a filling defect in the caudal vena cava signifying tumor infiltrating that vessel. Today's veterinary surgical oncologist is able to successfully resect the entire tumor mass, including the vascular component, in some patients.

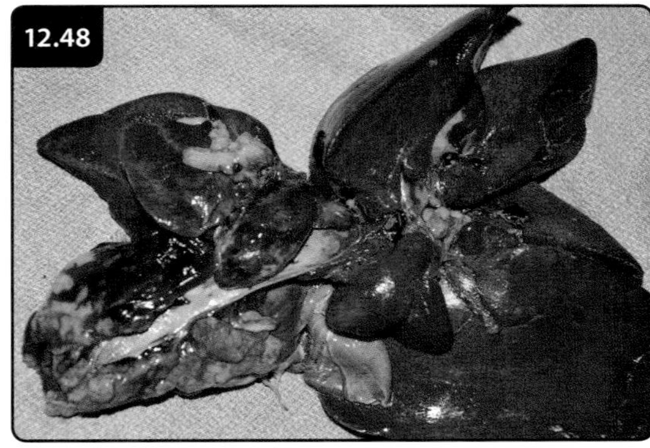

12.48. Postmortem specimen showing an adrenal tumor invading the posterior vena cava. This pathologic specimen from a different dog shows a large and invasive adrenal tumor. The definitive diagnosis on histopathology was pheochromocytoma.

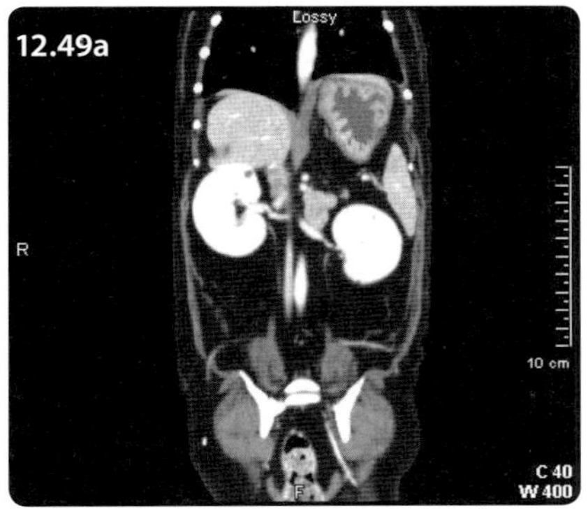

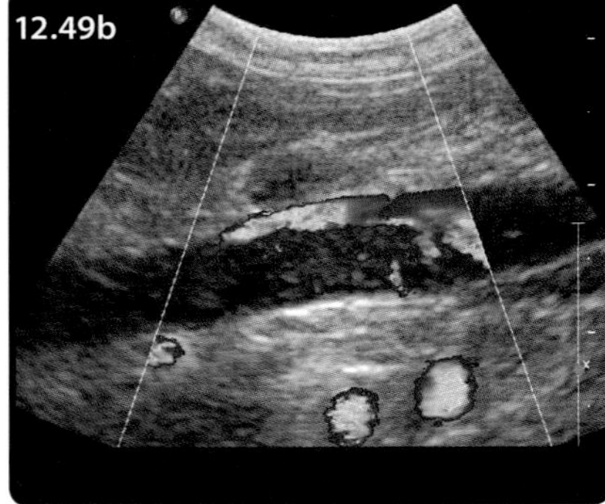

12.49a, b. Bilateral pheochromocytoma in a dog. The preoperative blood pressure in this dog peaked at 255 mmHg. The large bilateral masses on the CT image (Figure 12.49a) depict left- and right-sided pheochromocytomas. Note that the right-sided one is much larger than the left. Figure 12.49b is an abdominal color flow Doppler examination from the same dog showing the right-sided tumor invading the caudal vena cava. Both tumors were surgically resected, but the dog had ventricular fibrillation during surgery and died. Histopathology confirmed the diagnosis.

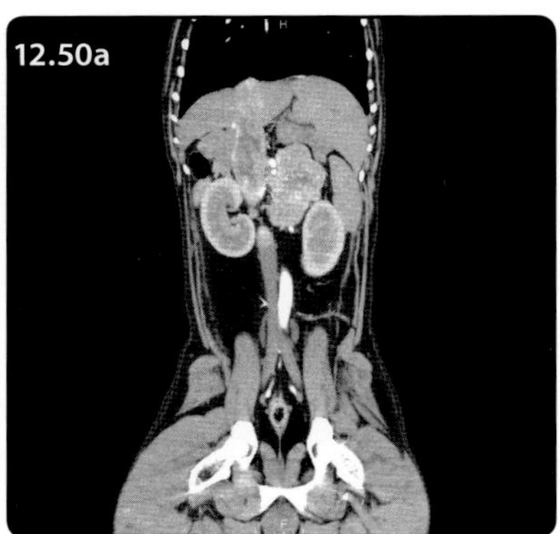

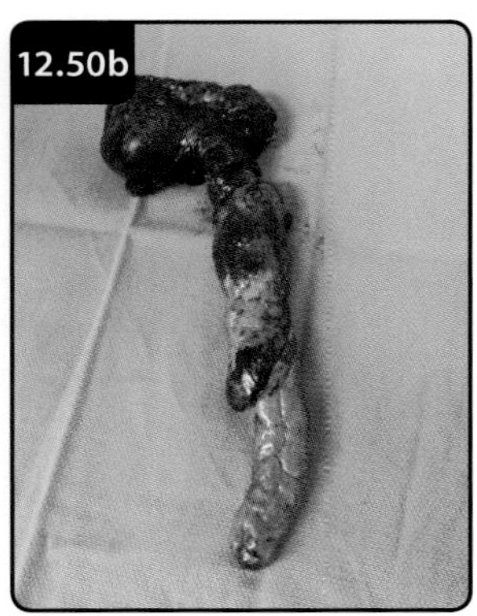

12.50a, b. Very large pheochromocytoma invading the vena cava. The abdominal CT scan shows a very large left-sided pheochromocytoma invading the caudal vena cava and extending cranially to the diaphragm. The tumor is shown with the segment that had invaded the caudal vena cava. (Courtesy Dr. S. Boston)

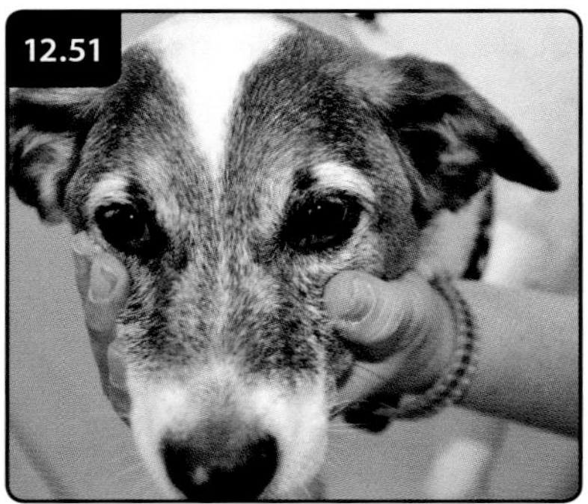

12.51. Hypertensive ocular hemorrhage associated with pheochromocytoma. This Jack Russel Terrier was evaluated for an acute onset of left-sided blindness caused by an acute ocular hemorrhage. Further evaluation found the dog to be very hypertensive, with the systolic blood pressure over 200 mmHg. Medical treatment consisted of oral phenoxybenzamine (an alpha adrenergic blocker), which gradually normalized the blood pressure.

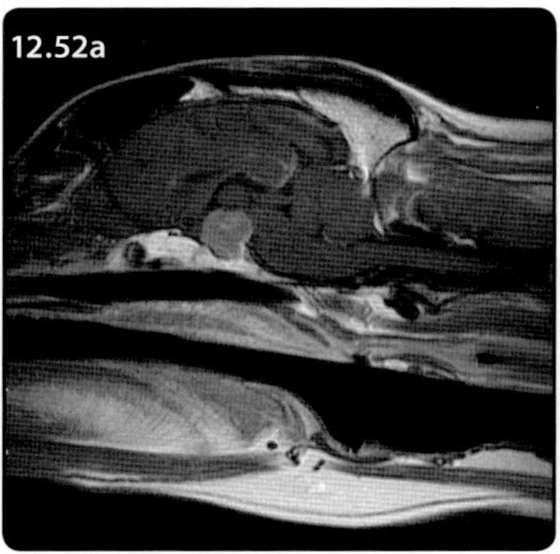

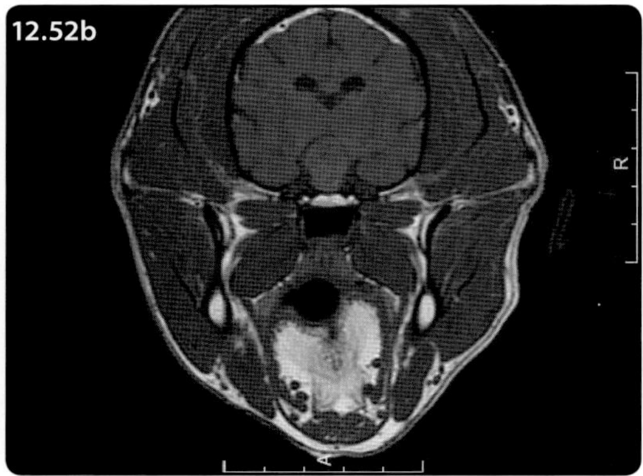

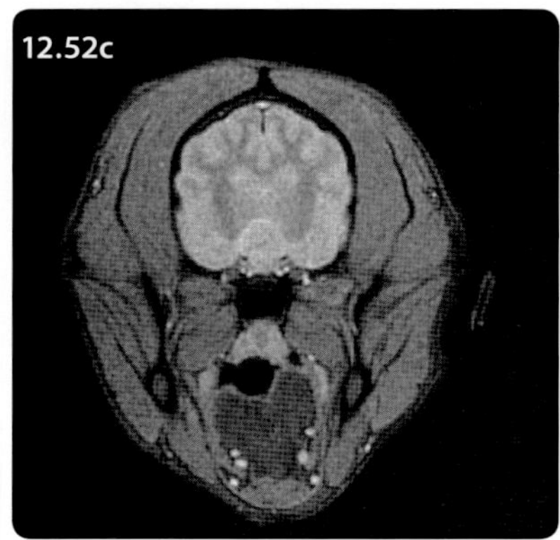

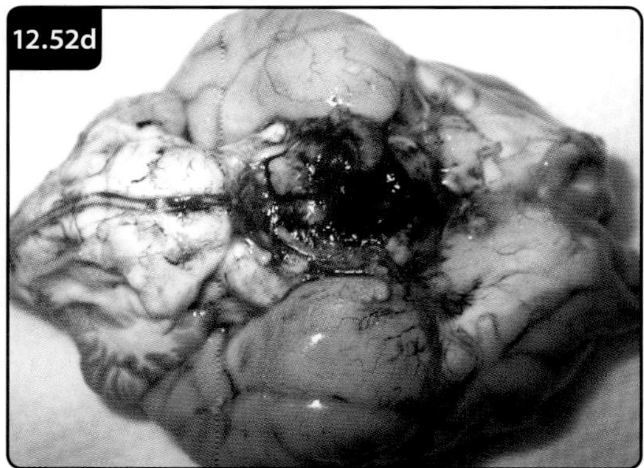

12.52a–e. Pituitary tumor on CT and at postmortem. Figures 12.52a–c are from a dog with Cushing's disease, showing a pituitary macroadenoma on the lateral and frontal views (with and without contrast enhancement). The postmortem images (Figures 12.52d, e) are from a different dog showing pituitary apoplexy, where the tumor is causing hemorrhage and sudden enlargement of the diencephalic mass, which can cause a previously normal acting dog to transition into one that has dementia and head pressing. Additional images demonstrating different perspectives can be found in Case 12.21.

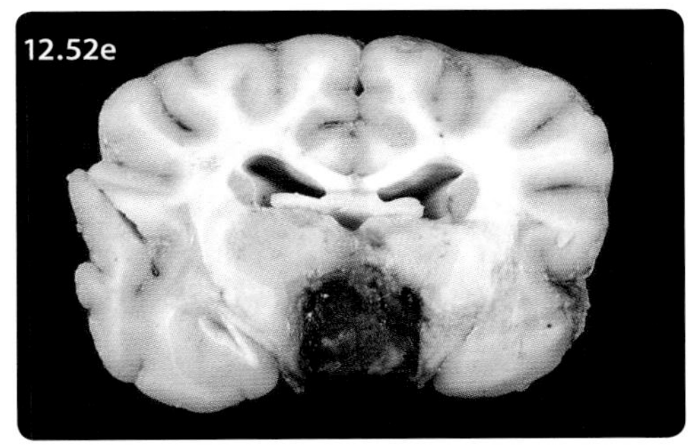
12.52e

12.53. Psychogenic polydipsia. This dog is obviously polydipsic (PD), and he would also be polyuric (PU) with hyposthenuria, thus calling for differentiation from diabetes insipidus after eliminating the other causes of PD and PU. In this case, a water deprivation test over 10 hours showed the urine SG increasing from 1.005 to 1.025, supporting the diagnosis of psychogenic PD. Treatment was then focused on treating the underlying compulsive–obsessive disorder with environmental modifications and concomitant administration of an anxiolytic drug, which worked to benefit this dog.

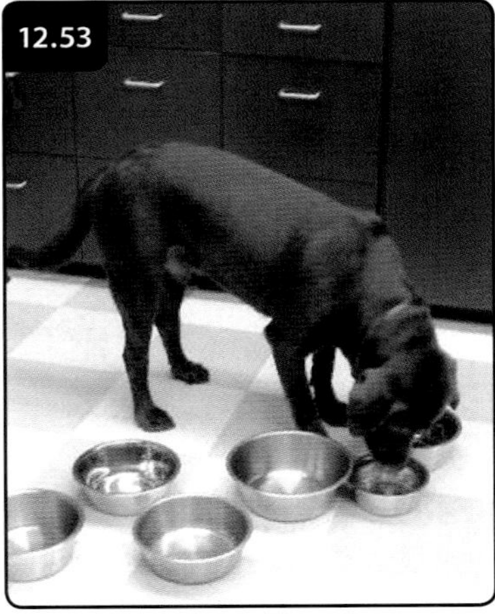
12.53

12.54a–c. Parathyroid adenoma. This ultrasound image (Figure 12.54a) shows a parathyroid adenoma that was discovered during evaluation of a dog for hypercalcemia and hypophosphatemia. Parathyroid adenoma is much more common than parathyroid adenocarcinoma, which therefore offers a favorable prognosis. Preferred treatment is surgical resection of the involved tissue, which often requires resecting the ipsilateral thyroid gland with the tumor (Figures 12.54b, c). Hypocalcemia is a potential complication for up to 72 hours postoperatively. In most cases, endogenous parathyroid hormone secretion resumes after several days. In rare situations, the endogenous resumption of normal parathyroid function might not occur for weeks or months, therefore requiring long-term calcium and or calcitriol supplementation.

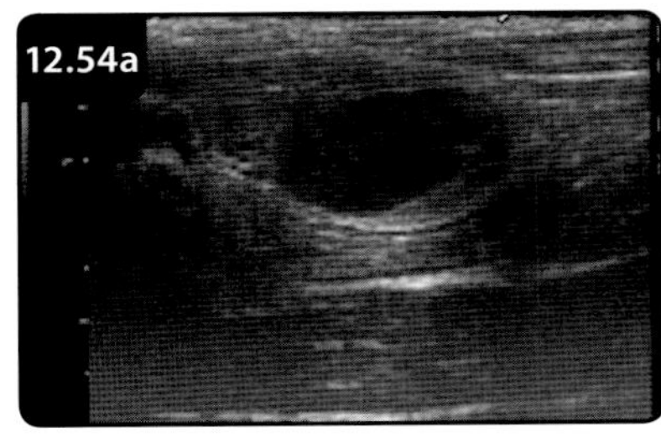
12.54a

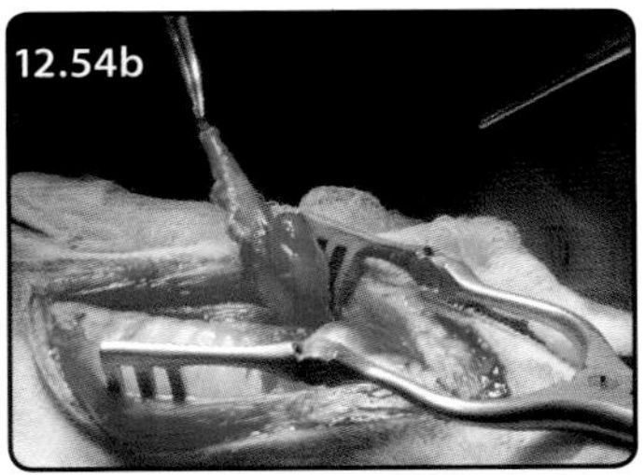
12.54b

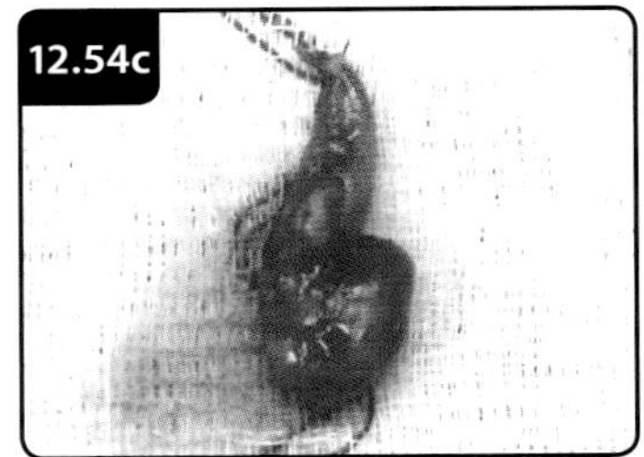
12.54c

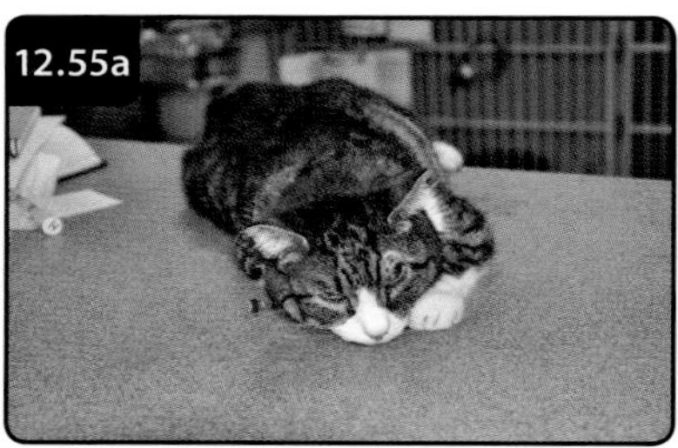
12.55a

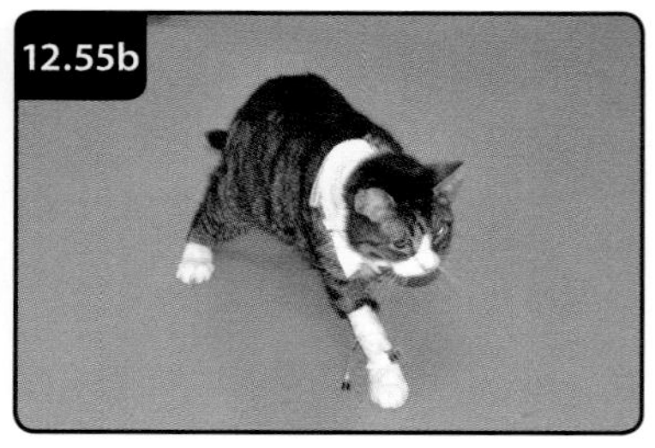
12.55b

12.55a, b. Diabetes mellitus with hypokalemia and thiamine deficiency. This domestic shorthair cat was diagnosed initially with diabetic ketoacidosis and hypokalemia. The cat's weakness was attributed to the hypokalemia. After potassium supplementation and return to eukalemia the cat still postured abnormally and had a mildly demented consciousness (Figure 12.55a). These signs suggested the possibility of thiamine deficiency, and the cat was given 100 mg of thiamine subcutaneously. This brought about a dramatic improvement over the subsequent 24 hours (Figure 12.55b), thus making thiamine deficiency diagnosis more plausible. Continued supplementation was provided orally for the next month. The cat's diet had ample amounts of thiamine according to the label, but deficiencies are still possible.

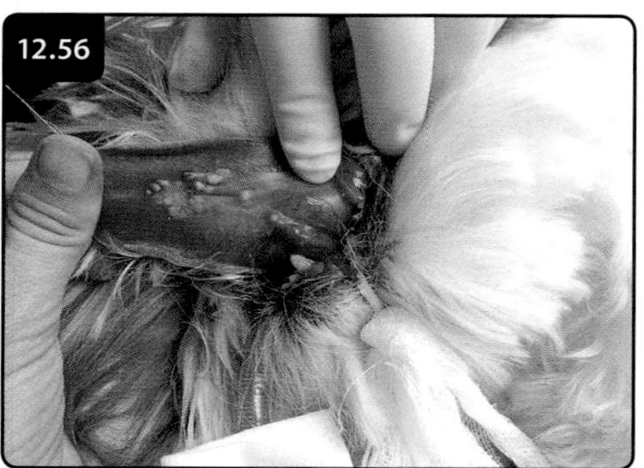
12.56

12.56. Calcinosis cutis involving the tongue. Calcinosis cutis commonly involves the skin of the Cushing's disease dog. However, this dystrophic change can involve other body areas as well. Shown are mineralized deposits on the tongue of a dog with hypercortisolism. There is no treatment for this lesion other than to treat the Cushing's disease. It might require weeks for the lesions to resolve. Lingual calcinosis is also shown in Case 12.18.

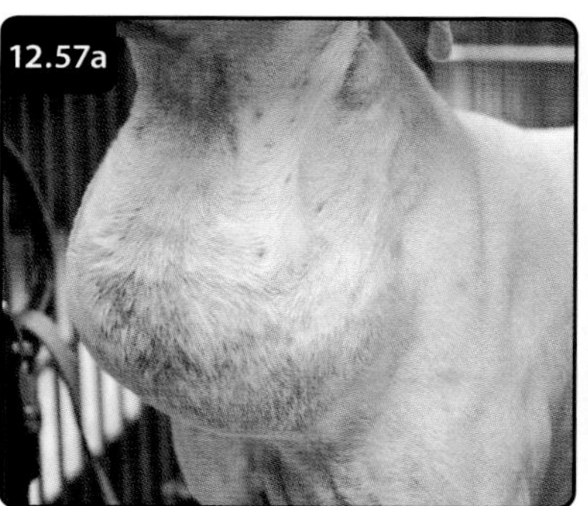
12.57a

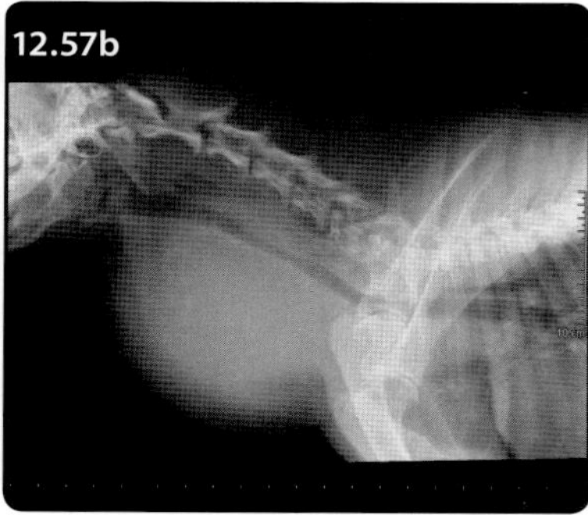
12.57b

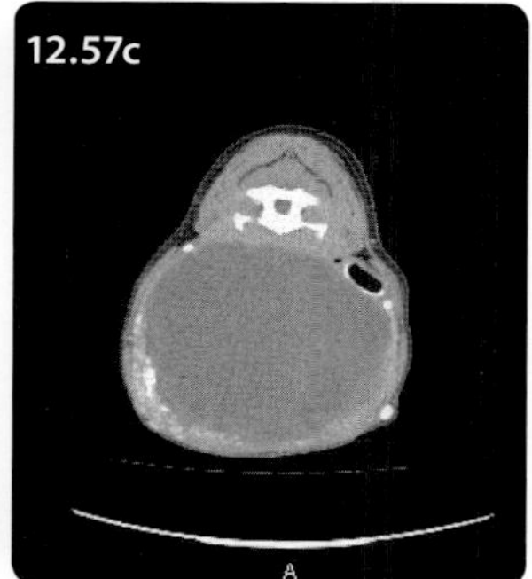
12.57c

12.57a–c. Thyroid carcinoma. This dog has a very large mass involving its ventral cervical region. The enlargement is firm and is indistinct at the base. The lateral radiograph shows the space-occupying mass effect with upward deflection of the trachea. The CT image shows the mass and the trachea deflected dorsally. In the USA, most dogs with malignant thyroid tumors do not hypersecrete thyroxine, although this effect is more common in Europe. The tumor can readily metastasize to the caudal cervical lymph nodes and the lungs. Surgery can be very helpful provided the tumor does not extend beyond its capsule and invade neighboring vital structures.

12.58a–d. Thyroid adenoma and parathyroid adenoma. Figures 12.58a, b are ultrasonograms of the cervical region of a dog depicting a parathyroid adenoma and a large thyroid adenoma, respectively. Surgery was successful in removing both tumors. Figures 12.58c, d show the large thyroid adenoma. Note the usual dark red color of endocrine tumors, which is caused by their rich blood supplies.

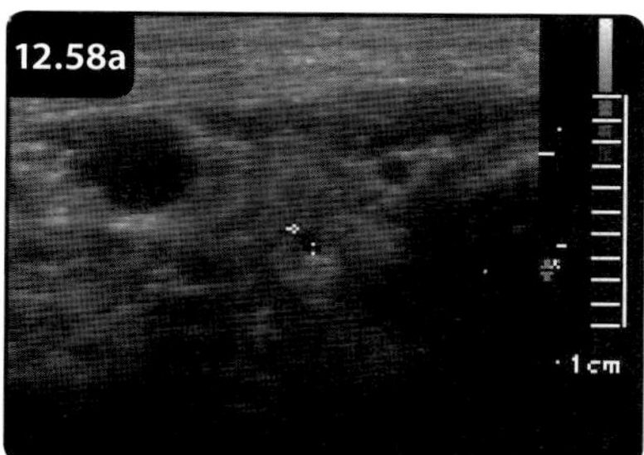

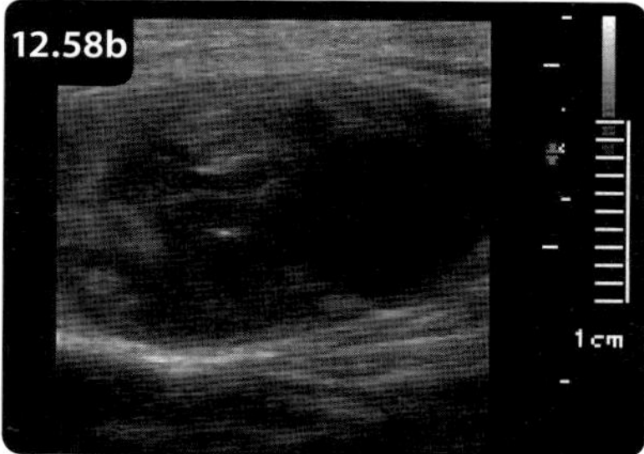

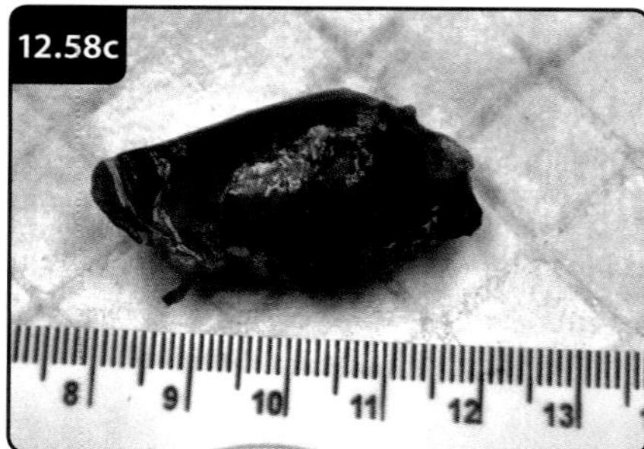

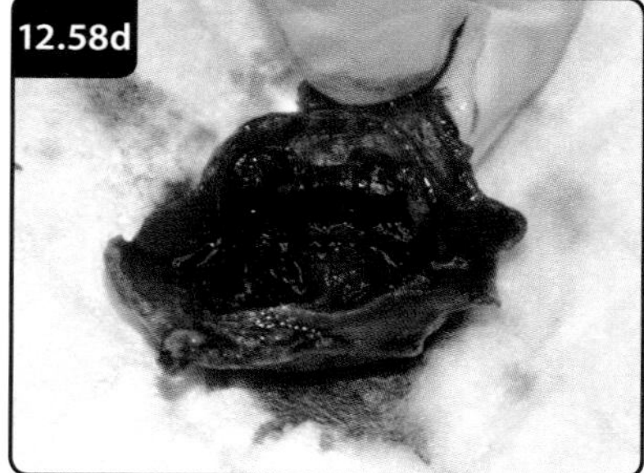

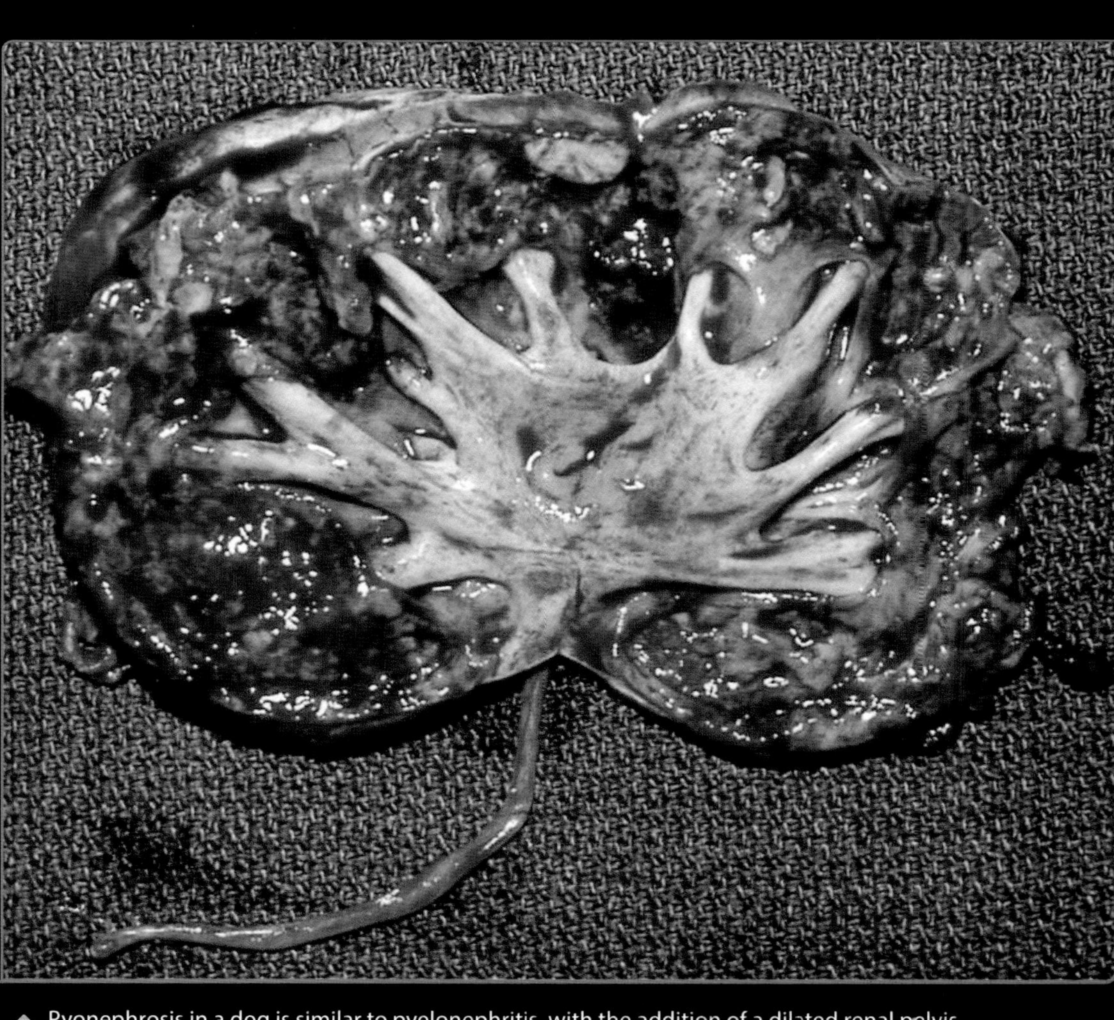

▲ Pyonephrosis in a dog is similar to pyelonephritis, with the addition of a dilated renal pelvis due to obstructive uropathy.

13

Urogenital disorders

UROGENITIAL is derived from the Greek words *ouron*, meaning urine, and the Latin word *genitalis*, pertaining to reproduction. This specialty includes a variety of clinical disorders, because it covers the entire urinary and reproductive systems. Although kidney disorders can be covered in their own nephrology specialty, they can also be included in the urogenital system. Several interesting clinical disorders can therefore be covered in this organ system. Certain diagnostic tests are essential for urinary disorders, including hematology and serum chemistry analysis, urinalysis, and various forms of diagnostic imaging, especially radiography and abdominal ultrasonography.

Abdominal ultrasonography is one of the most helpful diagnostic tools for evaluating the internal genital organs, while a thorough physical examination will be of particular diagnostic value. Some of the images that follow might not be that rare, but several of them might be considered to be highly interesting.

13 Urogenital disorders

- Rule out pyometra in any sick intact female.
- Never let the sun set on a pyo (Garvey, M).
- Murky urine can be caused by: pus, chyle, crystals.
- Bilateral renomegaly means very serious disease: lymphoma, hydronephrosis, pyonephrosis, granuloma, inflammation, subcapsular edema, polycystic.
- Cats: one big kidney plus one small kidney can mean one contracted fibrotic kidney and one compensatory hypertrophic and fibrotic kidney.
- Hematuria without stranguria – consider coagulopathy or renal bleed; however, a recent renal bleed plus clots in the urinary bladder can cause stranguria.
- Male dog plus stranguria – must examine as a possible emergency and radiograph or perform ultrasound in order to rule out obstructive uropathy.
- Cessation of polyuria in sick patient – consider oliguria/anuria – a bad sign.

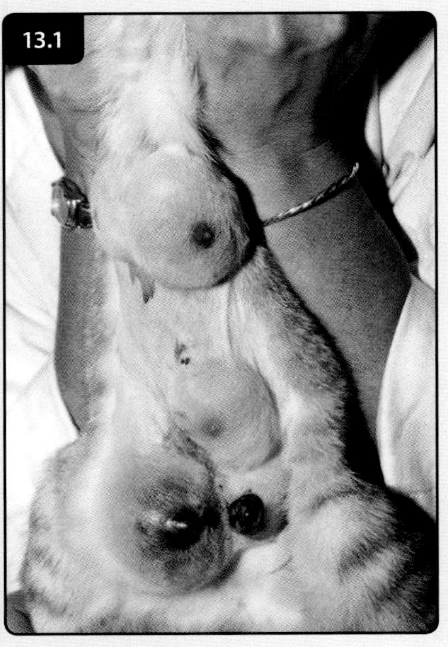

13.1. Mammary fibroadenomatous hyperplasia in a cat. This is a progesterone-mediated inflammatory disorder of young female cats that should not be confused with neoplasia. It can occur in the cycling cat or in one that has received progesterone by injection or tablet (megestrol acetate). The tissue can become quite inflamed, become necrotic, and cause discomfort. The condition can be treated by surgery or it can diminish with time if the progesterone source can be removed. Spaying the cat will solve the endogenous source.

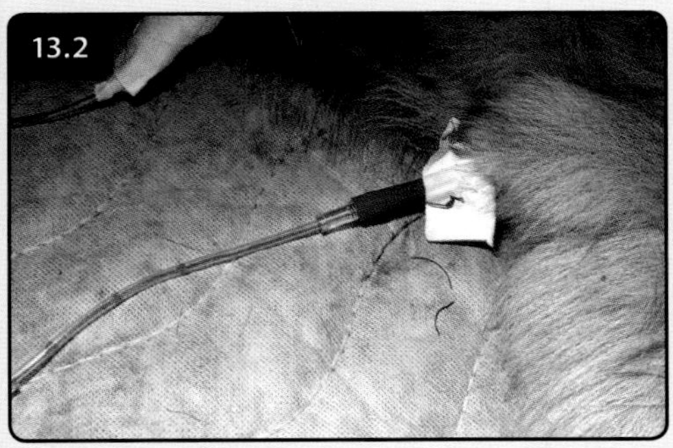

13.2. The empty urinary catheter line and collection bag. There are three causes of an empty urinary catheter line: (1) the collection bag was recently changed and the system emptied; (2) the catheter is kinked; and (3) the patient is anuric. The latter discovery would require a major adjustment in the intravenous fluid dose where the amount administered would equal actual urine production/hour, insensible losses amounting to 20 ml/kg/day, and on-going losses through vomiting and diarrhea. Therefore, it is best to rule out the easiest to fix conditions before concluding that the patient has the most serious problem.

13.3. Pyometra in a cat. Cats might be more subtle in their clinical signs of pyometra, and might not become clinically ill until the condition is well advanced, as seen in this pyometra from a cat. A large sized pyometra provides ample reason to be careful when undertaking a cystocentesis. Avoiding this procedure under this circumstance is a judicious choice.

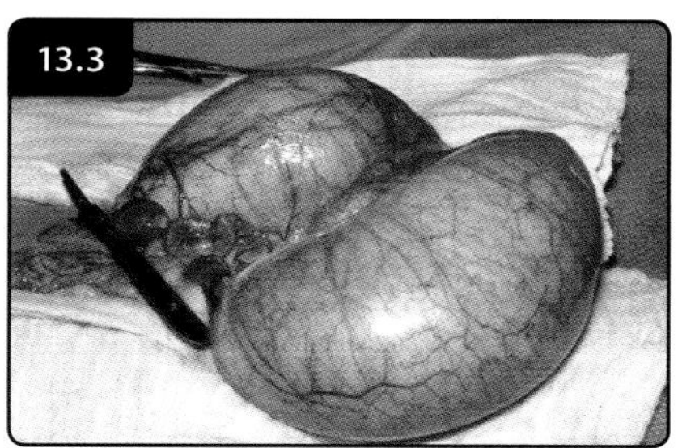

13.4a, b. Extraluminal cystic calculus. These radiographs show several cystic calculi that had eroded through the urinary bladder wall to lie free in the abdominal cavity. This condition is accompanied by uroperitoneum, which caused the dog to be azotemic and clinically ill. The white screen lines in 13.4a are the result of having to photograph the image from a computer screen.

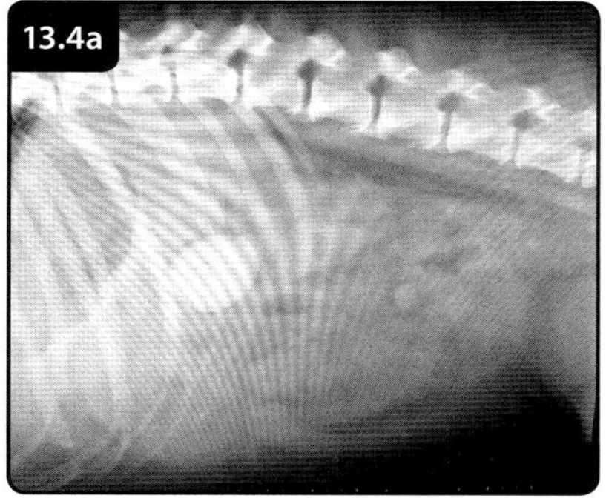

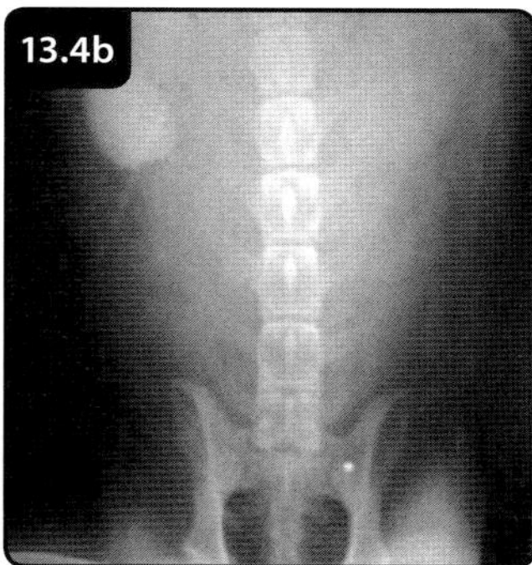

13.5a–c. Large blood clot in the urinary bladder of a cat. Figure 13.5a is an ultrasound image of a blood clot in the urinary bladder caused by the cat's hemorrhagic cystitis condition. Figures 13.5b, c show the clot during and after its surgical removal from the urinary bladder. Its exceptional large size and resistance to dissolving with irrigation measures made surgery necessary. (Courtesy Soft Tissue Surgery Service, University of Florida)

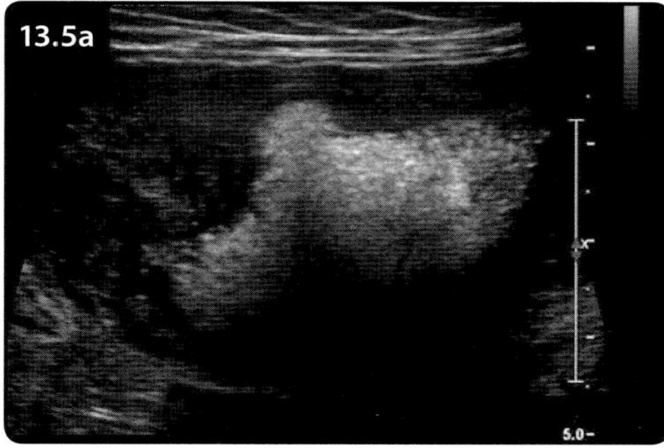

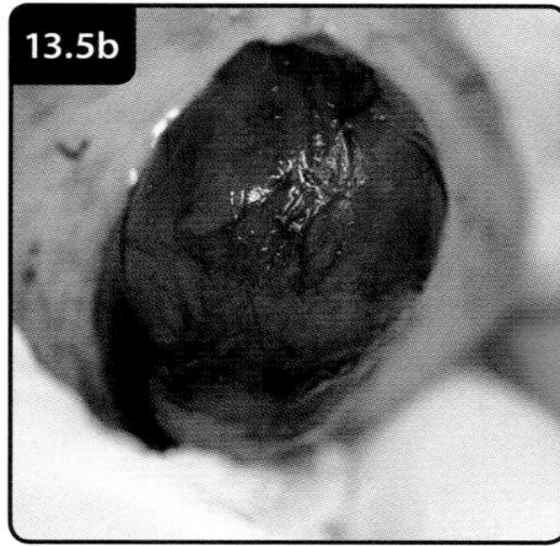

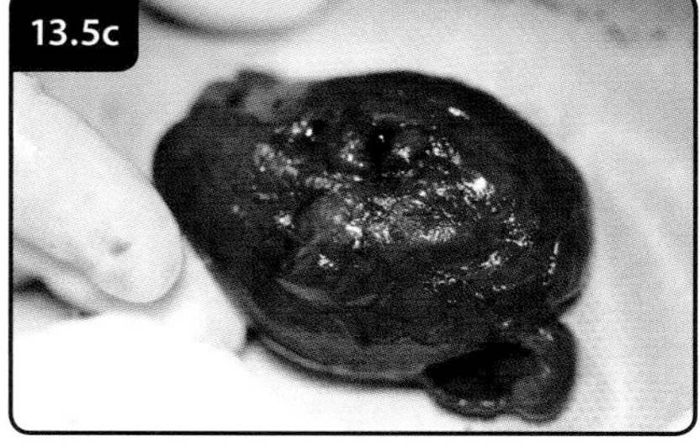

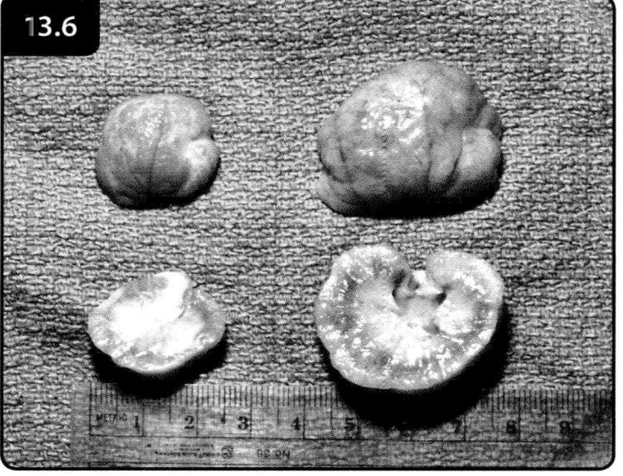

13.6. The big kidney–small kidney finding. This can be seen in aging cats with chronic kidney disease. While one kidney becomes small from contraction due to fibrosis, the other kidney might undergo tubular hypertrophy while it too becomes fibrotic. The difference in renal size will be apparent on physical examination and the urine SG will typically be isosthenuric.

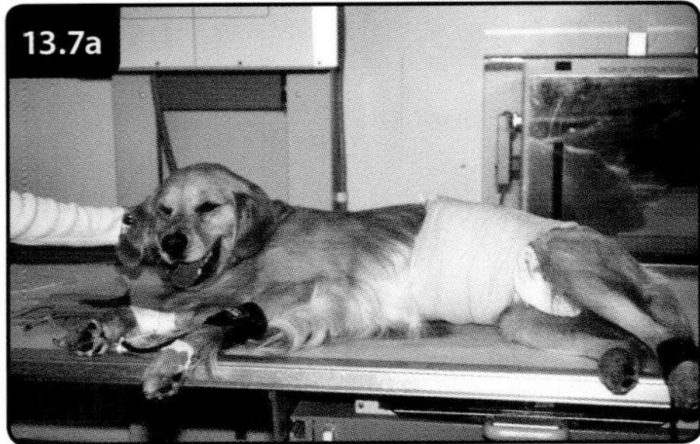

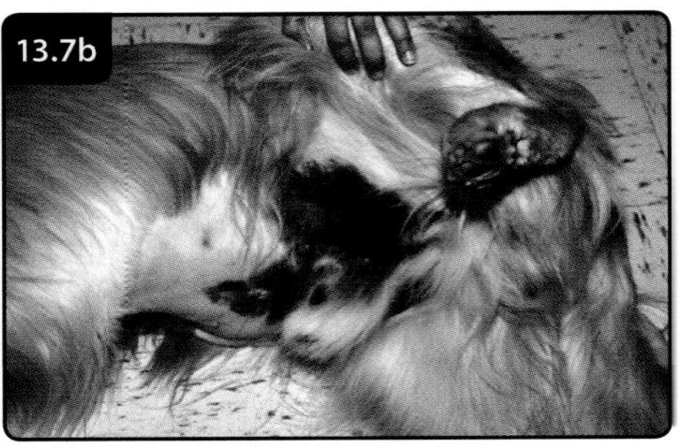

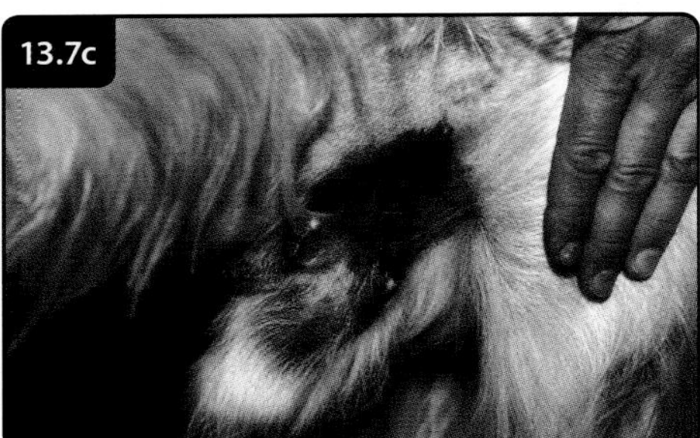

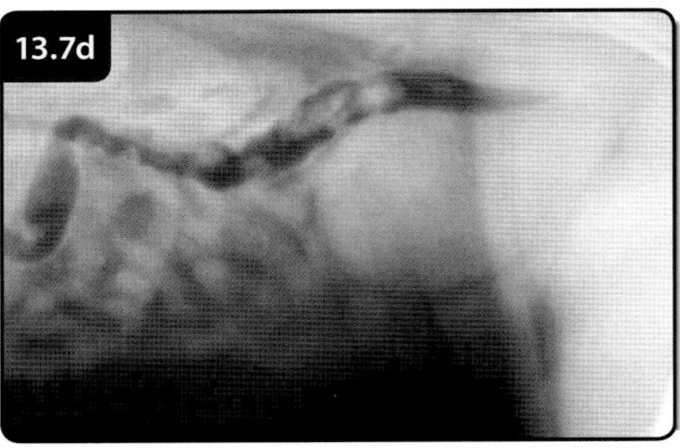

13.7a–d. Cystocentesis causing a tear of the caudal epigastric artery. This Golden Retriever began to bleed into his abdominal wall shortly after a cystocentesis procedure, during which time he became active while the needle was penetrating the abdominal wall. The shearing effect on the artery occurred while the dog resisted being placed in position for the procedure. A pressure bandage was used to stop the bleeding (Figures 13.7a–c) while intravenous crystalloid was necessary to treat the hypovolemia. The lateral abdominal radiograph (Figure 13.7d) shows thickening of the ventral abdominal wall caused by the hemorrhage.

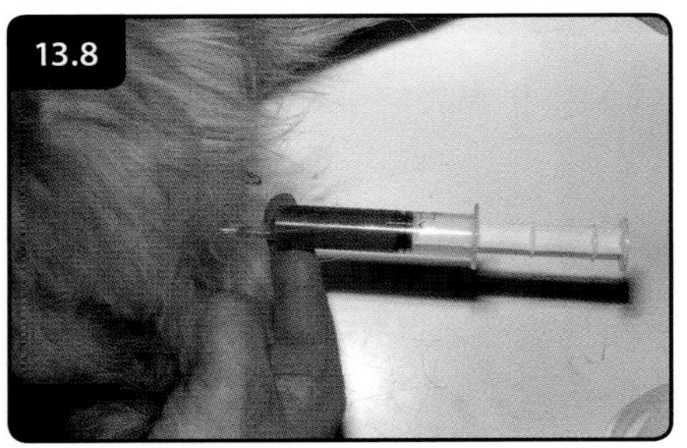

13.8. Cystocentesis: aspiration of pus while attempting the procedure. Although cystocentesis is a commonly used diagnostic procedure, there are times when complications can occur, as seen in the above case, where the fluid coming into the syringe is pus from an inadvertently tapped pyometra. The benefits of the procedure are certainly beyond question, but these two examples (Figures 13.7a–d and 13.8) illustrate why no procedure should be viewed as 'routine'.

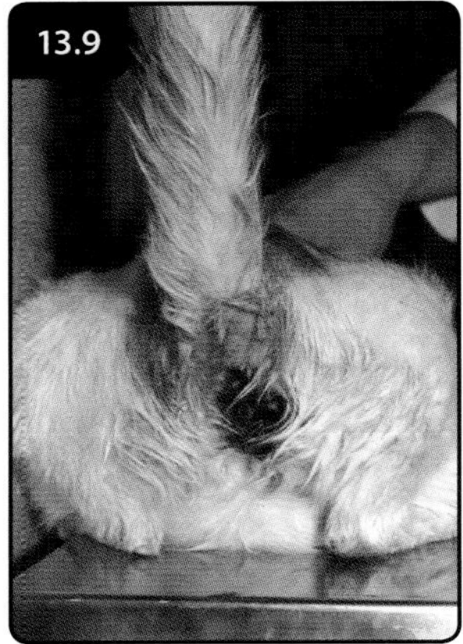

13.9. Pyometra in the cat. The diagnosis of pyometra in the cat might not be easy compared with dogs because the clinical signs might not be overt, as shown by the rather clean perineum of this cat with a draining pyometra, made possible by the cat's meticulous cleaning behavior. The polydipsia/ polyuria might not be so apparent either when compared with dogs.

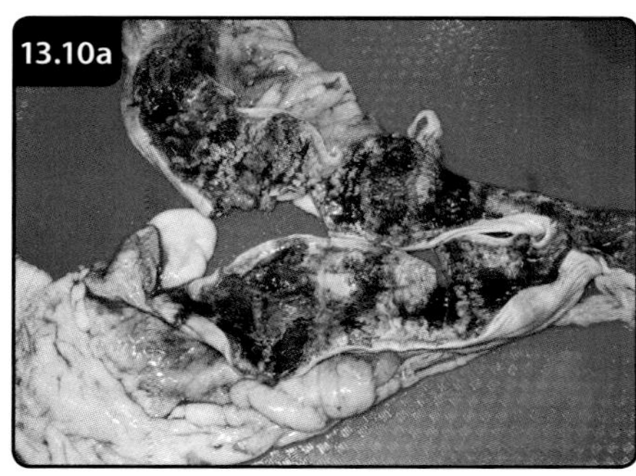

13.10a

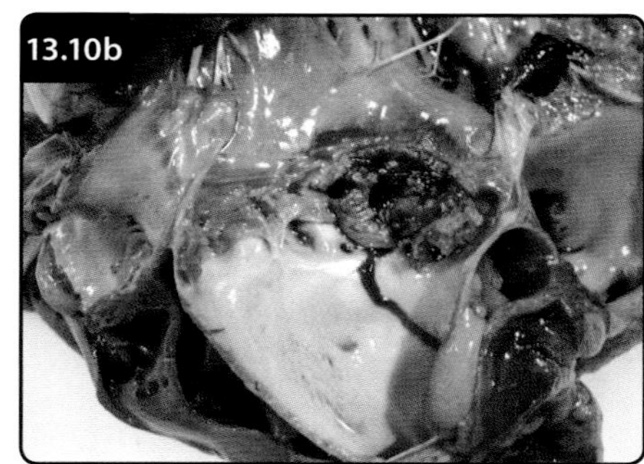

13.10b

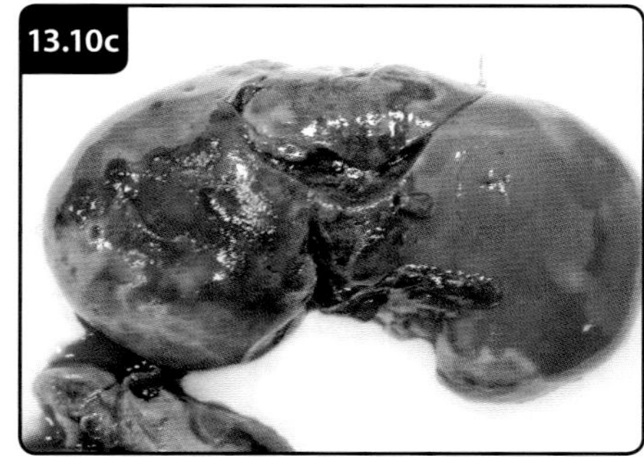

13.10c

13.10a–c. Renal infarction, bacterial endometritis, and vegetative endocarditis. Figure 13.10a depicts a dissected uterus from a Great Dane that became critically ill and died shortly after admission to the ICU. The dog had clinical features of sepsis, which was caused by postparturient endometritis. The dog also had fulminating congestive heart failure, tachyarrhythmias, and a bounding pulse, which was caused by severe vegetative endocarditis (Figure 13.10b). The vegetations fragmented into emboli and heavily showered the kidney, causing multiple renal infarcts (Figure 13.10c). Acute kidney injury caused by the massive embolic event was evident on the initial laboratory test evaluation.

13.11. Feline urethral obstruction with urethral abscess. Feline urethral obstruction can have many complications including infection, ruptured urethra, and systemic illness caused by azotemia and metabolic abnormalities such as acidosis and hyperkalemia. The urethral abscess in Figure 13.11 is a rare complication that would require culture and sensitivity, commencement of antibiotic treatment, and surgical drainage and débridement.

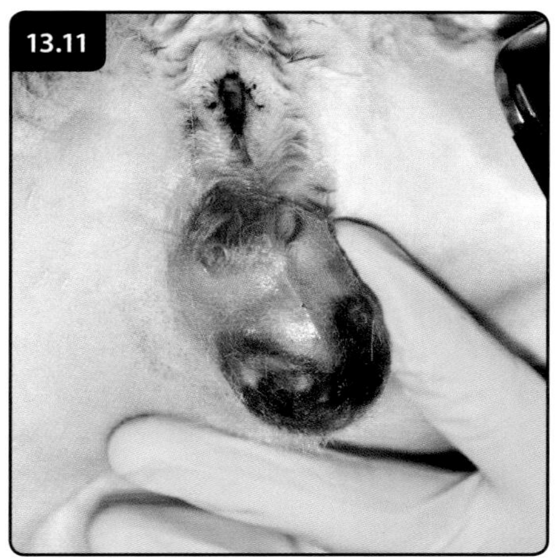

13.11

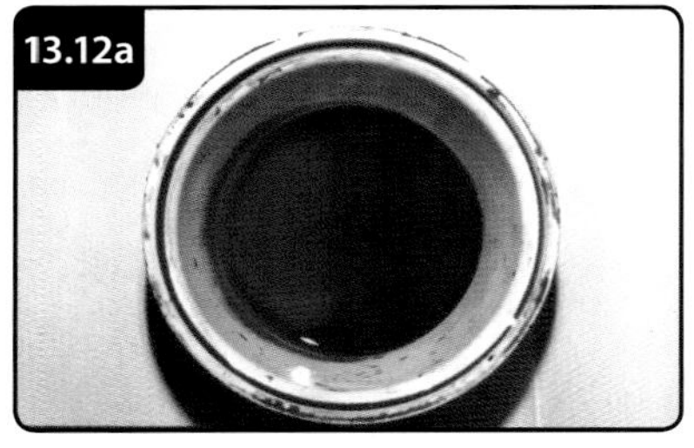

13.12a

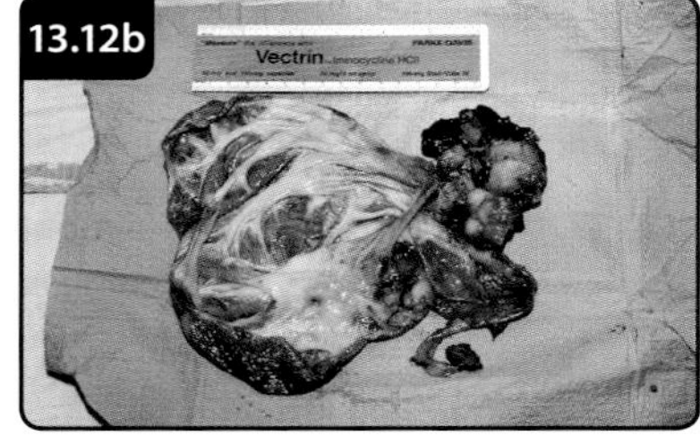

13.12b

13.12a, b. Hydronephrosis with spontaneous hemorrhage. This rare condition has been reported in the dog. It entails a dog with asymptomatic hydronephrosis that has a sudden onset of a renal blood vessel tear producing hemorrhagic urine. An abdominal radiograph can usually show the abnormally enlarged kidney, but an abdominal ultrasound evaluation would be more informative. Treatment entails nephrectomy after first confirming that the patient has a functioning contralateral kidney (usually done by contrast pyelography). Note that the clot within the kidney has both acute (dark red clot) and chronic (organized and white) features.

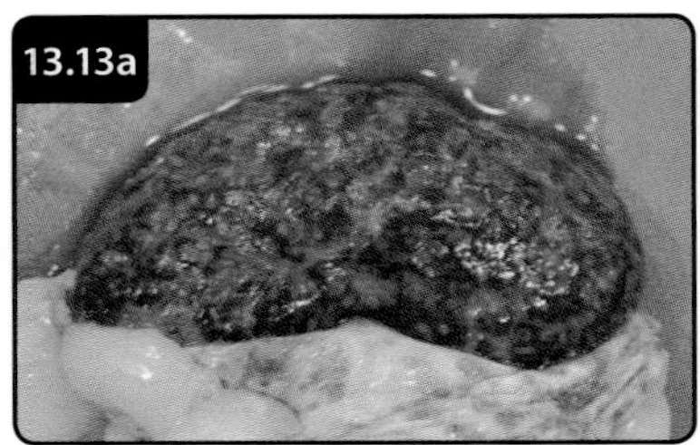

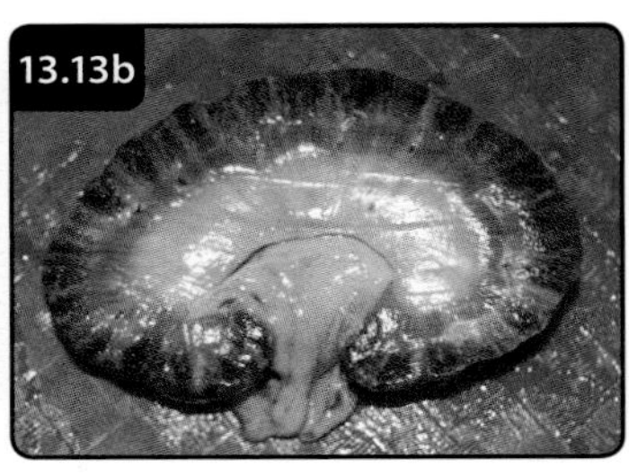

13.13a, b. Renal interstitial fibrosis and glomerulosclerosis. The dog with these kidneys had progressive chronic kidney disease with both tubular and glomerular abnormalities. Representing the tubular dysfunction in life would be azotemia, hyperphosphatemia, and metabolic acidosis. The clinical consequences of glomerular disease would have been hypertension and proteinuria. All of the pathology resulted in severe glomerulotubular imbalance for this dog and eventually complete renal decompensation. The irregular surface on the kidney is a result of the fibrosis. The abnormal glomeruli are evident as small white dots amongst the fibrous tissue striations on the cut section.

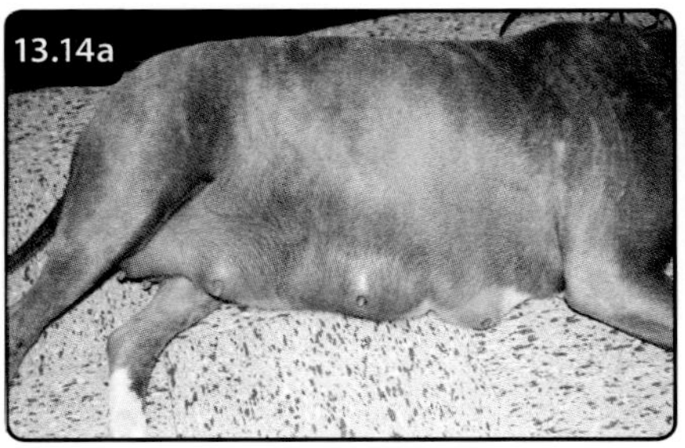

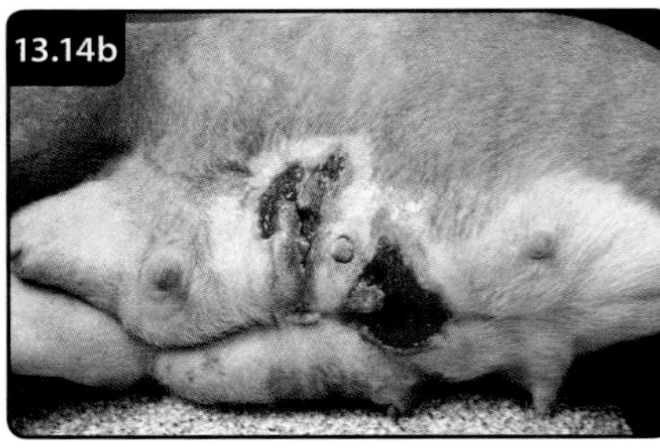

13.14a, b. Mastitis and mammary abscess formation. This condition typically occurs during the postpartum period during nursing. The mammae initially become warm and painful (Figure 13.14a) and the bitch is reluctant to nurse her pups. Treatment consists of warm compresses and antibiotics. An abscess that is ready to be lanced will characterize as a darkened surface with palpable subsurface cavitation. Surgical lancing and débridement should be done at that time. Any mammary inflammation in a female dog outside of diestrus should be suspect for inflammatory mammary carcinoma.

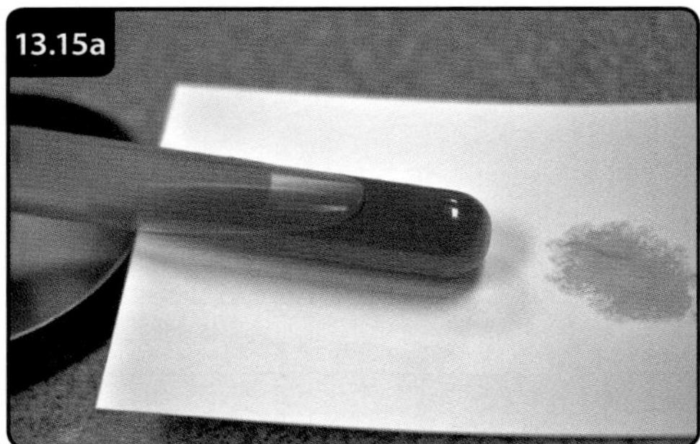

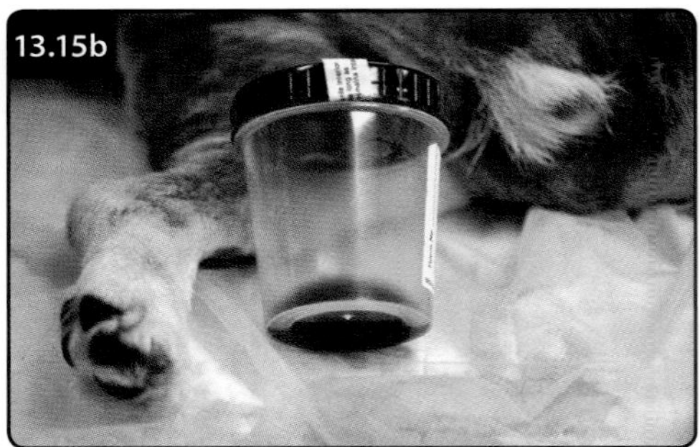

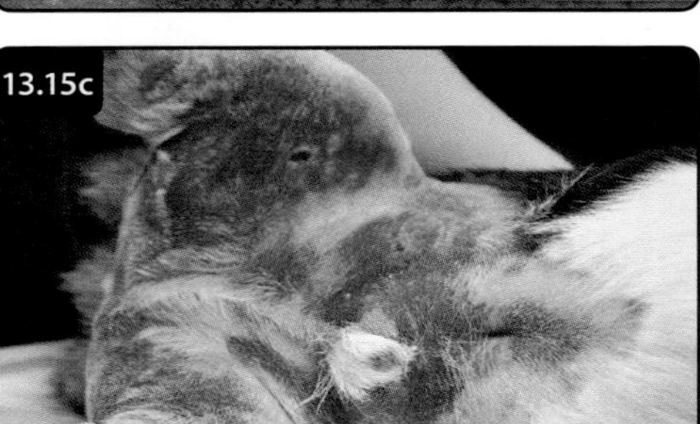

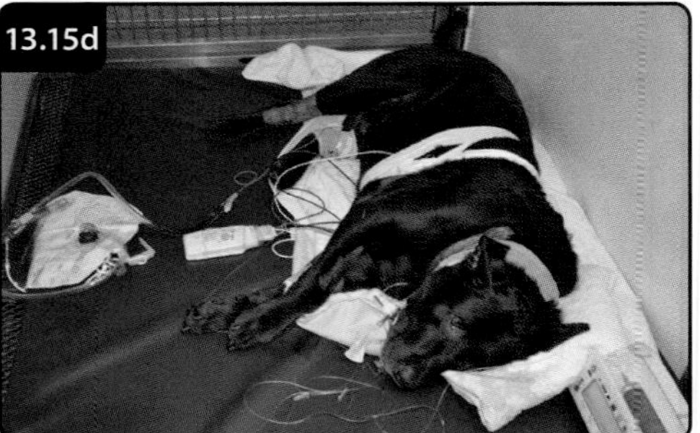

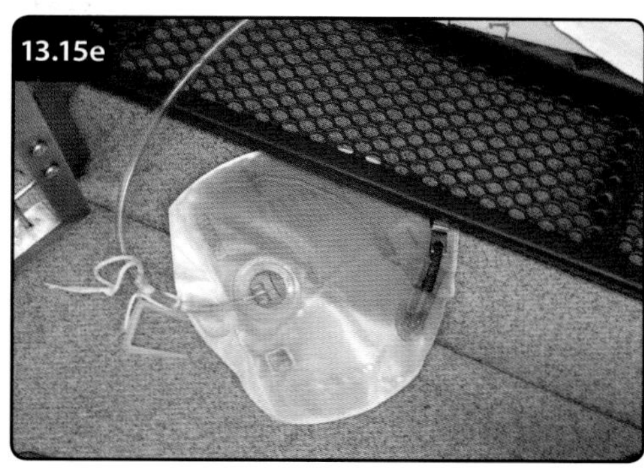

13.15a–e. Myoglobinuria. This urinary pigment follows skeletal muscle destruction. It has a green tea appearance but it can also be a light brown color, as shown in Figures 13.15 a, b. It can occur with traumatic injury (Figure 13.15c) and with certain types of envenomation. Myoglobin is tubulotoxic and acute kidney injury can be of consequence. Various treatments have been recommended including urine alkalinization, which can be accomplished by the administration of sodium bicarbonate solution. Alternatively, providing ample intravenous crystalloid solutions can also be of benefit, as shown by the improvement in urine color between days 1 and 2 in Figures 13.15d, e.

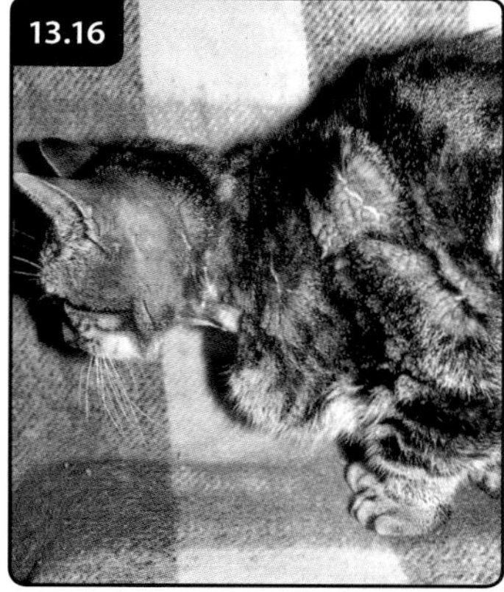

13.16. Glomerulopathy in a cat. This cat has nephrotic syndrome. It had proteinuria, hypoprotinemia, edema (as shown in the cranial thorax), and hypertension, and it eventually became azotemic. There are several causes of glomerulopathy in cats and dogs. Those caused by antigen–antibody complex formation are potentially treatable with immunosuppressive drugs, especially if the cause can be eliminated. Most of the other types cause progressive deterioration of the kidney and commonly lead to end-stage disease.

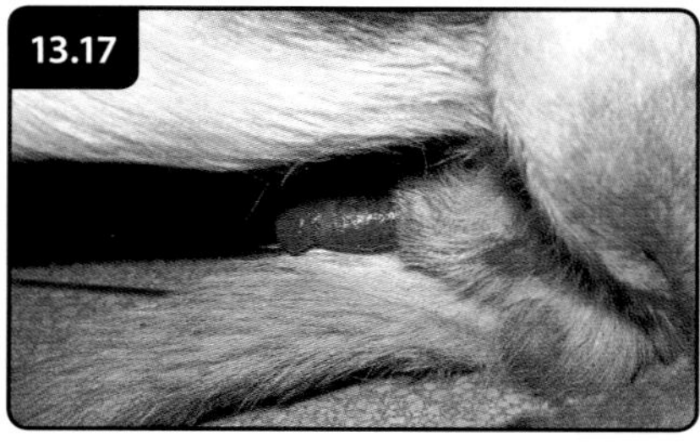

13.17. Paraphimosis. This condition occurs when the penis cannot be retracted into the prepuce. It can be caused by hypoplastic prepuce, constriction of the prepuce by hair or string while the penis is exposed, ineffective prepucial musculature, neurologic disorders, tumors or masses at the bulb of the penis, and others. Treatment is usually surgical depending on the cause.

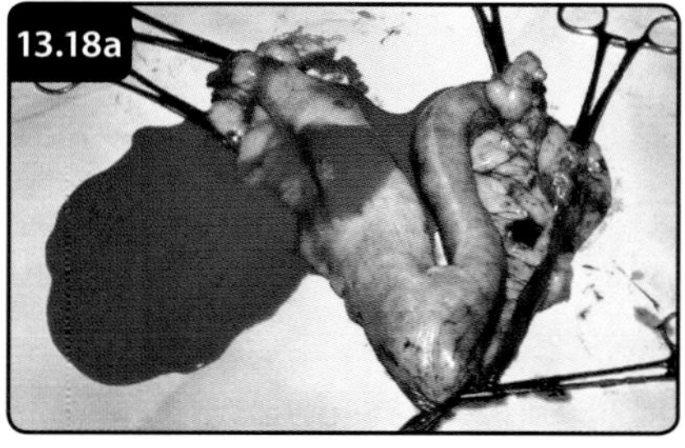

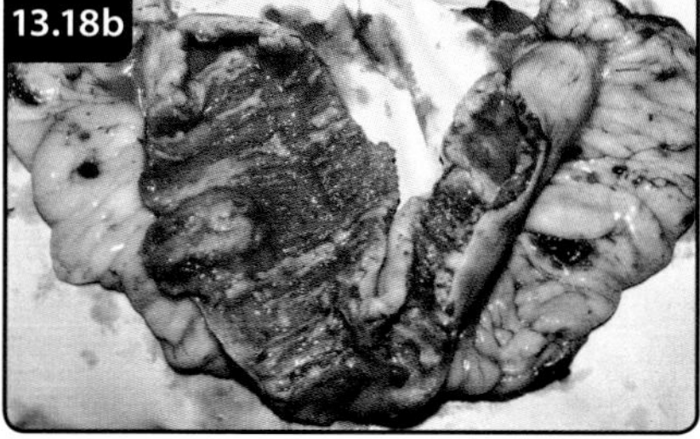

13.18a, b. Pyometra. The earliest uterine pathology with pyometra is endometrial hyperplasia, which then becomes secondarily infected to become a pyometra. *Escherichia coli* is usually the associated bacteria. The polydipsia and polyuria complex associated with this condition is thought to occur from bacterial endotoxin binding to the vasopressin V2 receptor in the distal renal tubule epithelium to cause resistance to antidiuretic hormone. The images show the suppurative uterine contents and the endometrial hyperplasia. The mucosal proliferation occurs under the influence of progesterone.

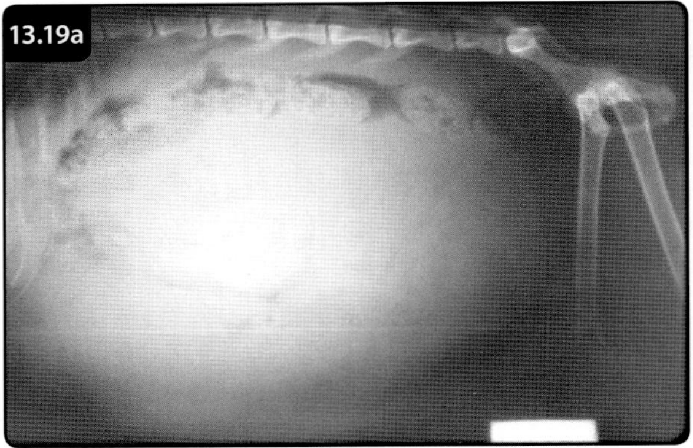

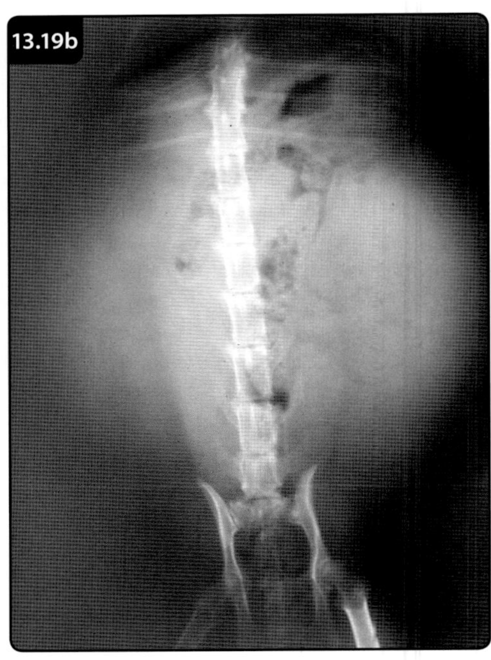

13.19a, b. Radiographs of a large pyometra in a cat. At first glance, the clinician might think that the cat has a large amount of ascites. Note how the distended uterine horns displace the abdominal viscera cranially and dorsally while displacing the bowel toward the center of the abdomen. The enlarged uterus makes the cystocentesis procedure foreboding.

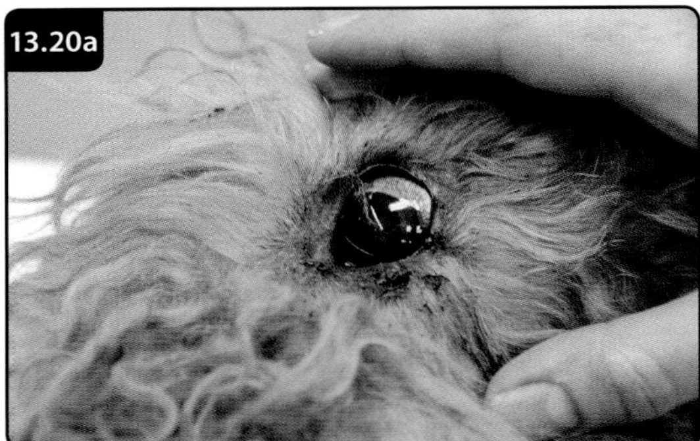

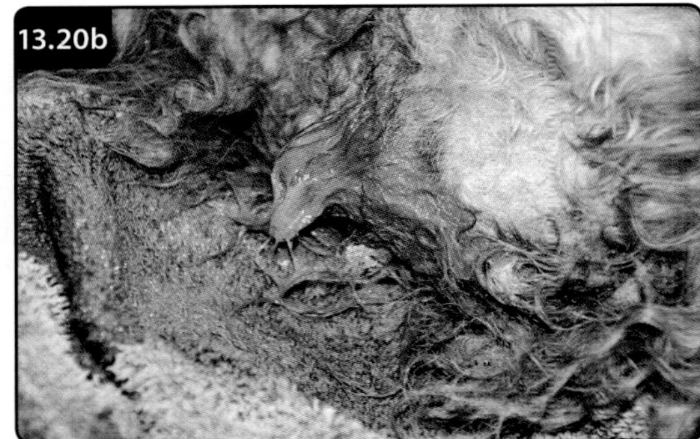

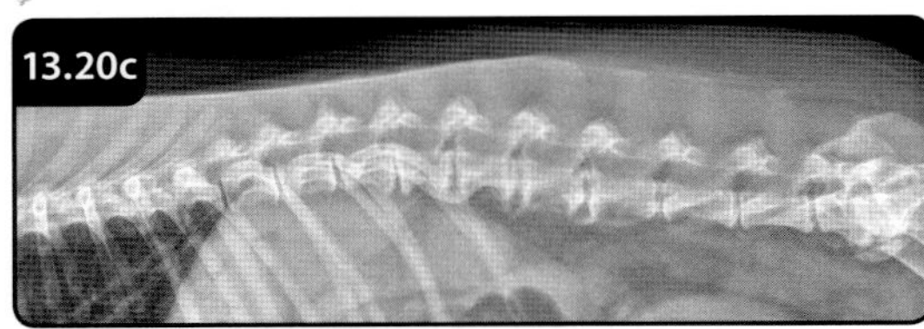

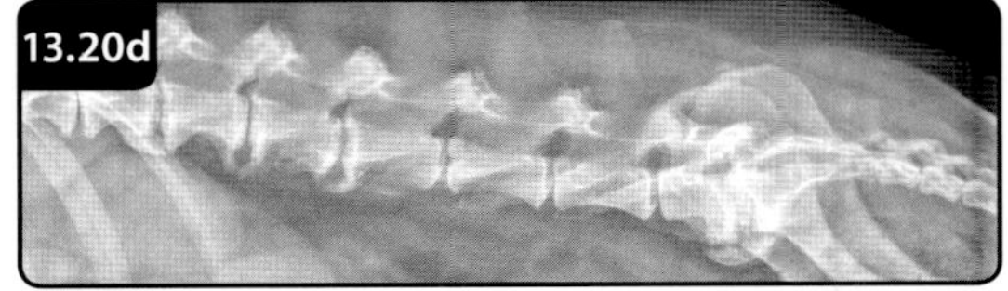

13.20a–d. Pyometra and diskospondylitis in a female Airedale dog. This dog presented with the typical signs of pyometra, but she also showed lumbar pain that was localized to her thoracolumbar and lumbosacral vertebral regions. On physical examination, she showed considerable scleral injection (Figure 13.20a), reflecting her endotoxemia, a suppurative vaginal discharge (Figure 13.20b), and exquisite hyperpathia over her back. The radiographs show eroded endplates at L1–L2 and L7–S1 compatible with diskospondylitis (Figure 13.20c, d). Extended antibiotic treatment was necessary for an additional 6 weeks or more pending re-evaluation findings.

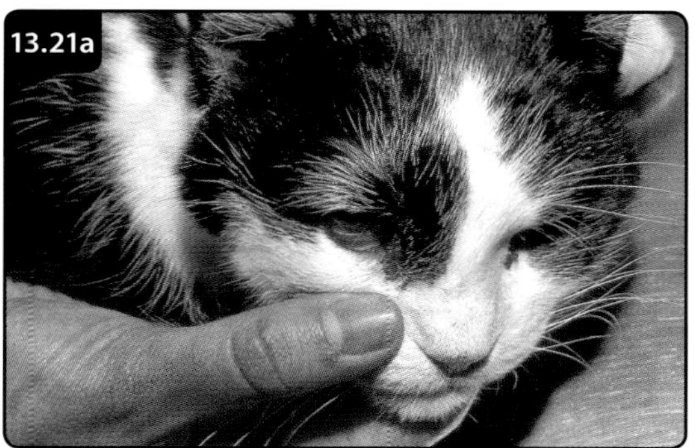

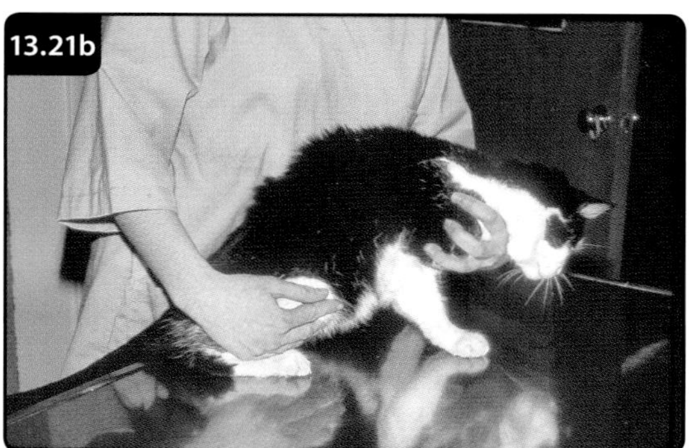

13.21a–c. Common signs of dehydration in a cat. This cat had chronic decompensating renal failure. He was estimated at 8–10% dehydration, as shown by the eye globe regression and obvious skin tenting (Figures 13.21a, b). As expected in a cat with chronic kidney disease, this cat had dilute urine (isosthenuria) (Figure 13.21c), indicating a loss of 70% or more of nephron function. Cats tend to feel remarkably improved after euhydration is restored with intravenous crystalloid solution.

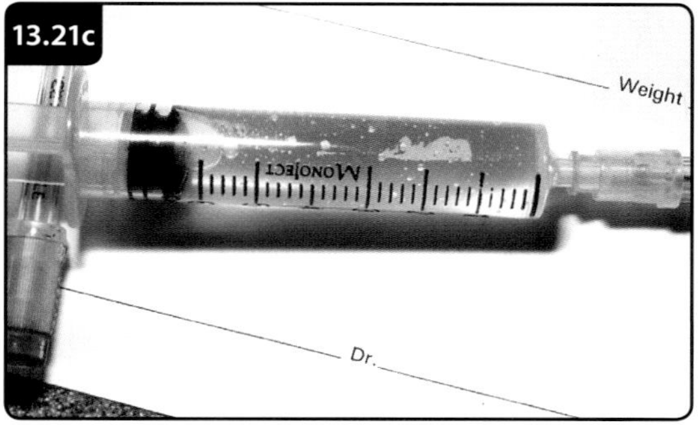

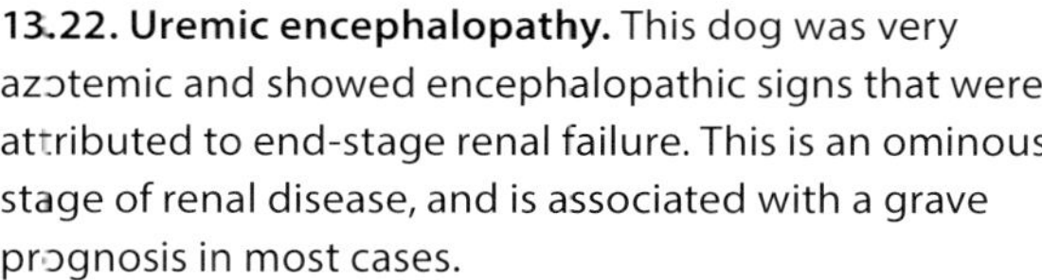

13.22. Uremic encephalopathy. This dog was very azotemic and showed encephalopathic signs that were attributed to end-stage renal failure. This is an ominous stage of renal disease, and is associated with a grave prognosis in most cases.

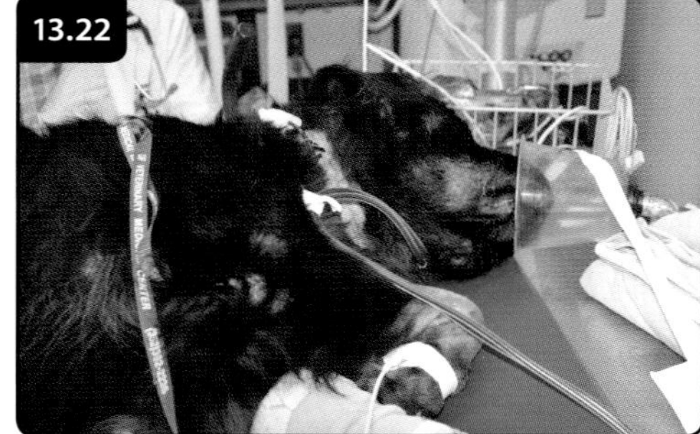

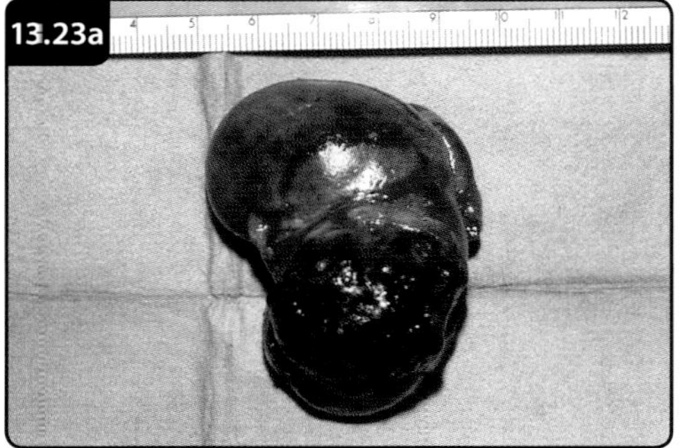

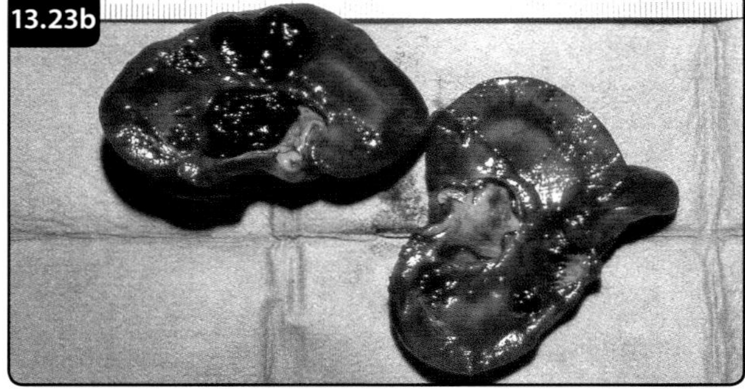

13.23a, b. Renal hemangioma. These images show a renal hemangioma that was diagnosed after the dog urinated on the snow. If left undetected, this dog would have eventually suffered from iron deficiency anemia or spontaneous hemorrhage, which might have occurred if the dog lived in a more temperate climate devoid of snow.

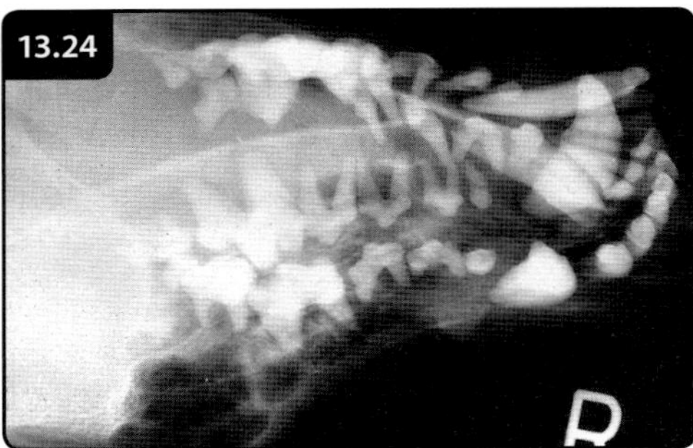

13.24. Renal osteodystrophy. This skull radiograph is from a dog with chronic kidney disease and renal osteodystrophy. Of note is the absence of the lamina dura dentes, which is necessary to anchor teeth into their sockets. Its absence causes the teeth to become loose and 'float', which can be detected on physical examination.

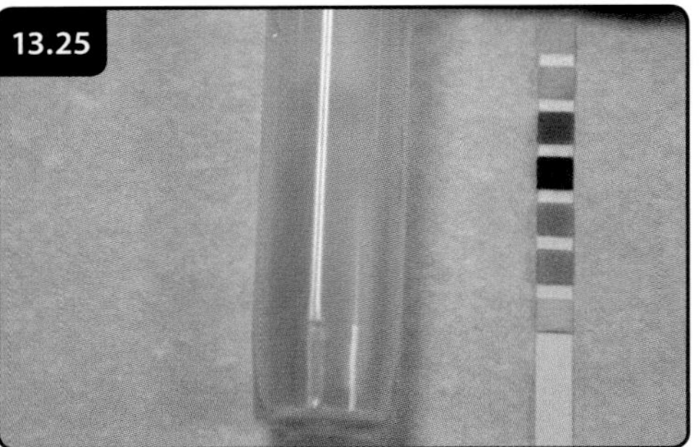

13.25. Green pigmenturia. This urine sample had a greenish appearance. It was from a dog with traumatic liver tears and hemoabdomen. The urine reagent stick was strongly positive for hemeprotein and bilirubin (3rd and 5th reagent pads from the top). The green hue was probably due to degraded heme pigment.

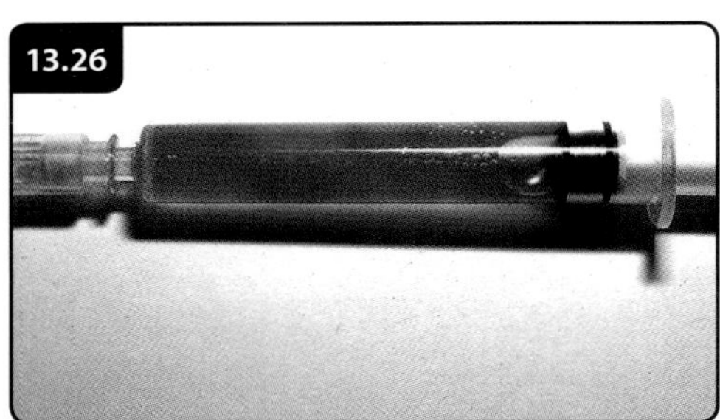

13.26. Pyuria. This urine sample is opalescent due to the large number of white blood cells present. In this case, it was due to pyelonephritis. Opalescent urine can also accompany chyluria and abundant crystalluria.

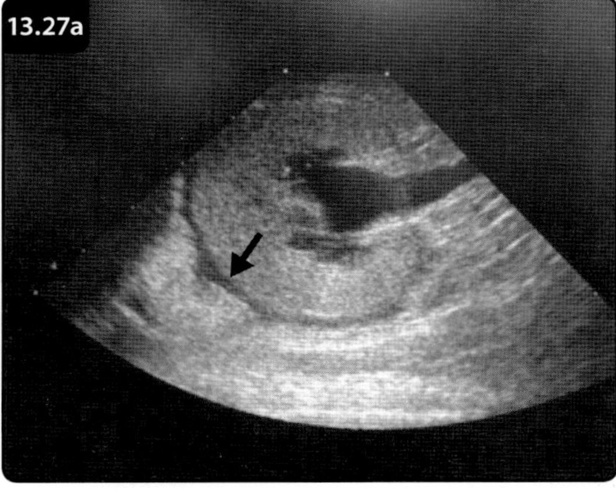

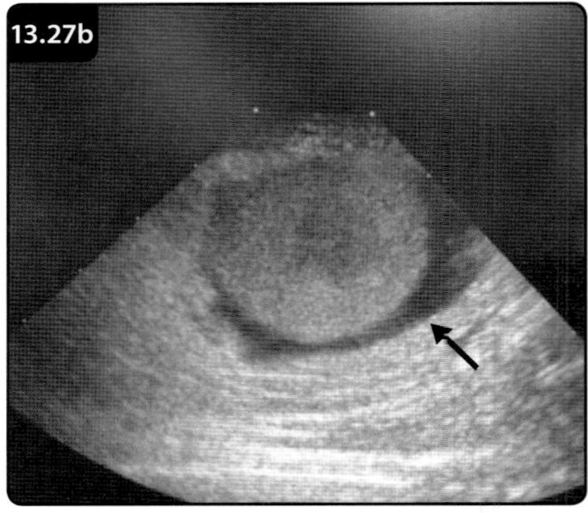

13.27a, b. Renal pericapsular edema with acute kidney injury. The hypoechoic rim surrounding the kidney is edema (arrows). Pericapsular edema can occur with acute kidney injury and is due to swelling of the renal parenchyma causing the renal lymphatics to become obstructed.

13.28. Renal subcapsular edema on radiography. This ventrodorsal radiographic view of the abdomen shows a halo-like pattern around the kidney that represents renal subcapsular edema. It is more clearly seen around the left kidney (arrow).

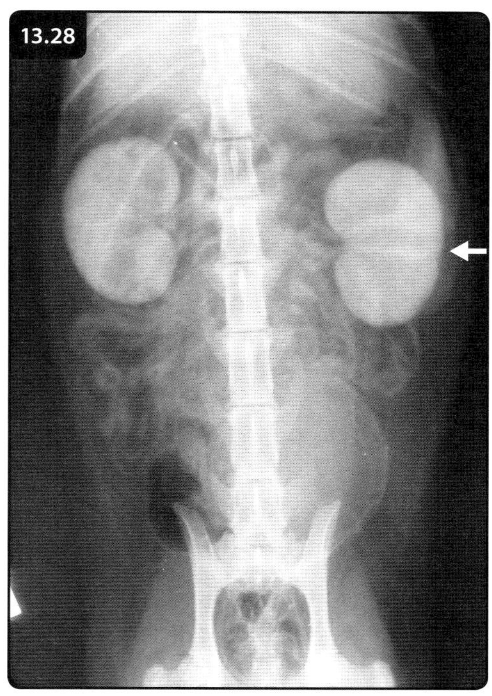

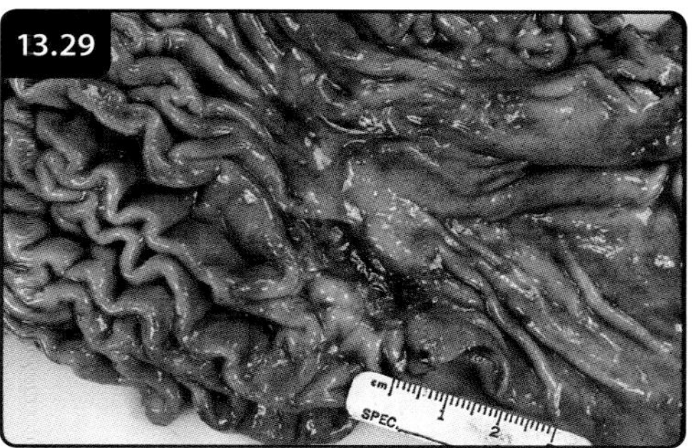

13.29. Uremic gastritis. This postmortem view shows foci of renal hyperemia, small hemorrhages, and a gastric ulcer, all components of uremic gastritis, which occurs because of the accumulation of uremic toxins (ammonia), hypergastrinemia, and in some cases (in humans) *Helicobacter* sp.

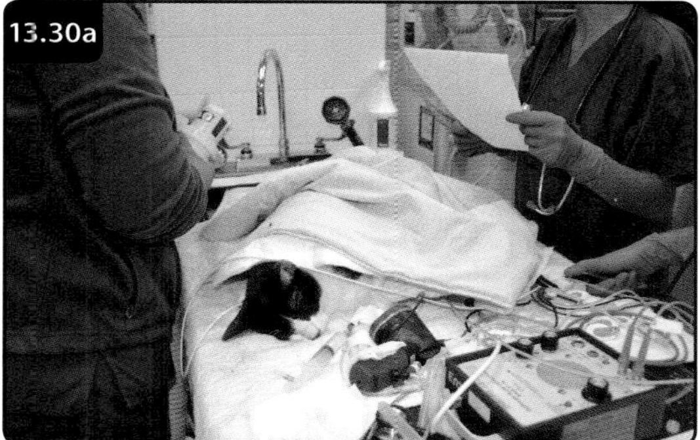

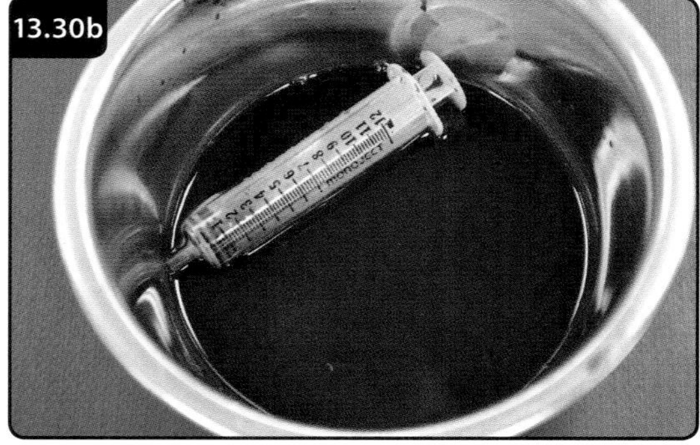

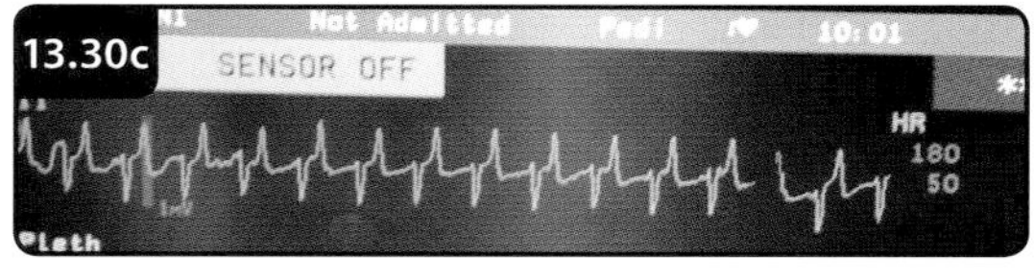

13.30a–c. Urethral obstruction in a cat. This very sick cat is a medical emergency with a BUN of 200 mg/dl (71.4 mmol/l), creatinine 16 mg/dl (141.4 µmol/l), serum bicarbonate 9.5 mEq/l (9.5 mmol/l), and serum potassium of 9.7 mEq/l (9.7 mmol/l). Characteristically, the urine is red colored. The ECG shows a life-threatening idioventricular rhythm calling for emergency treatment with 10% calcium gluconate (1.0 ml/kg) and insulin and dextrose (1–2 units of regular insulin with 2–4 ml of 50% dextrose solution intravenously). Sodium bicarbonate at 1.0 mEq/kg can also be given to counteract the hyperkalemia and metabolic acidosis, respectively, although it is not currently popular in human medicine because of the large doses needed and the unpredictable results. Intravenous buffered isotonic crystalloid solution and insertion of a urethral catheter are done in tandem with the other emergency measures.

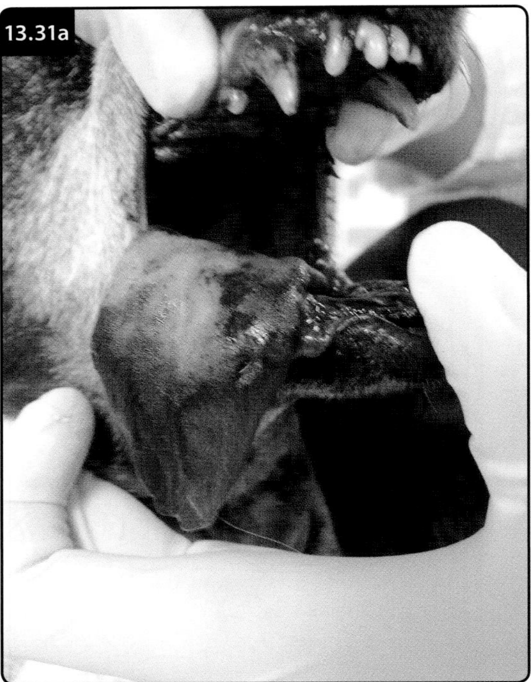

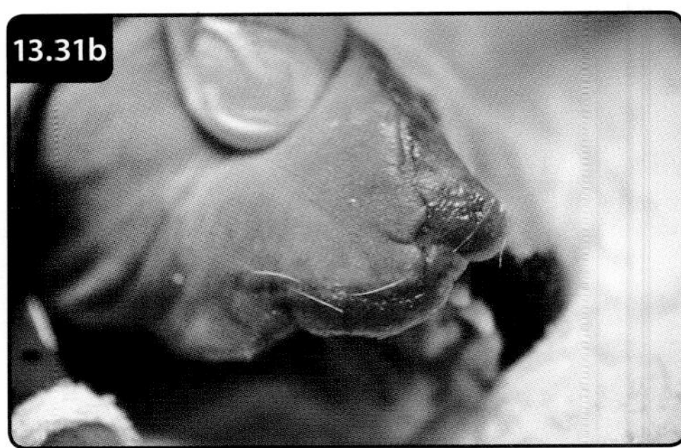

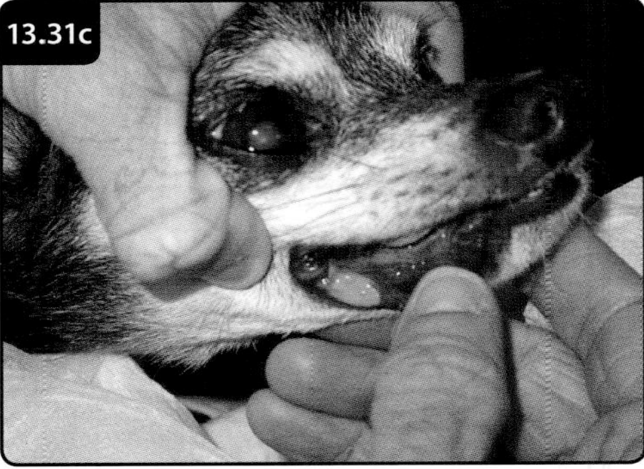

13.31a–c. Uremic oral ulcers. This lesion is shown in three different forms. Figure 13.31a shows uremic glossitis with a distinct area of necrosis that was likely due to an accompanying vasculitis. The other lingual ulcers (Figure 13.31b) and the oral labial ulcer (Figure 13.31c) are not as impressive, but they reflect the high levels of azotemia that can occur with both acute kidney injury and chronic kidney disease. The uremic toxins, including ammonia, are thought to cause the mucosal irritation.

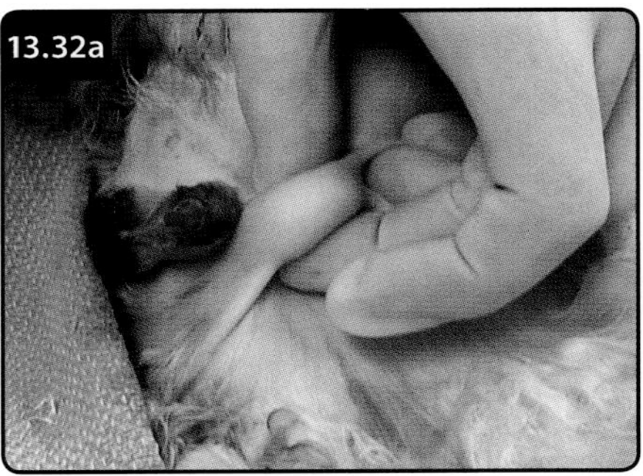

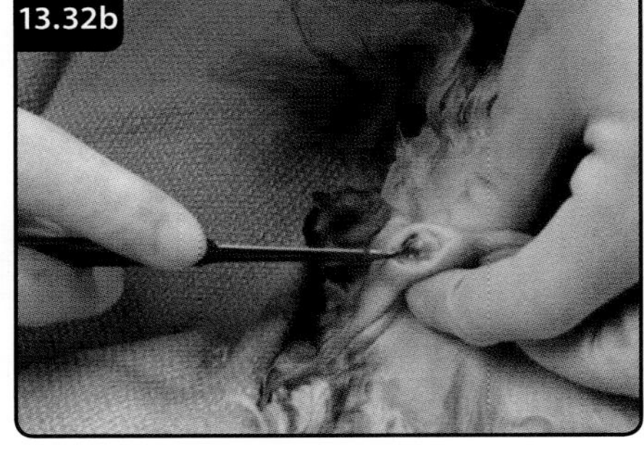

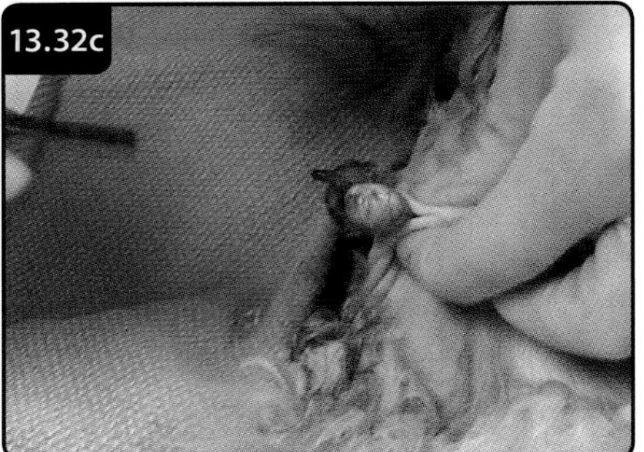

13.32a–c. Inguinal cryptorchid in a cat. Cryptorchidism occurs less commonly in cats compared with dogs. The procedure for removal of the 'hidden' testicle is the same. Although retained testicles in the dog are associated with testicular neoplasia, there is no documentation that this is the case in the cat, probably because of its low incidence in this species. Figures 13.32a–c show an inguinal testicle being removed surgically.

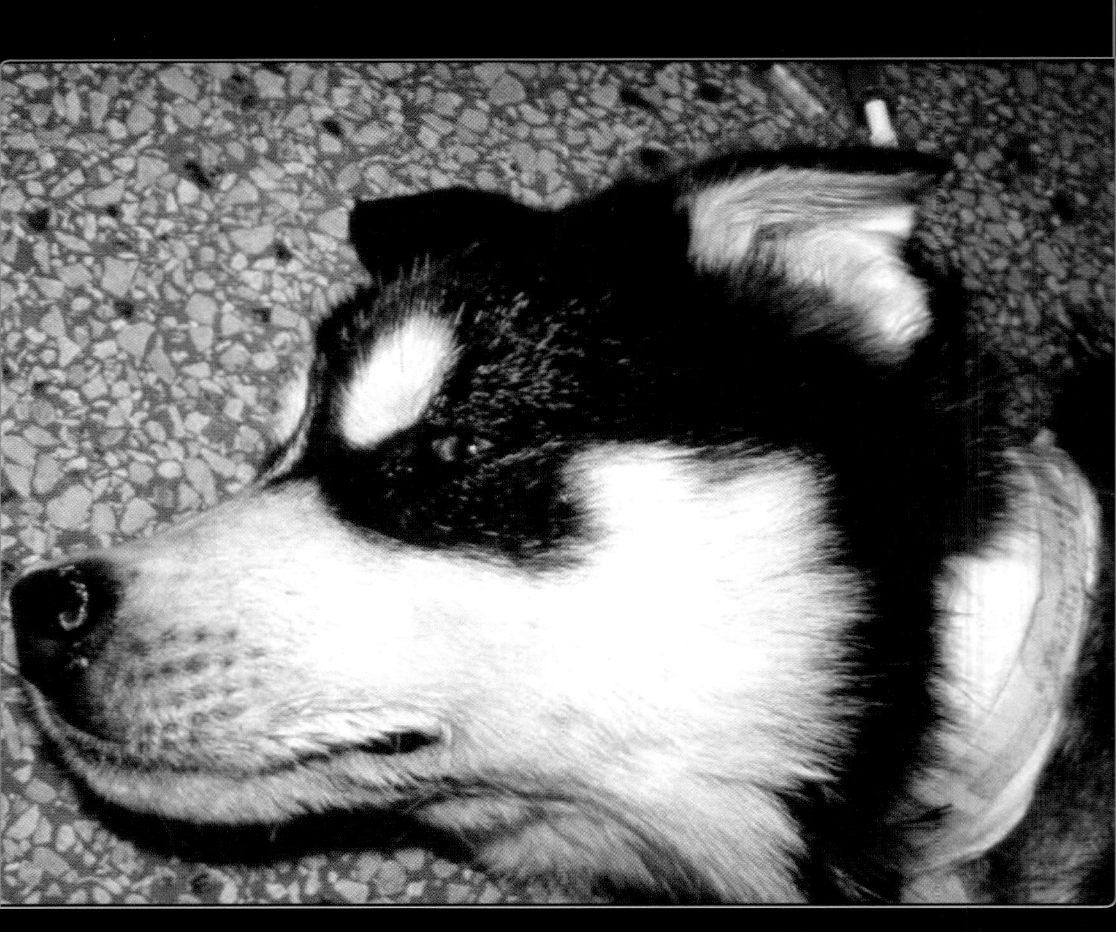

This young Malamute with tetanus shows the 'sardonic grin' typical of this disease.

14

Neurologic disorders

NEURO is derived from the Greek word *neuron*, meaning 'sinew'. The competent practice of internal medicine is almost impossible without a firm understanding of clinical neurology. This is because many patients can present to the clinician with one disease, only to be complicated by another disorder that can involve the nervous system; for example, a dog or cat with a bleeding disorder that suffers a hemorrhagic stroke or hypoxia causing an epileptogenic focus in the cerebrum.

My mentor taught me that neurology is the queen that shows mastery of a clinician's history taking and physical examination skills. This is the one main discipline where 'A picture is worth a thousand words' comes to life, because it demands the cognitive skills of the clinician. The images that follow will illustrate this well.

14 Neurologic disorders

- Rapid onset lower motor neuron paralysis – think ticks, organophosphate, botulism, polyradiculoneuropathy, metronidazole or some other adverse drug reaction, coral snake or other source of neurotoxin.
- Cats with dilated pupils and blank stare – think thiamine deficiency.
- Coma: diffuse cerebral, brainstem, but don't forget metabolic.
- Animal brains have amazing recuperative ability with time and good patient care.
- Loss of the oculocephalic reflex is very concerning and a sign of a very guarded prognosis.

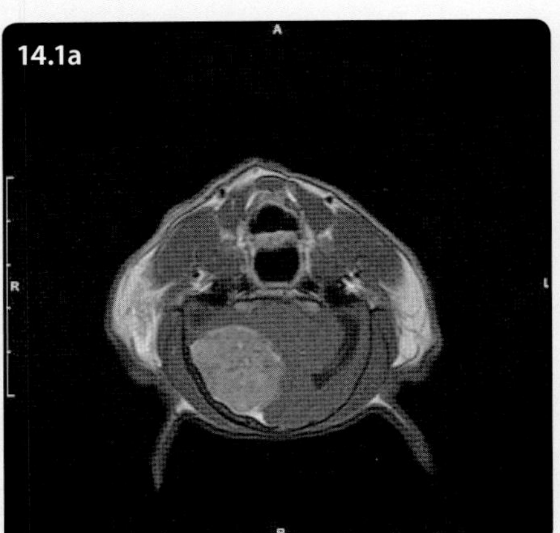

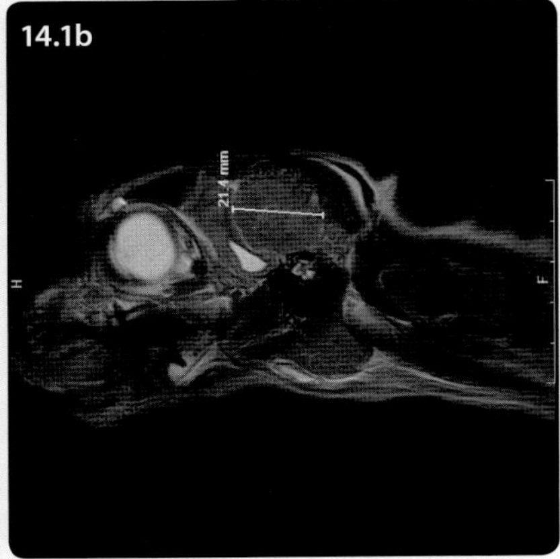

14.1a, b. Meningioma in a cat. These CT views show a very large meningioma in a cat. Many dogs and cats can accommodate slow growing large brain tumors, sometimes with a paucity of abnormal signs. Any surgical attempt to remove this mass could lead to anterior–posterior syndrome because of a herniation that already looks likely at the occipital foramen. Osmotic agents such as mannitol would be essential to help lessen the potentially fatal consequences.

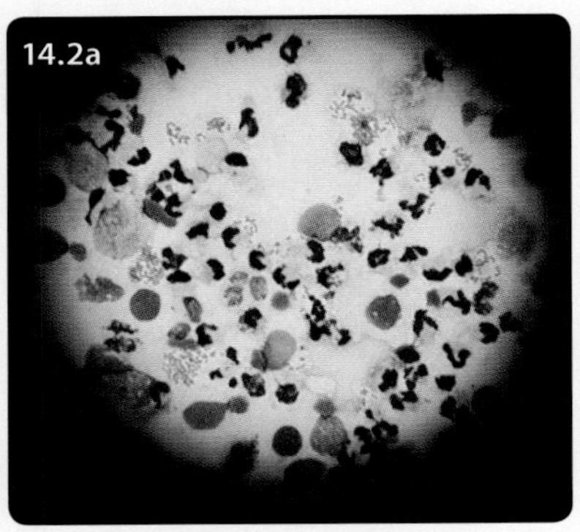

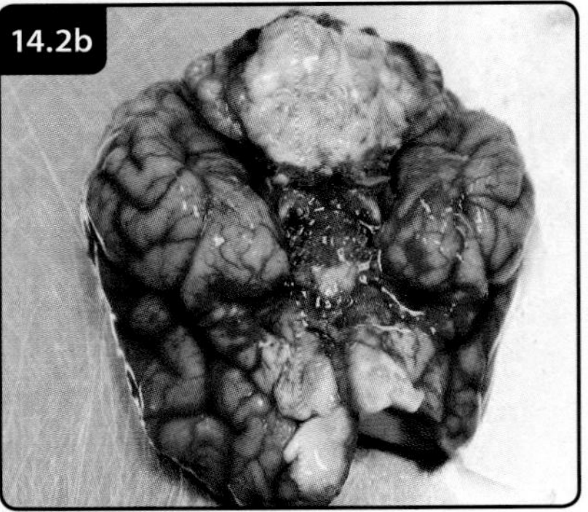

14.2a, b. Streptococcal meningitis in an English Bulldog. Pure bacterial meningitis is an uncommon disorder in the dog. The signs include neck pain and guarding, fever, and generalized systemic illness, as was the case in this dog at the time that the cerebrospinal fluid cytology (Figure 14.2a) showed this septic involvement. The dog died and the accompanying image shows the diffuse inflammation of the meninges (Figure 14.2b).

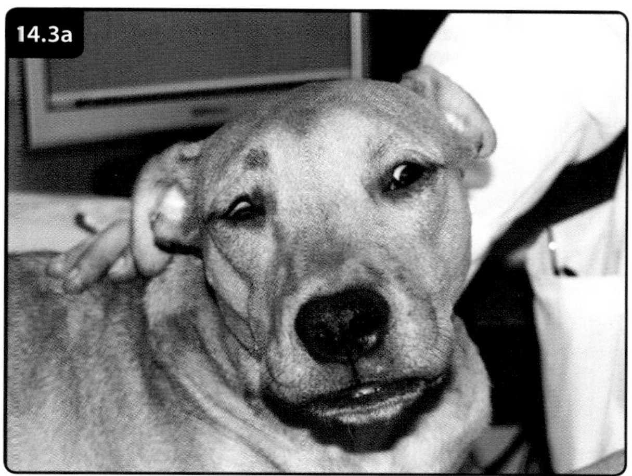

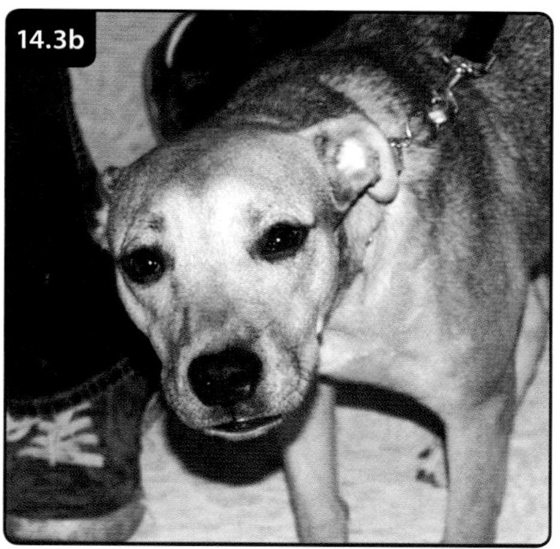

14.3a, b. Ciprofloxacin-associated polyneuropathy. This dog was receiving ciprofloxacin for an unusually long duration (approximately 8 weeks) for a respiratory infection. It then had slow-onset generalized weakness and cranial nerve abnormalities, as seen in Figure 14.3a (note the ventral deviation of the eyes and the abnormal mouth appearance). This has been reported in humans and in other animals, albeit uncommonly. The respiratory disease was in remission so the drug was discontinued. All of the abnormal neurologic signs disappeared over the next 2 weeks, and the dog returned to normal, as shown in Figure 14.3b.

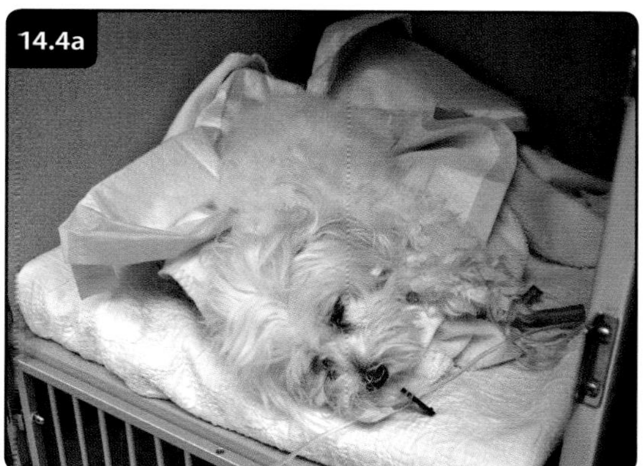

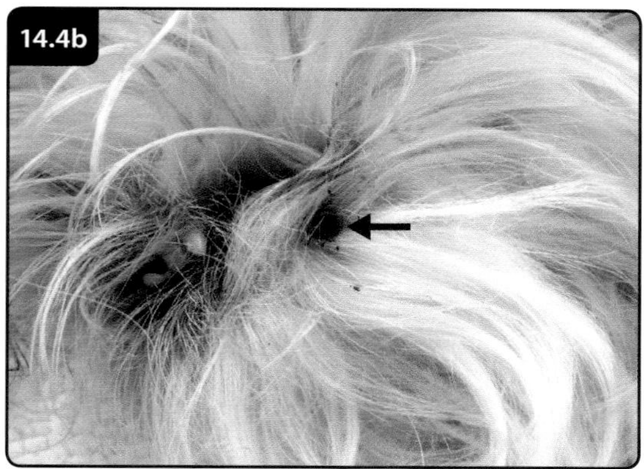

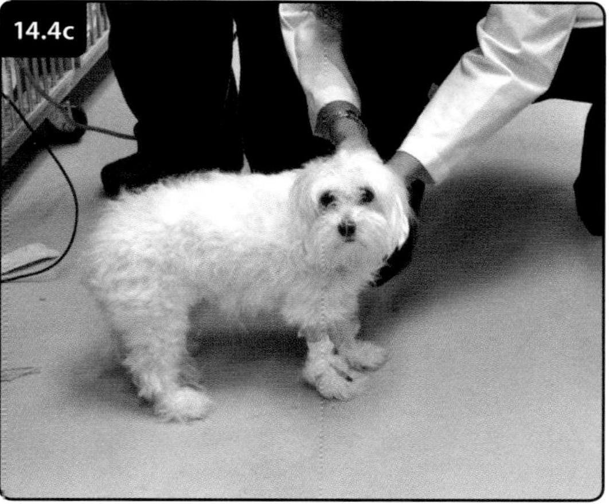

14.4a–c. Tick paralysis. Tick paralysis was diagnosed in this dog when it presented with an acute lower motor neuron neuropathy (Figure 14.4a) and an engorged tick attached to its body (Figure 14.4b, arrow). The dog returned to normal over the next 12 hours after the tick was removed (Figure 14.4c). The detrimental effects of tick paralysis will vary in different regions of the world. This case is typical of what occurs in the USA. The tick paralysis syndrome in Australia is much more severe because of its tendency to compromise ventilation and require ventilatory assistance. It would be prudent to warn owners of possible tick transmittable diseases should clinical signs arise over the subsequent 2 weeks following a tick bite.

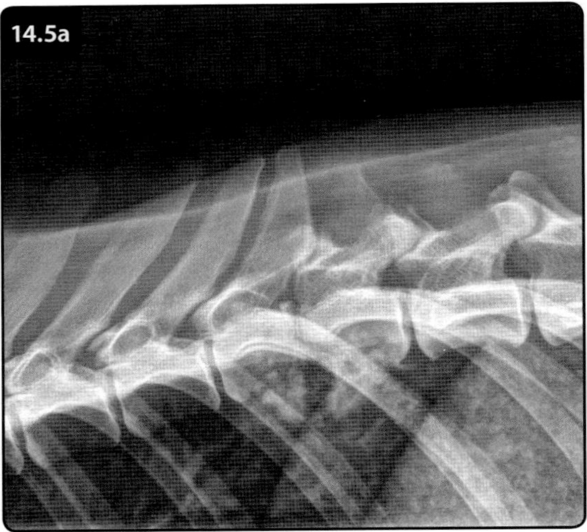

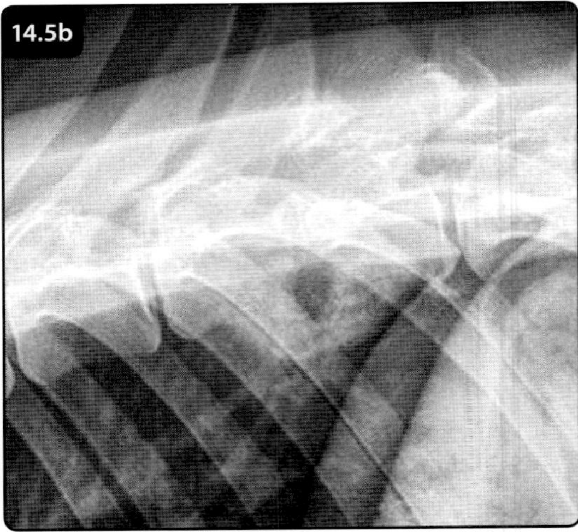

14.5a, b. Diskospondylitis. These spinal radiographs are from a dog that showed signs of fever, generalized pain, and focal hyperpathia over the thoracolumbar spine. The fever and the focal back pain put diskospondylitis high on the list of differentials. The radiographs show the typical subacute and more chronic changes of diskospondylitis osteolysis of the vertebral body and the endplates. These gross changes require approximately 3 weeks to become apparent on a radiograph. The cause can be either bacterial or fungal, with the latter having a worse prognosis. Fungal disease often involves other bones and body parts such as the eyes, where one would expect to find uveitis and chorioretinitis. If the dog is actively breeding, it would be helpful to search for *Brucella* organisms as a possible cause, although *Staphylococcus* spp., *Escherichia coli*, and *Streptococcus* spp. are more common bacterial causes.

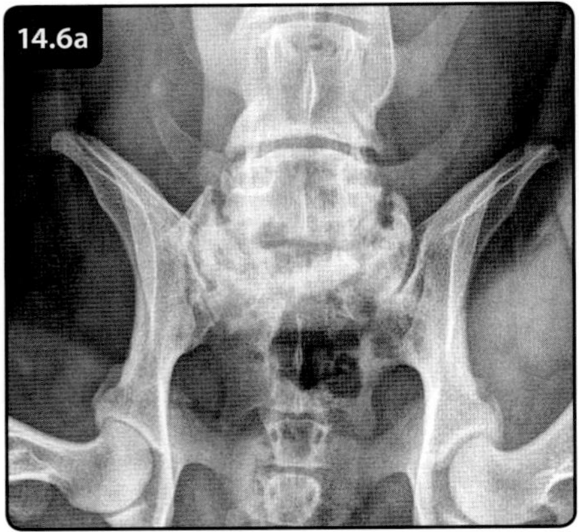

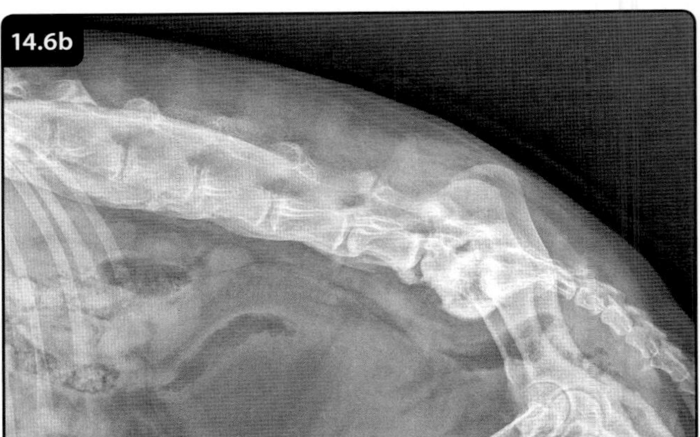

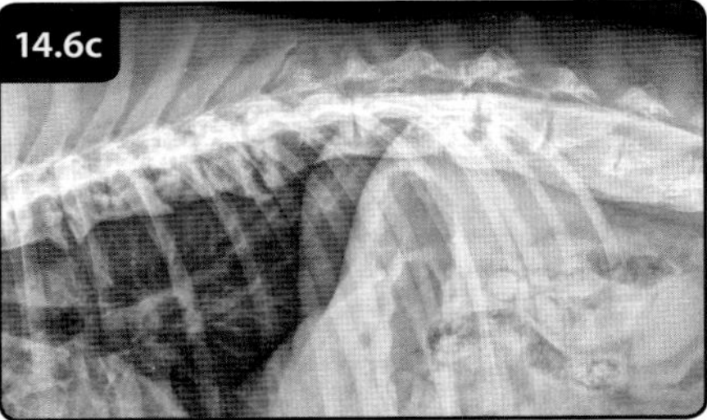

14.6a–c. Multifocal *Brucella suis* diskospondylosis in a dog. This dog had a history of chronic lumbar pain. The radiographs show L6-L7 endplate erosion and vertebral osteolysis of L7. The same lesions are evident in the caudal thoracic spine. Further medical evaluation of this dog should include a urinalysis and culture and sensitivity. A CT-guided aspiration biopsy of the involved spine for culture and cytology and serum *Brucella* titers would also provide important information. The dog's titer result was *Brucella suis* positive.

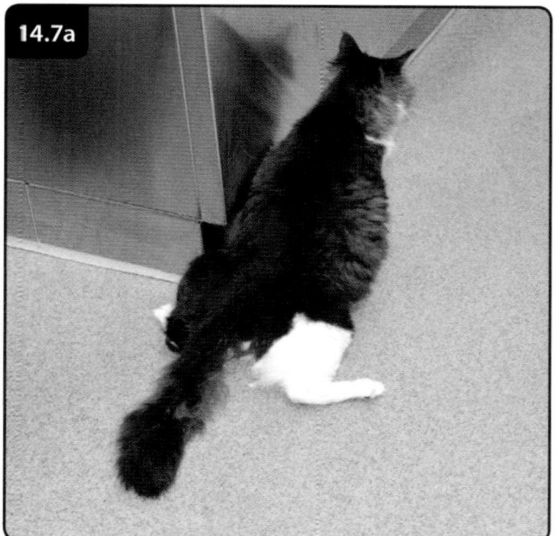

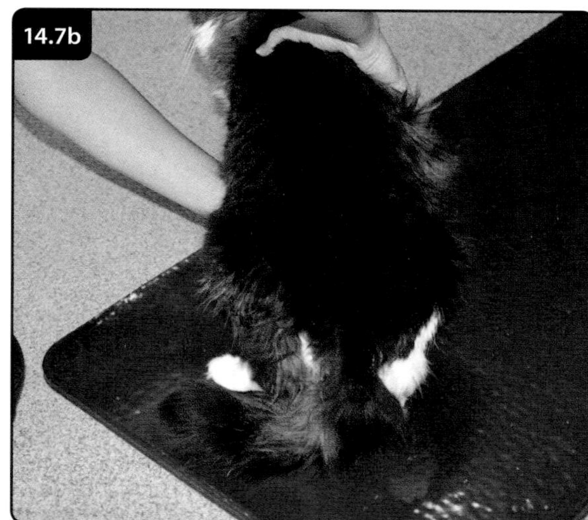

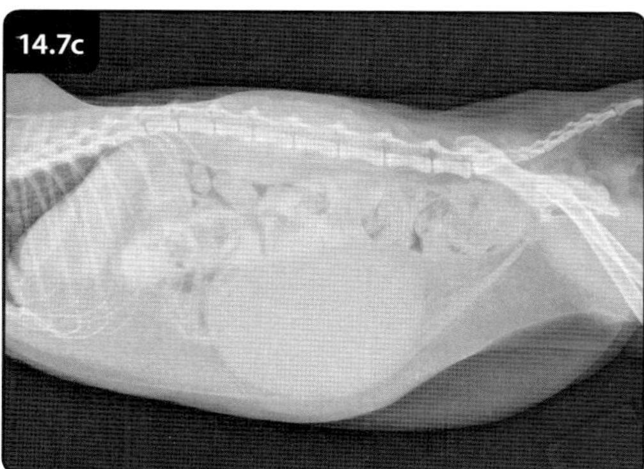

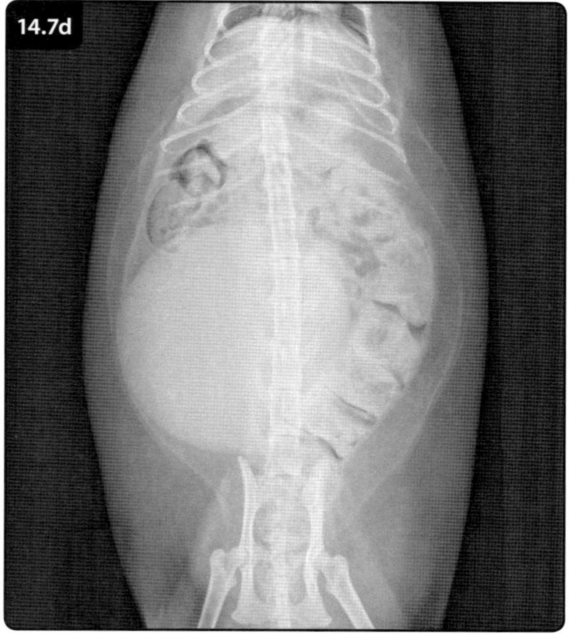

14.7a–d. Caudal spine neuropathy with involvement of the pelvic plexus. This cat is showing hindlimb abduction (compatible with obturator nerve dysfunction) in addition to its bilateral hindlimb weakness. The cat also had marked constipation and a very distended urinary bladder, indicating dysfunction of the pelvic plexus. This combination of signs would likely be associated with a guarded to grave prognosis.

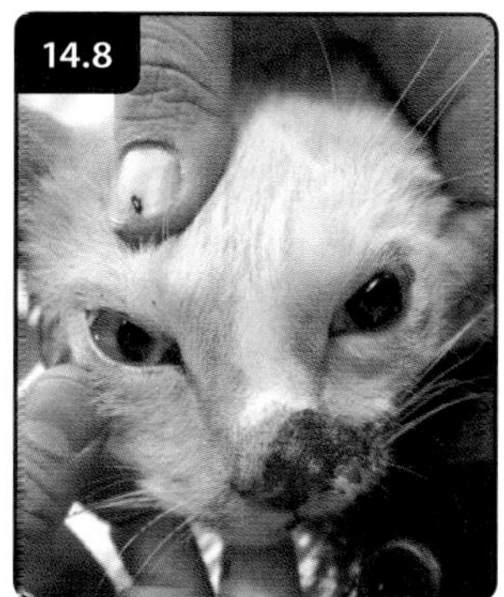

14.8. Severe brainstem trauma. This cat sustained brain injury after it was hit by a car. The clinical signs included quadriparesis, epistaxis, coma, absent oculocephalic reflex, anisocoria, and left-sided Horner's syndrome, which were compatible with midbrain damage and was indicative of a guarded to grave prognosis. The cat deteriorated and died despite supportive treatment that included hypertonic saline treatment for the brain swelling.

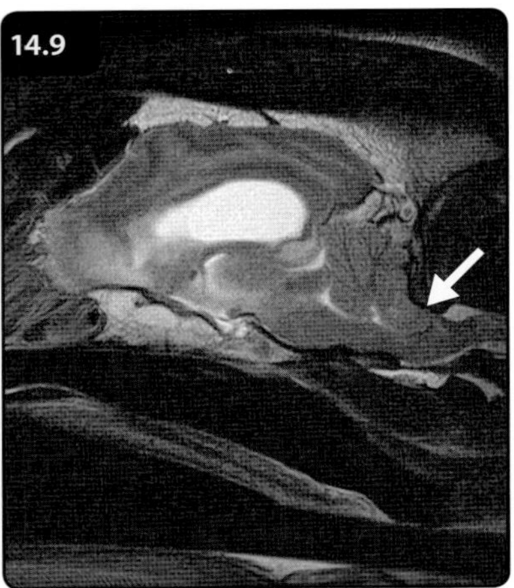

14.9. Brain herniation through the occipital foramen. This MR image shows dilated lateral ventricles and a caudally displaced cerebellum and medulla through the occipital foramen (arrow). Brainstem compression in this area can be life-threatening and would discourage any plans for a cerebrospinal fluid tap through the cistern for fear of pithing the medulla.

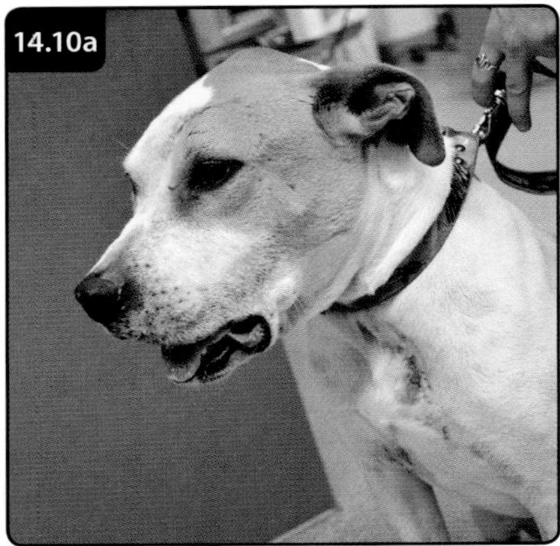

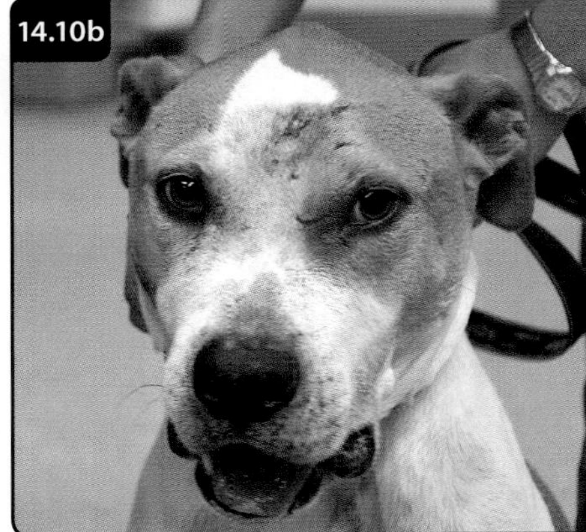

14.10a, b. Trigeminal palsy. This dog was hit by a car and suffered head wounds. Note the dropped jaw, which in this case was attributed to injury to the motor branch of the mandibular nerve. Other causes, such as mandibular bone fracture or temporal mandibular joint trauma, were not present. A traumatic lesion such as this can improve with time.

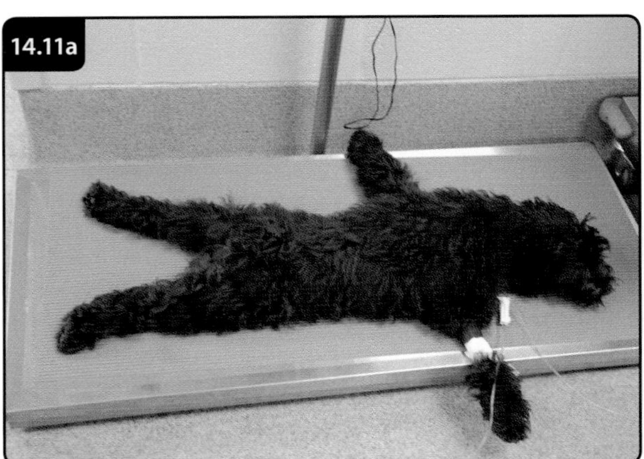

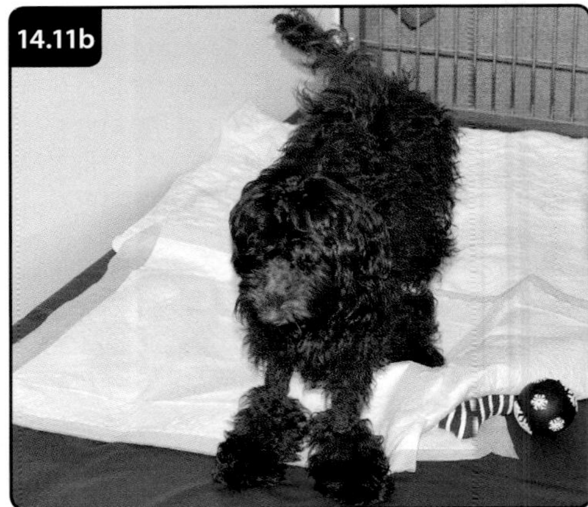

14.11a, b. Severe tetanus in a dog. This 4-month-old Golden Doodle puppy had a severe form of tetanus that included complete spastic paralysis, autonomic dysfunction of temperature and heart rate regulation, and loss of voluntary ventilation. He required approximately 10 days of ventilator support and 2 months of intensive care for complete recovery.

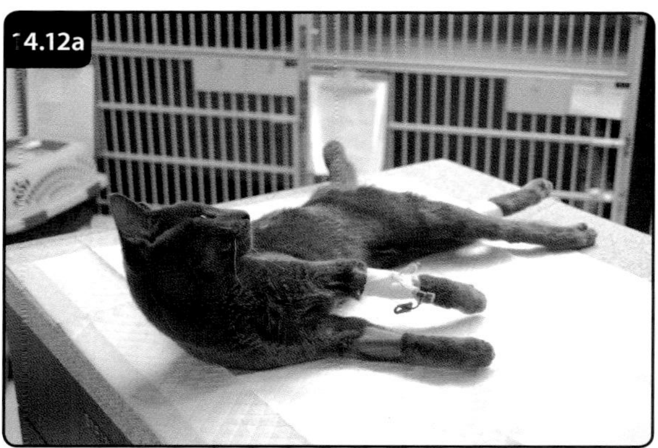

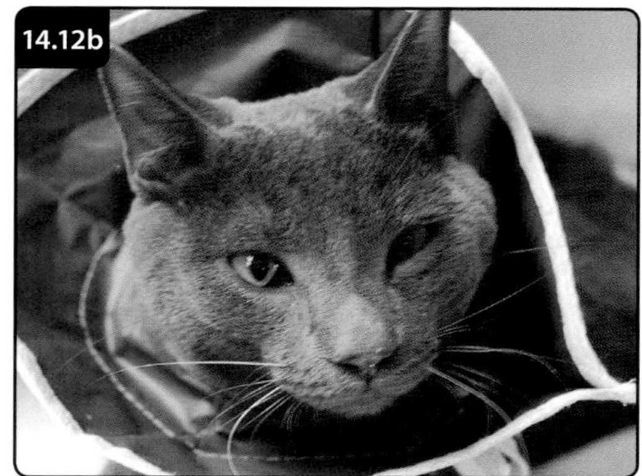

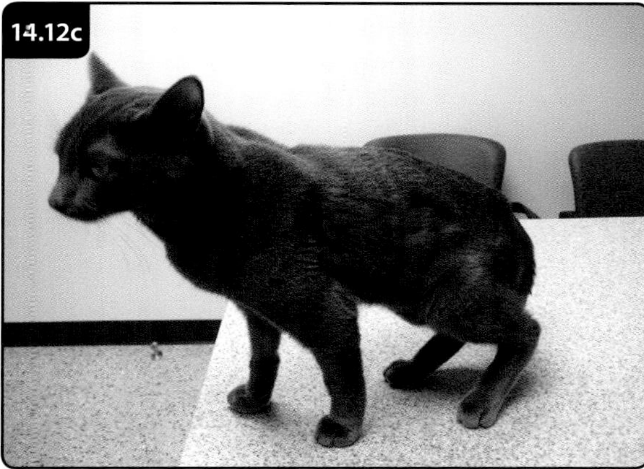

14.12a–c. Tetanus in a cat. Cats are not as susceptible to tetanus as dogs. Infection commonly causes spastic paralysis of both hindlimbs and spasticity involving the muscles of facial expression (Figures 14.14a, b). Most cats will need an indwelling urinary catheter until they regain functional use of their hindlimbs, with normal function requiring approximately 2 weeks (Figure 14.12c).

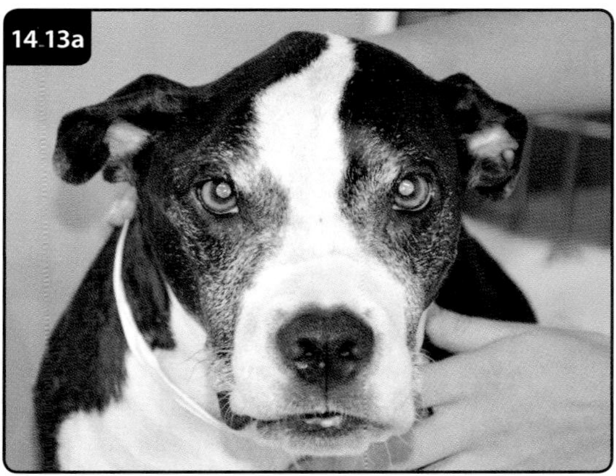

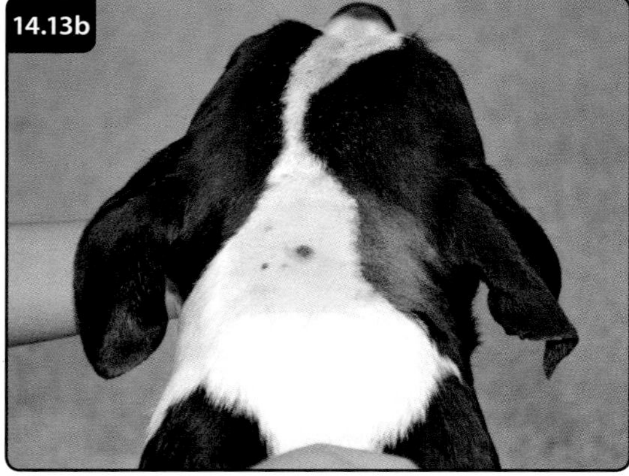

14.13a, b. Masseter atrophy in a dog. The unilateral right-sided masseter muscle atrophy in this dog was due to pathology involving the right trigeminal nerve. Various causes include trauma, neoplasia, and polyradiculoneuropathy.

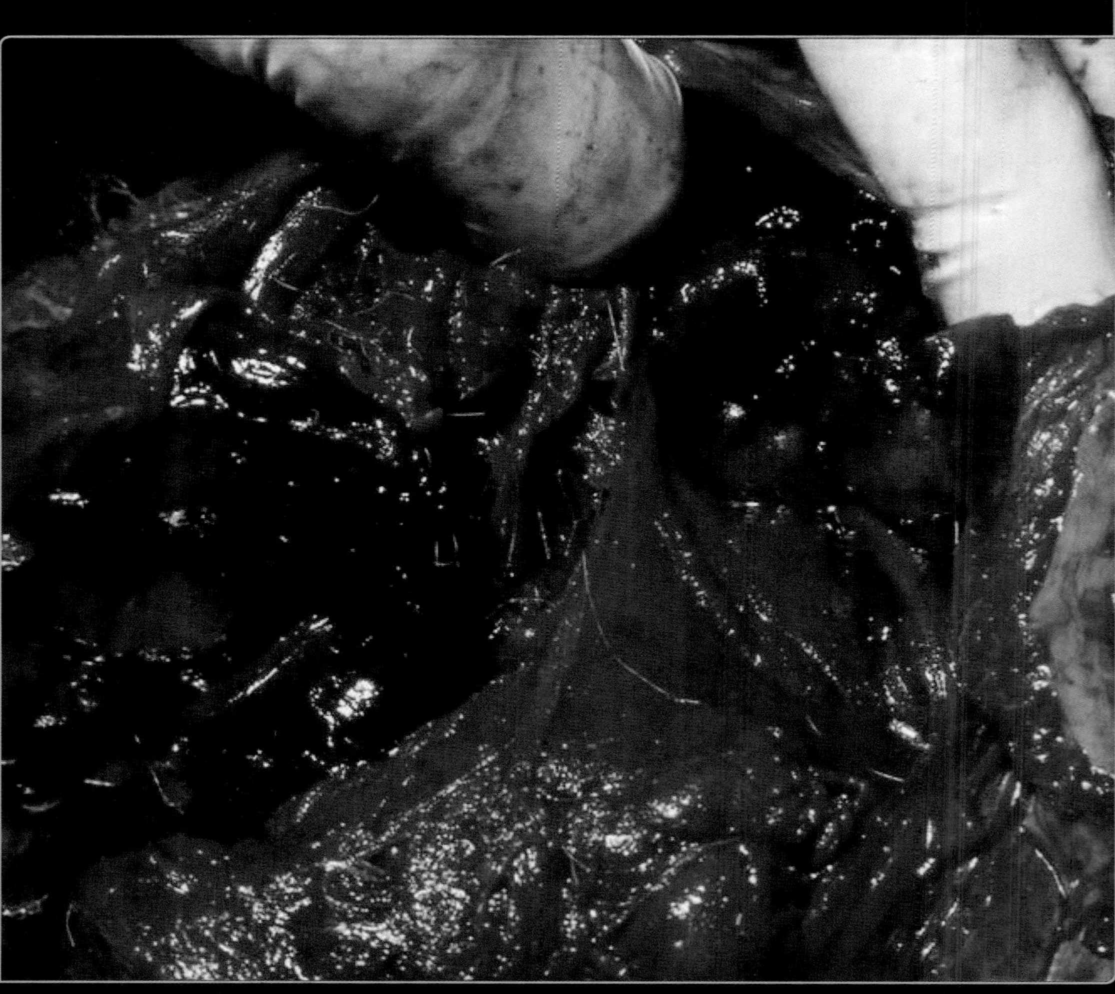

▲ Hemangiosarcoma involving the thigh muscles seen at necropsy.

15

Neoplastic disorders

NEOPLASIA comes from the Greek words *neo*, meaning new, and *plasis*, meaning molding. Cancer has reached epidemic proportions in human and veterinary medicine and it should come as no surprise that close to 40% of the cases that come into a veterinary referral facility are cancerous disorders. Therefore, it behoves the clinician to know when to biopsy a tissue that might be neoplastic. Cancer can involve any tissue of the body and this, therefore, offers a clinician the opportunity to observe several interesting disorders. The two main diagnostic modalities are imaging and biopsy, but it is still essential to evaluate the entire patient in order to appreciate the full scope of the disease at hand. Many of the lesions illustrated will be available to visualization and palpation, thus making a thorough physical examination an essential part of the diagnostic evaluation.

15 Neoplastic disorders

- Cutaneous mast cell tumors can mimic any type of skin growth.
- Mammary tumors – 'Don't stick it, cut it'.
- Don't miss lymphangitic inflammatory mammary carcinoma.
- Copious mucoid nasal discharge – think nasal adenocarcinoma.
- Try gastric biopsy forceps for nasal biopsy.
- Cancer can cause elevated temperature, increased white blood cells, and fever.

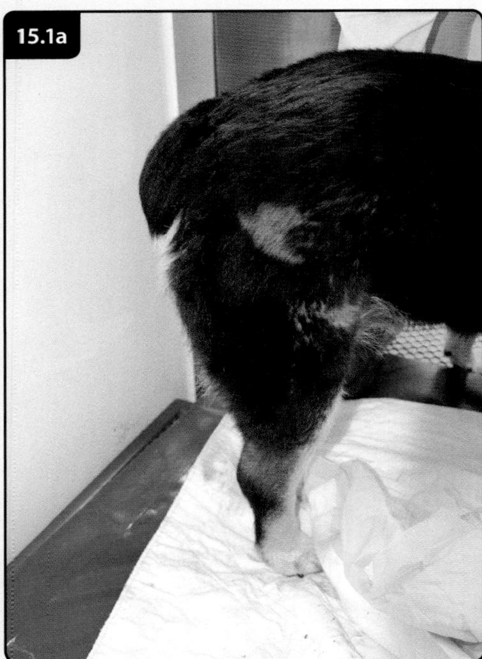
15.1a

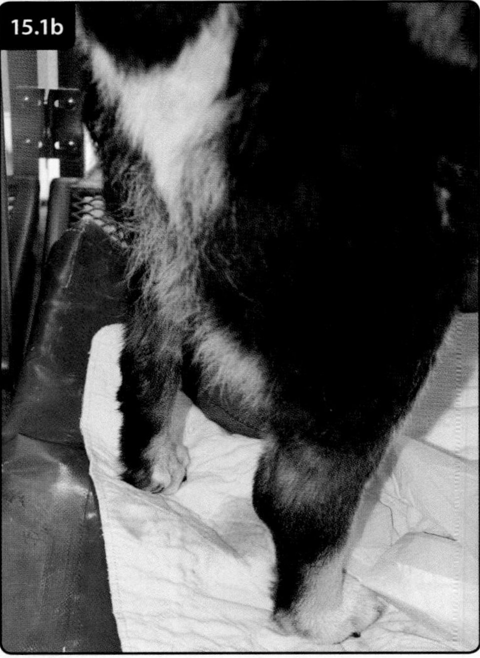
15.1b

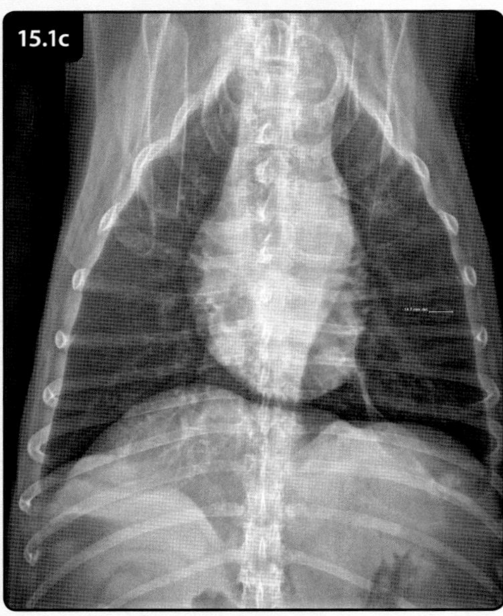
15.1c

15.2. Bronchogenic carcinoma in the dog. Many animals with diffuse lung cancer do not cough when the cancer is distributed mainly to the periphery. However, if the tumor causes tracheal–bronchial compression, coughing will be a primary clinical sign because the cough reflex has its sensory fibers in the bronchi and the trachea. This is a bronchoscopic view of a bronchogenic carcinoma causing compression to the secondary airways. Coughing would be associated with this type of lesion.

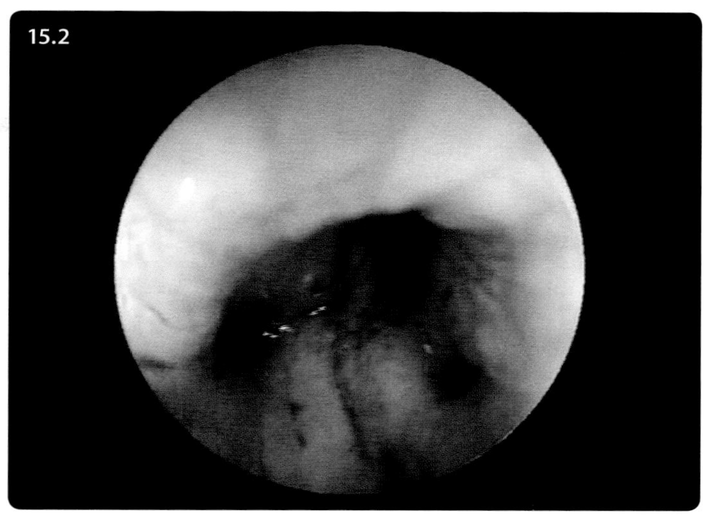

15.3. Lymphosarcoma of the liver and kidneys at necropsy. This cat would likely present with weight loss and an absent appetite. The extent of tumor involvement would allow for detection of hepatomegaly and renomegaly on abdominal palpation. Diagnosis could be made with a fine needle aspirate and cytology of either organ.

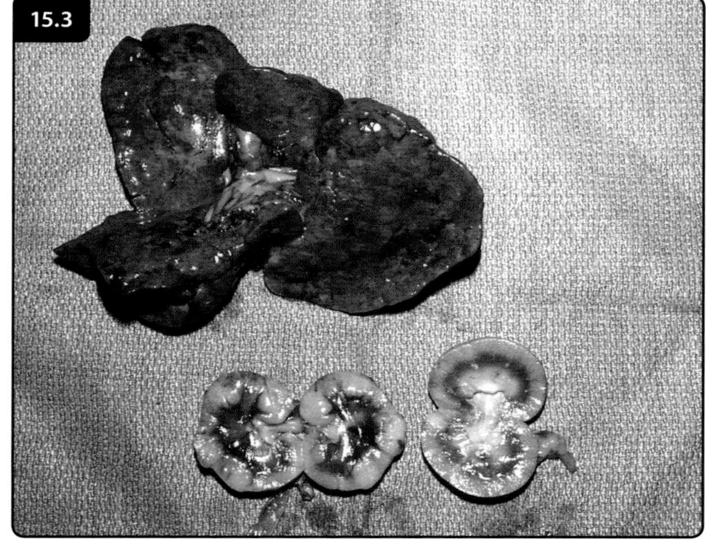

15.1a–c. Inflammatory mammary carcinoma causing lymphatic obstruction. This female mixed breed dog was evaluated for inflamed mammary masses that were diagnosed on biopsy as inflammatory mammary carcinoma. The cancer had invaded the lymphatic drainage nodes and vessels, which caused lymphatic obstruction and resulted in swelling of the dog's hindlimbs, especially the right hindlimb. Radiography revealed metastatic nodules in the lungs (Figure 15.1c). The lesions were not amendable to treatment and the dog was subsequently euthanized.

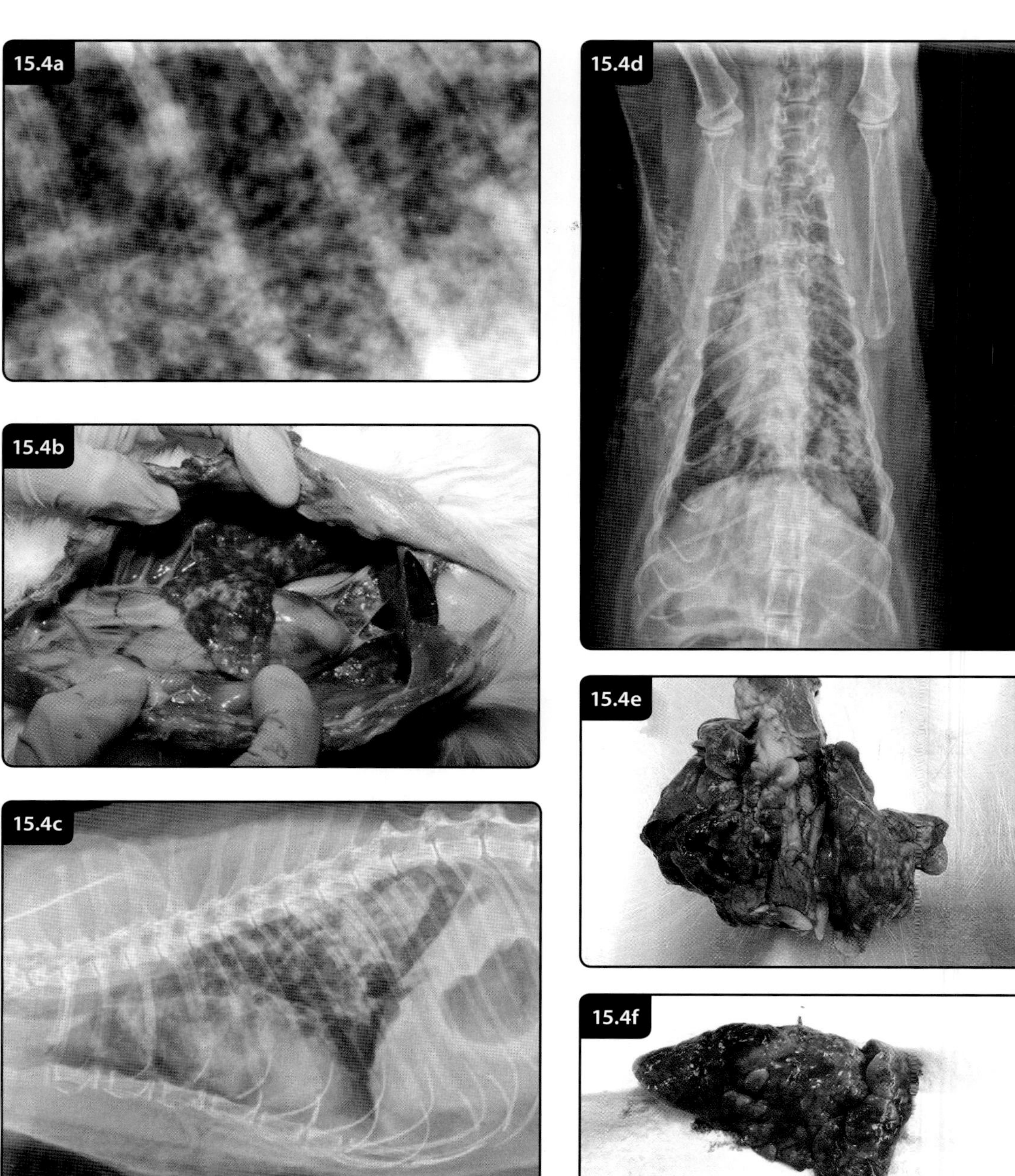

15.4a–f. Pulmonary carcinoma in two cats. Figures 15.4a, b and Figures 15.4c–f are from two different cats that had each been diagnosed with pulmonary adenocarcinoma. The radiographs (Figures 15.4a, c, and d) show diffuse pulmonary infiltrate as an alveolar–interstitial infiltrate. Clinically, these cats will become progressively dyspneic and cachechtic. Diagnosis is made by surgical lung biopsy and histopathology. These tumors are not easily accessed with tracheal wash cytology unless they directly infiltrate the tracheal lumen. Shown are radiographic, surgical (Figure 15.4b), and pathologic (Figures 15.4e, f) features.

15.5a–c. Hemangiosarcoma involving the thigh muscles. Hemangiosarcoma is a ubiquitous tumor because it can arise from blood vessels located almost anywhere in the body. It most commonly involves the spleen, liver, and right auricle, but it can also involve other tissues as well. Primary hemangiosarcoma of the thigh muscles can grow to a fairly large size (Figure 15.5a) before it eventually bleeds and causes rapid distension of the thigh tissues. At this point the dog becomes lame, and physical examination will show the swollen and reddish discolored tissues. When the leg is opened at necropsy, the cancer tissue appears as clots, as shown in Figures 15.5b, c. This is the tissue that should be taken for histopathology. Some of these patients have disseminated intravascular coagulation.

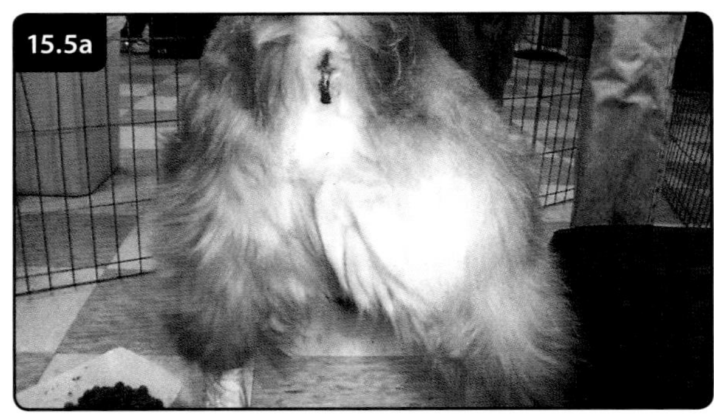
15.5a

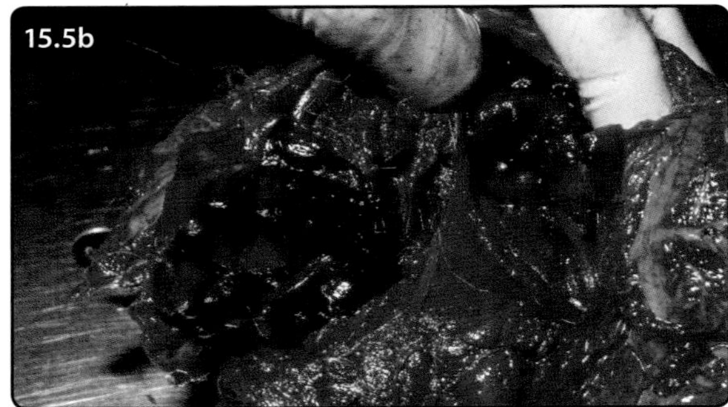
15.5b

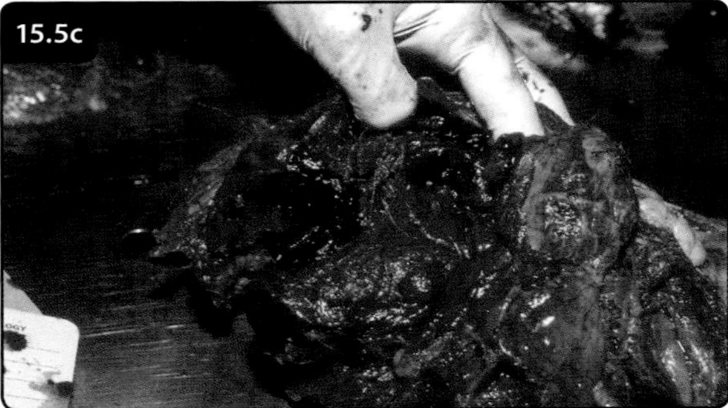
15.5c

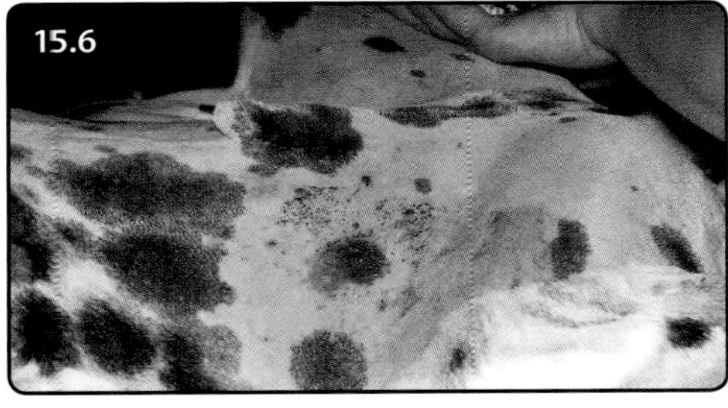
15.6

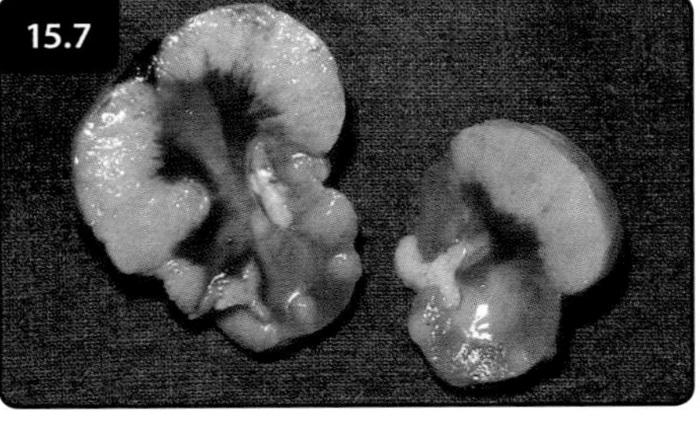
15.7

15.6. Cutaneous hemangiosarcoma. This tumor affects both dogs and cats. Surgical delay will eventually lead to nonresectable disease. Any suspicious lesion should be biopsied and then staged for a second surgery with clean margins. Thoracic radiographs are indicated during the initial patient evaluation.

15.7. Renal lymphoma. This cancer occurs as a bilateral disease and it will cause renomegaly. Progressive disease will impair kidney function. Bilateral renomegaly is usually detectable with abdominal palpation. Prognosis is guarded to grave because of the progressive nature of the disease.

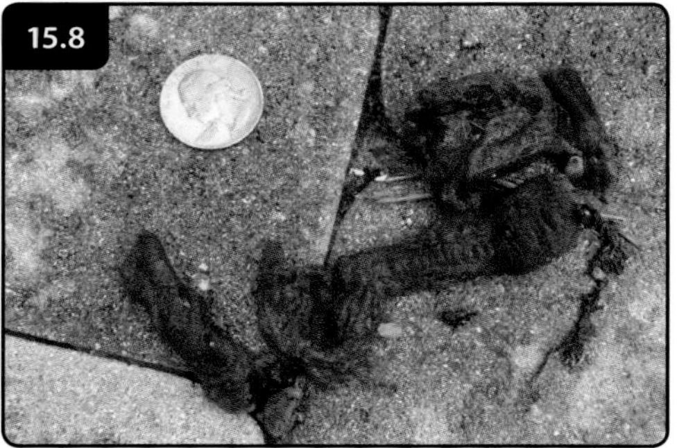

15.8. Gastrointestinal lymphoma in a dog. The sloughed intestinal cast shown is bowel mucosa from a dog with gastrointestinal lymphoma following chemotherapy. This can potentially lead to bowel perforation and sepsis because of the lost bowel mucosal barrier. The owner placed a 25 cent piece beside the cast for size comparison. This case is also discussed in Chapter 9 (9.46).

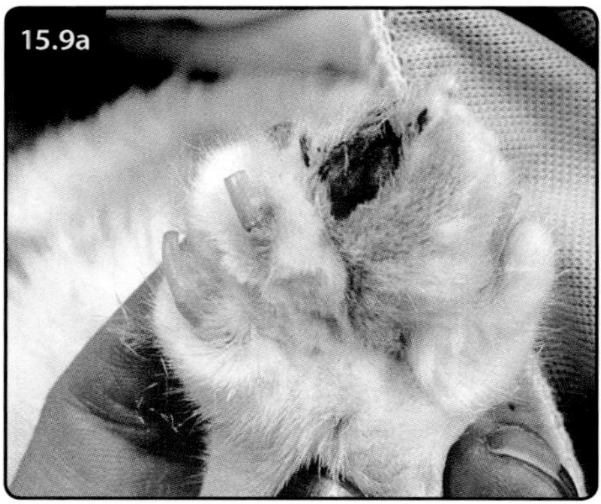

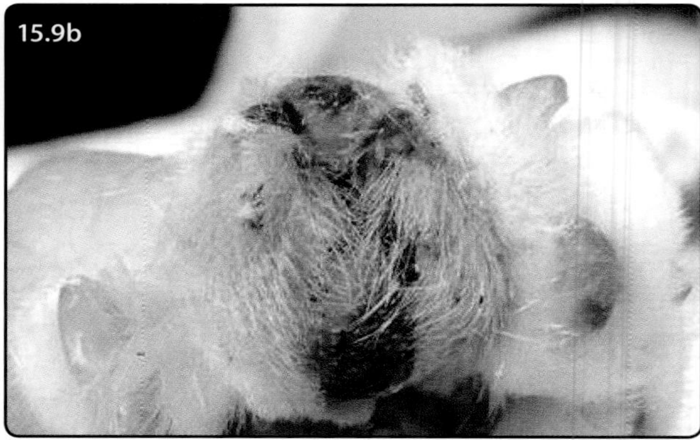

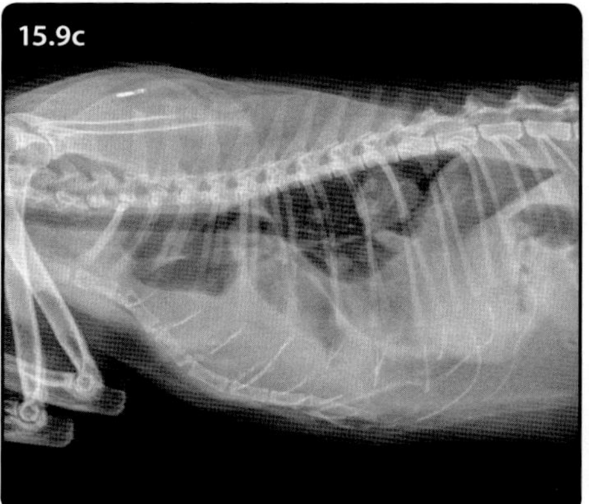

15.9a–c. Pulmonary carcinoma in a cat with digit metastasis. Primary lung tumors in the cat are rare. Pulmonary carcinomas tend to send off metastatic tumor emboli to the digits (Figures 15.9a, b). Figure 15.9c shows a lateral radiograph with pleural effusion and pulmonary infiltrate representative of lung carcinoma. The cytology of the chest fluid aspirate showed abnormal cells with features of a carcinoma. The cat was euthanized.

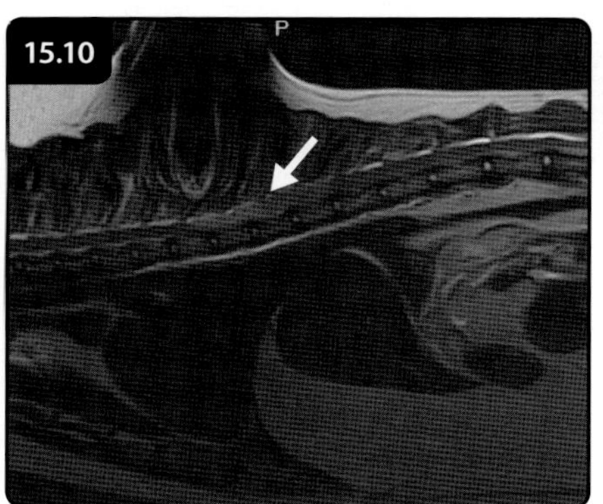

15.10. Lymphoma in the spinal canal. This MR image shows an abnormality spanning four vertebrae in the mid-thoracic spinal cord (arrow). The cytology on the cerebrospinal fluid sample showed malignant lymphocytes.

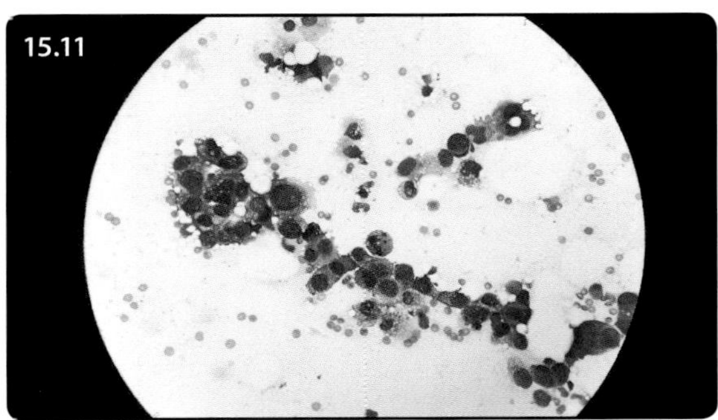

15.11. Cytology of mammary carcinoma in a dog. This cytology slide was taken from a dog with the inflammatory form of mammary carcinoma. The cells have abnormal nuclear cytoplasmic ratios, anisocytosis and anisokaryosis, vacuolated cytoplasm, bi-nucleate cells, and other features of atypia. The prognosis is usually grave because of the high tendency for metastasis.

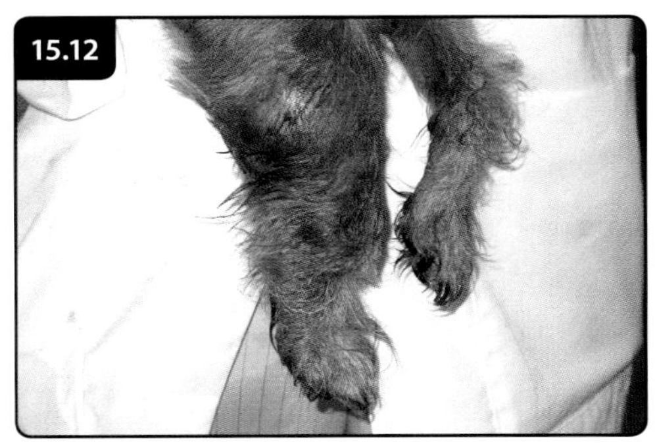

15.12. Mast cell tumor (MCT) in a dog. This tumor involves the soft tissues of the right forelimb. A fine needle aspirate cytology sample identified the mass as an MCT. These tumors can resemble many different types of neoplasms. When the index of suspicion is high for the presence of an MCT, the patient would benefit from receiving diphenhydramine 30 minutes prior to aspirating to help avoid any adverse effects caused by mast cell degranulation associated with manipulation of the mass.

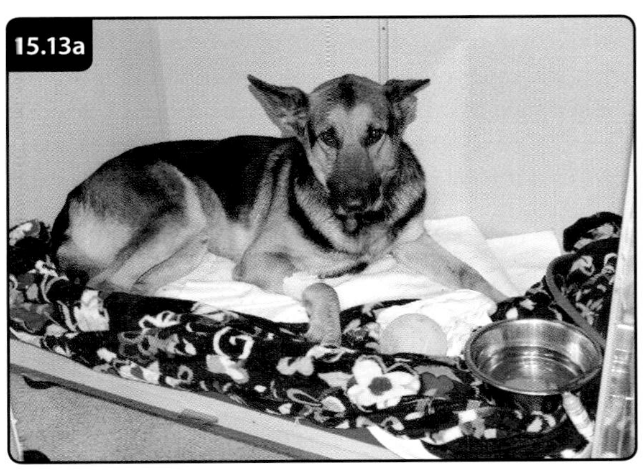

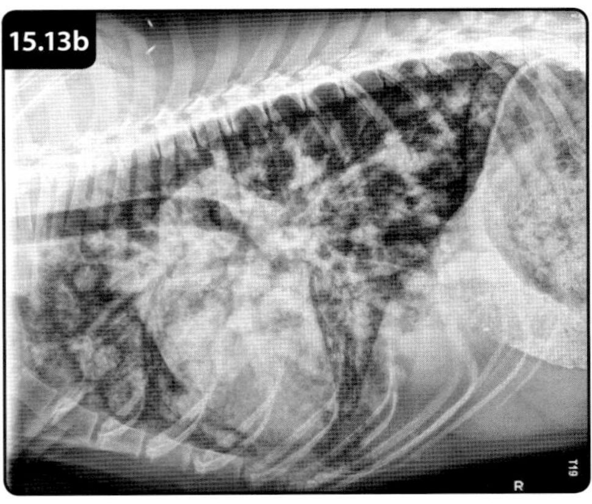

15.13a–c. Pulmonary adenosquamous cell carcinoma. Most primary lung tumors in the dog occur in the older age group. This dog, a 3-year-old neutered male German Shepherd Dog, presented with labored breathing from lung masses that were diagnosed with thoracoscopy and biopsy as adenosquamous cell carcinoma. The majority of primary lung tumors in dogs are adenocarcinomas.

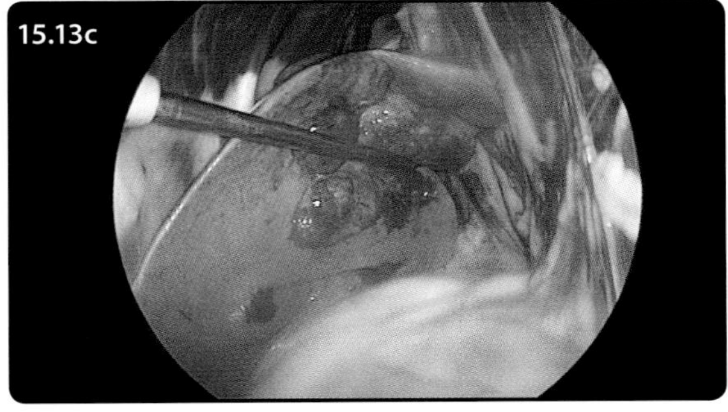

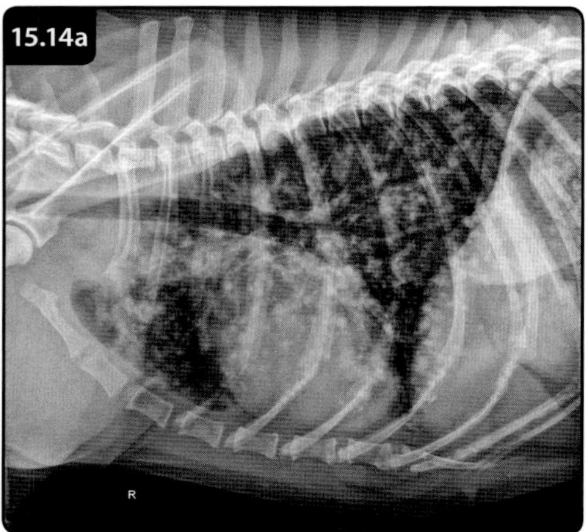

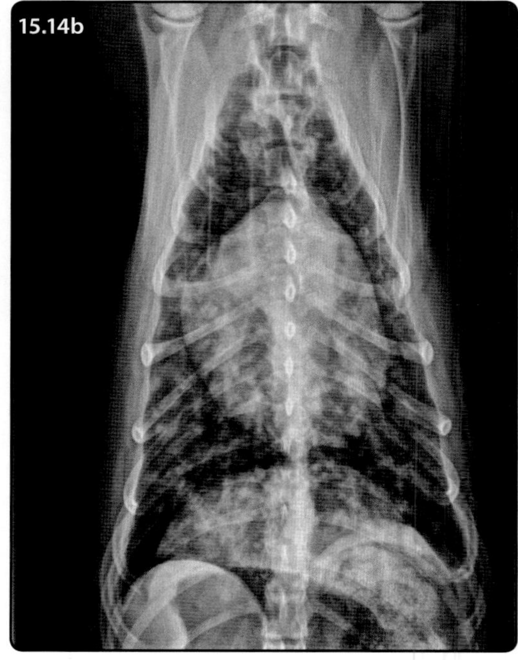

15.14a, b. Metastatic skeletal muscle hemangiosarcoma in a dog. As noted earlier, hemangiosarcoma can appear as a primary neoplasm originating in skeletal muscle (see Figures 15.5b, c). These thoracic radiographs show diffuse metastasis to the lungs.

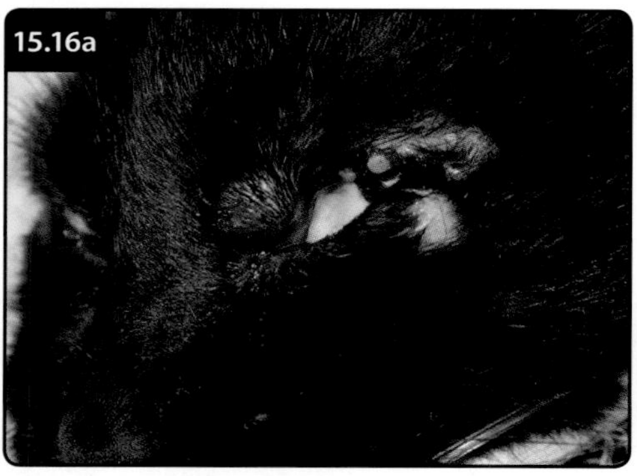

15.15. Pancreatic carcinoma with carcinomatosis in a cat. This necropsy image shows the pancreas on the right side and diffuse nodularity throughout the abdominal organs and mesentery (carcinomatosis). Pancreatic carcinoma is well known for this metastatic tendency. It is associated with a grave prognosis in most species. Ascites, weight loss, anorexia, and sometimes icterus are typical signs of this disease.

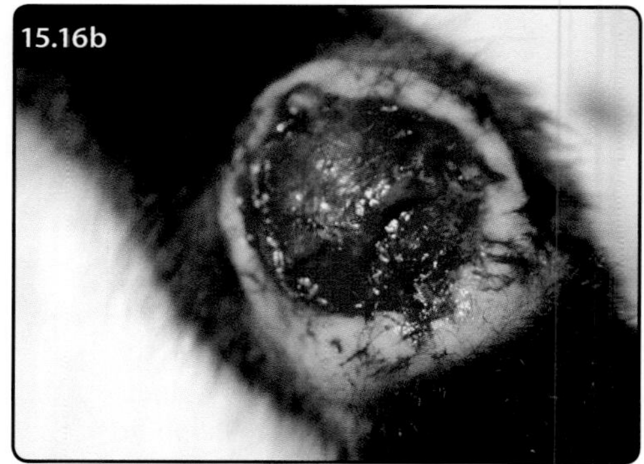

15.16a, b. Plasmacytoma in a cat. The incidence of plasmacytoma is comparatively less in cats than in dogs. It affects skin mostly, but it can also involve other organs. It usually has a benign course, but has malignant potential, so surgical removal is recommended. This cat had multiple site involvement, as shown in these two images showing periocular and forelimb involvements.

15.17. Squamous cell carcinoma in a dog. Squamous cell carcinoma (SCC) is a fairly common skin tumor, comprising 15% of all skin tumors in the cat but only 5% in the dog. In the dog, SCC is found most commonly in the nail beds, scrotum, nasal planum, legs, and anus. This dog has SCC of the nasal epithelium, and because it is bilateral, surgery would involve removal of most if not all of the anterior nose.

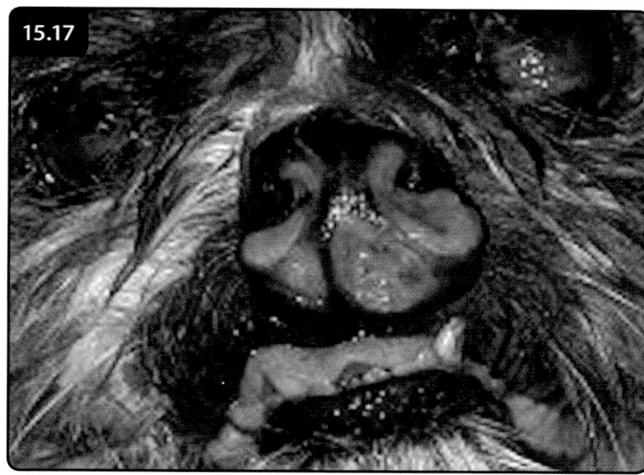
15.17

15.18a, b. Metastatic Sertoli cell tumor. These postmortem images are from a German Shepherd Dog that had a testicular Sertoli cell tumor removed 1 year prior. The dog had done well up until 2 weeks prior to examination, at which time he presented for progressive difficulty in breathing. The radiographs showed lesions compatible with metastatic disease. Figure 15.18a shows advanced metastasis to the chest while Figure 15.18b shows intra-abdominal spread to the external iliac lymph node and other caudal abdominal structures.

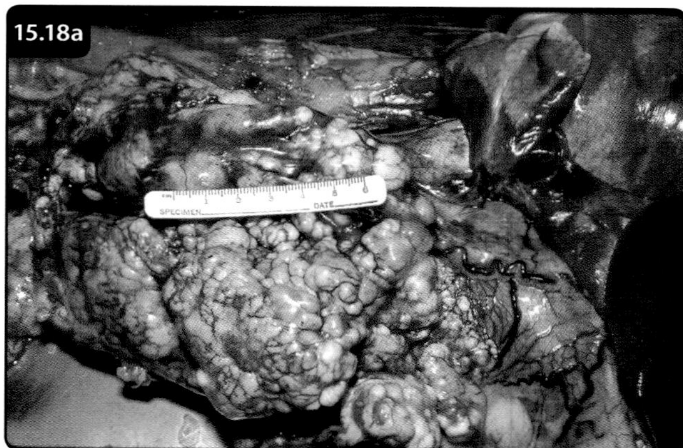
15.18a

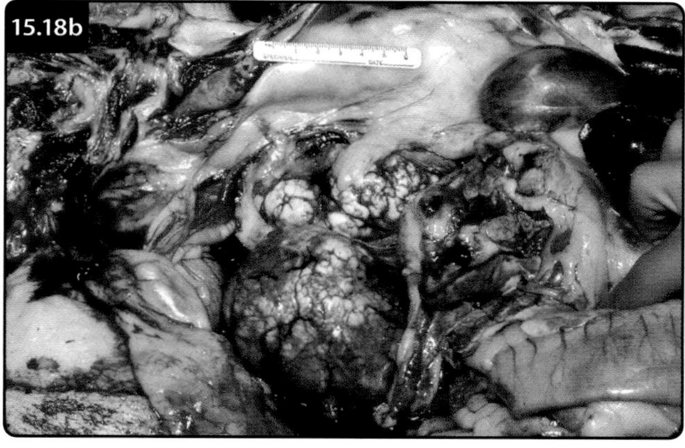
15.18b

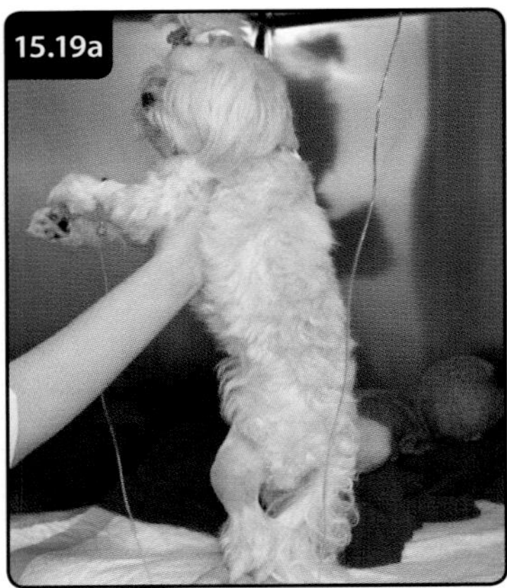

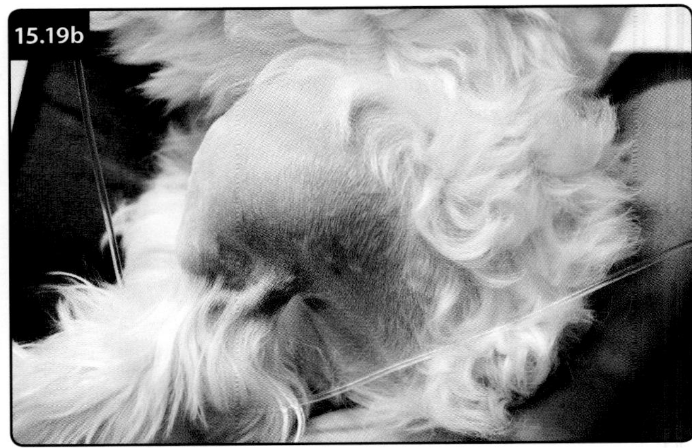

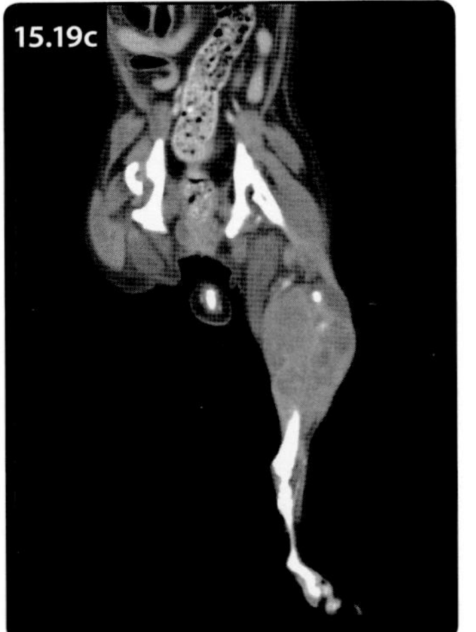

15.19a–c. Synovial cell sarcoma in a dog. This Maltese dog has had a progressive swelling of its right hindlimb characterized as firm and involving the distal femur and the proximal tibia (Figures 15.19a, b). The CT scan (Figure 15.19c) shows a soft tissue mass that crosses the joint, which is very characteristic of synovial cell sarcoma. Amputation would be the appropriate treatment option in the absence of gross metastatic disease.

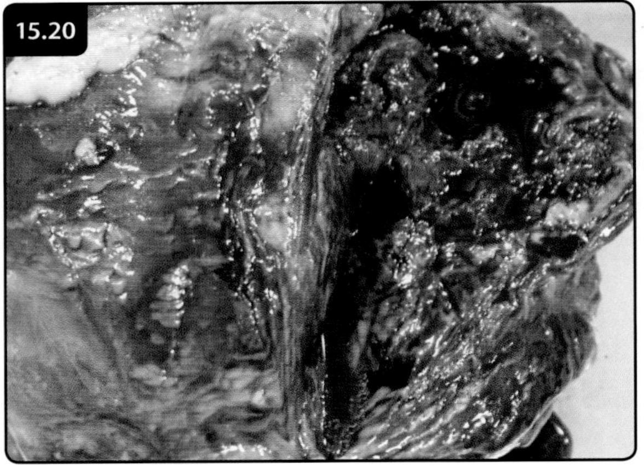

15.20. Telangiectatic osteosarcoma in a dog. This necropsy specimen is from a dog that presented with progressive disease that was ignored by the owner until the pathologic fracture made the dog immobile. Telangiectatic osteosarcoma is a highly malignant bone tumor that has a very grim prognosis. It is very vascular and causes profuse hemorrhage in the involved limb.

15.21. Cutaneous hemangiosarcoma in a dog. As with all hemangiosarcomas, this is a malignant tumor with a strong tendency to metastasize. The tumor should be treated with wide surgical excision and be deep enough to enable all of the neoplasm to be resected. Cutaneous hemangiosarcoma is best handled surgically in its earliest stages, unlike the lesion in Figure 15.21, which shows large infiltrative spread. This tumor also occurs in the cat with the same degree of severity. Thoracic radiography should precede surgery.

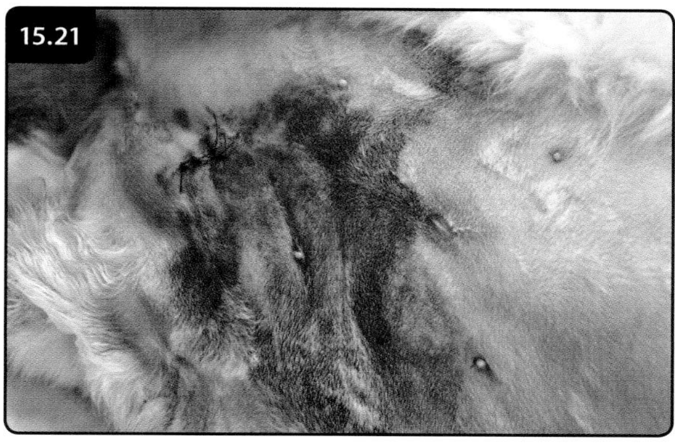

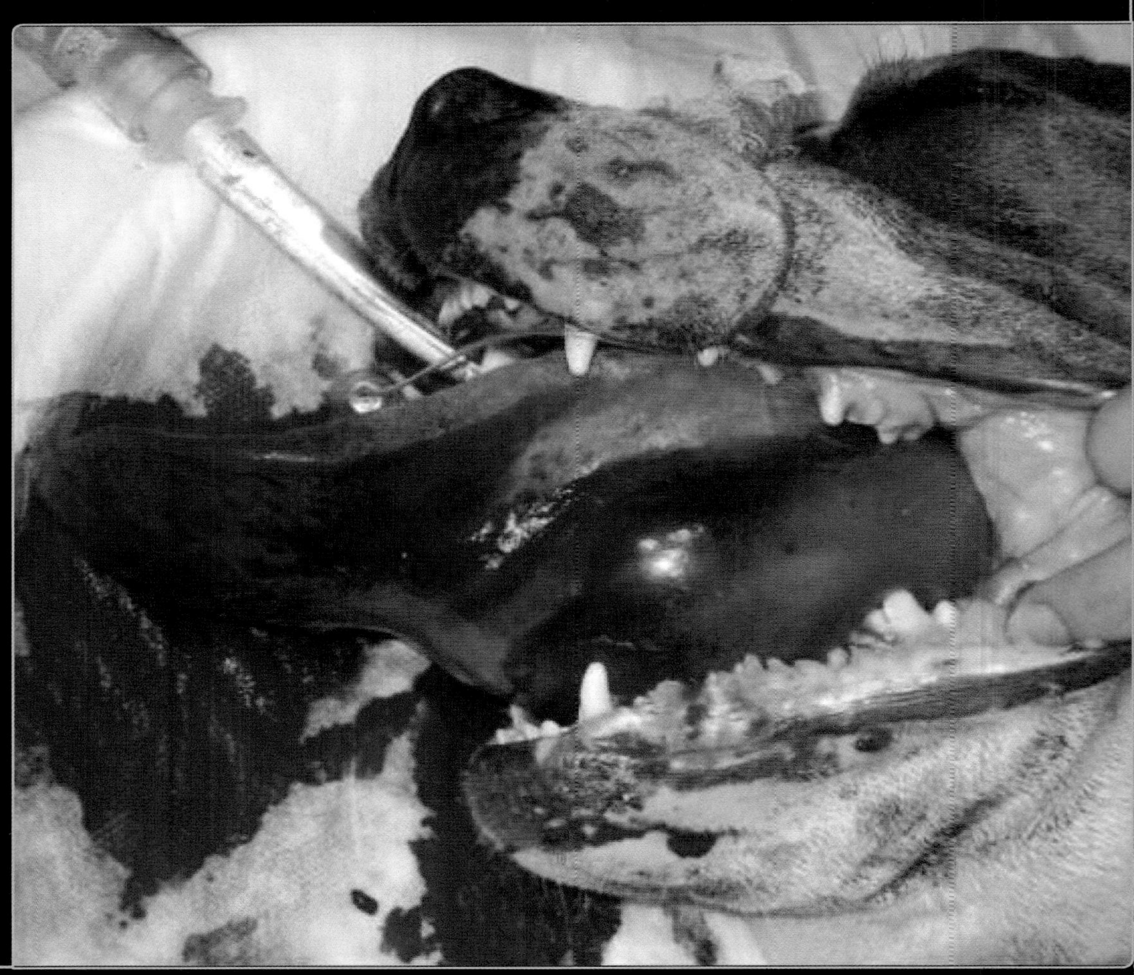

This massive sublingual hematoma was caused by an intraoral pit viper bite.

16

Toxicologic disorders (including snake bite envenomation)

TOXICOLOGY is derived from the Latin word *toxicon*, meaning poison. In small animal veterinary clinical practice, toxicology cases will often present as medical emergencies. The diagnosis and medical treatment are often fairly routine when the history provides the knowledge of exposure, but when that information is unavailable, the diagnosis will pose a definite challenge to the clinician. This is why the recognition of the characteristic signs of certain toxins is essential for making a timely and often life-saving diagnosis. The images that follow are all from true life cases representing the more common clinical toxicologic disorders. The clinician should also remember the antidotes for the various toxins and have them readily available in the hospital or close-by, where access can be expedient.

The reader will hopefully excuse the author for including snake bite envenomation in this 'picture book', but the nature of my practice in the State of Florida has offered me the opportunity to witness the devastating consequences that can occur when dogs and cats are envenomated by certain species of snakes. Although the examples that follow are due to bites from snakes indigenous to the Southeast United States, there are various other related snakes in other parts of the world that can cause similar pathology. Here again, modern day travel can bring animals from afar to parts of the world where these poisonous snakes prevail, thereby justifying some familiarization with these very interesting disorders.

16

Toxicologic disorders (including snake bite envenomation)

- Unexplainable radiodense particles in the bowel – think lead.
- Newly acquired bleeding – think anticoagulant rodenticide intoxication.
- Dimercaptosuccinic acid (DMSA; succimer) – an oral treatment for lead poisoning.
- Lipid infusions might help avermectin intoxication.
- Acetylcysteine for acetaminophen intoxication.

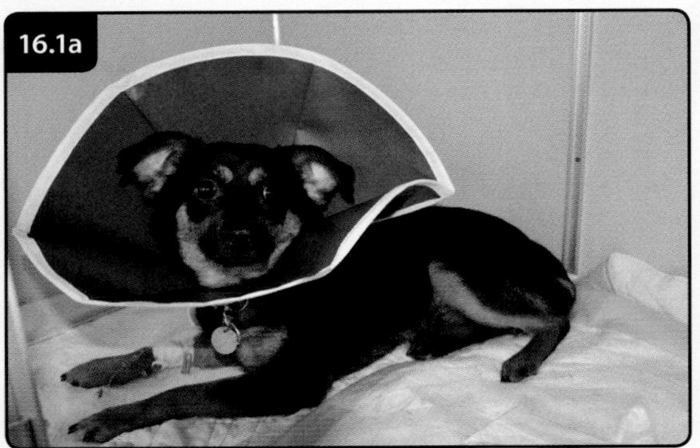

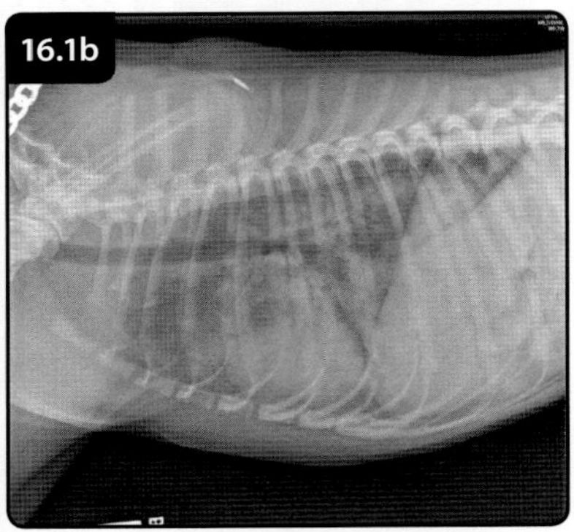

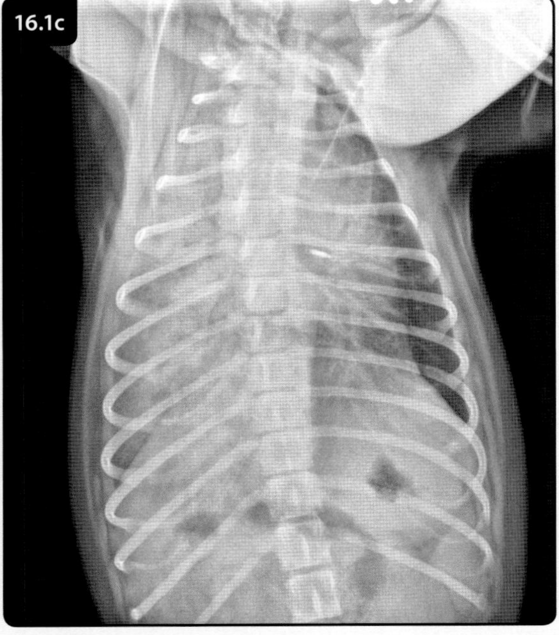

16.1a–c. Young dog with difficulty breathing that had developed gradually over the past 24 hours. The physical examination found the dog to be dyspneic with some abnormal lung sounds. There was a small amount of blood in a sample of sputum. The radiographs show a diffuse alveolar pattern that can represent pneumonia, edema, or blood (Figures 16.1b, c). The second history indicated exposure to an anticoagulant rodenticide. Subsequent blood tests showed prolonged prothrombin and partial thromboplastin times, establishing the clinical diagnosis of anticoagulant rodenticide intoxication. The dog was treated with vitamin K1 and did well.

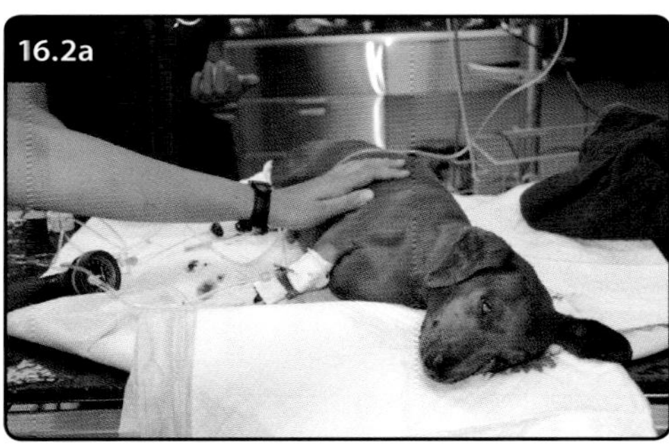

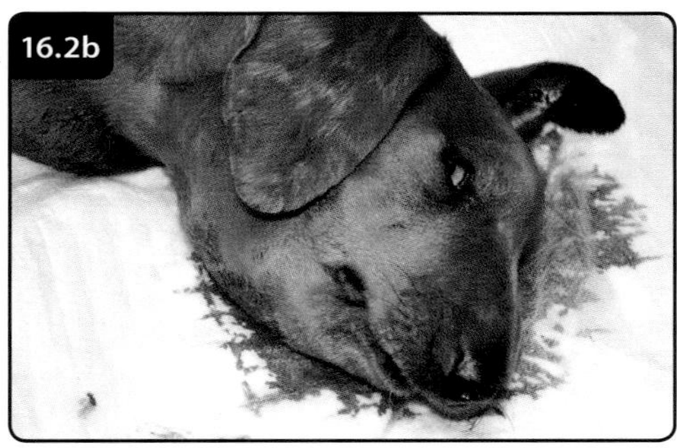

16.2a, b. Rattlesnake envenomation. This Dachshund was envenomated by an eastern diamondback rattlesnake. The venom is highly coagulopathic, hematoxic, sometimes neurotoxic, vasculotoxic, and necrogenic. Initial signs in a severe case can include spreading hemorrhagic lymphedema from the bite site, hypovolemia, active bleeding, and sometimes hemolysis. Treatment calls for ample amounts of antivenom and intravenous crystalloid fluids, close monitoring, and other drugs such as cardiac antiarrhythmics, vasopressors, sometimes blood products, opioid analgesics, and additional antivenom as indicated. This dog was classified as severe but he survived with intense treatment. The severity of the envenomation will depend on the specific snake, the amount of venom injected, initial health of the victim, and time delay before antivenom administration.

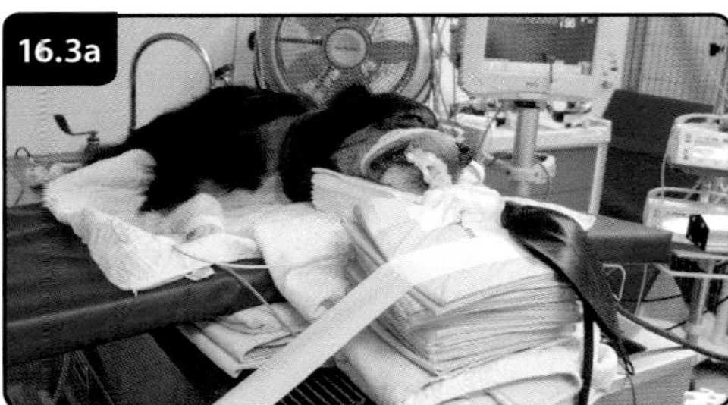

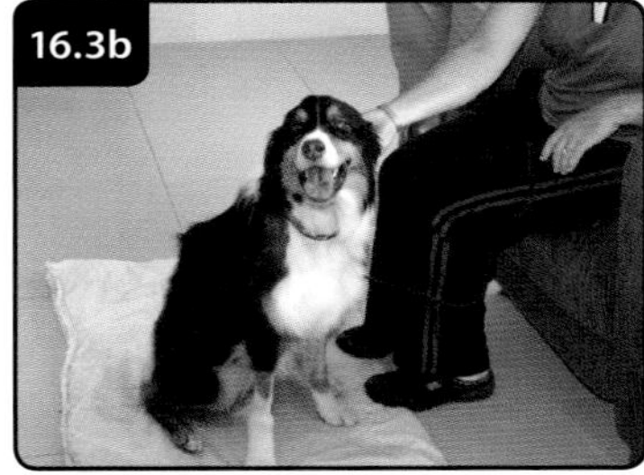

16.3a, b. Ivermectin intoxication in dog. This Sheepdog ingested ivermectin that was in horse feces. He became severely neurologically impaired and went apneic. He required ventilator assistance for 3 weeks in the ICU and survived. Ivermectin is known to be potentially toxic to the dog's nervous system, and particularly so to the Sheepdog group, because they have the multidrug resistance gene mutation (*MDR1*) that allows the ivermectin to remain longer in the system and potentiate its effects on GABA, a potent neurotransmitter inhibitor. There is no antidote other than maintain life support.

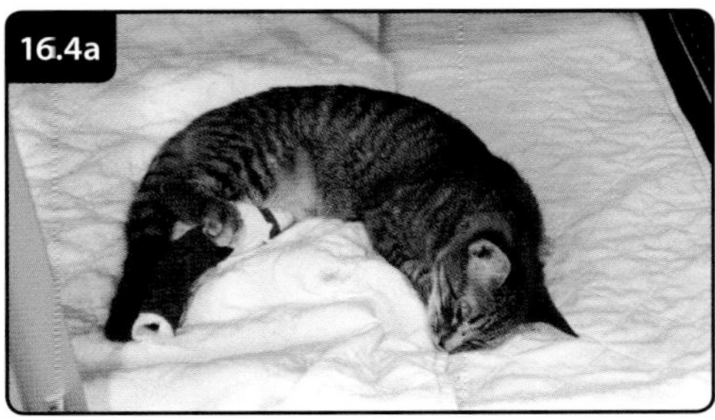

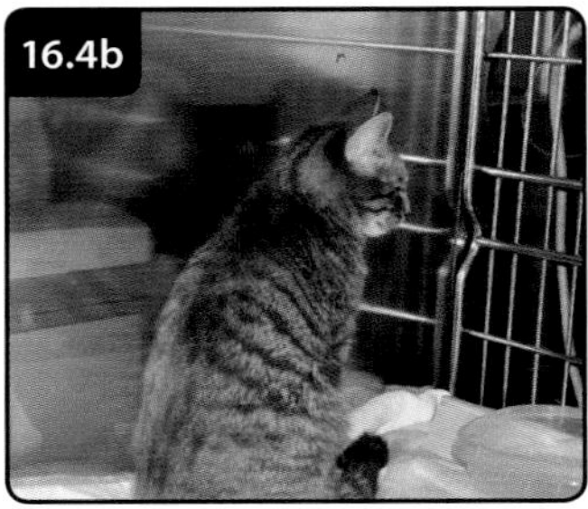

16.4a, b. Ivermectin intoxication in cat. Cats can also become neurotoxic from ivermectin intoxication. They can respond to supportive treatment. Shown is an intoxicated cat before and after 2 days of supportive treatment.

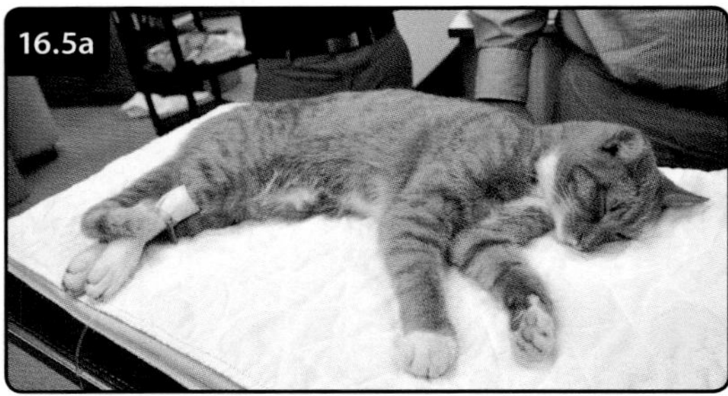
16.5a

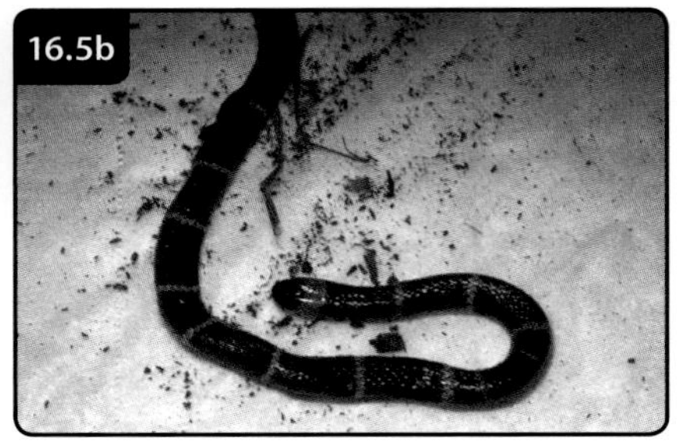
16.5b

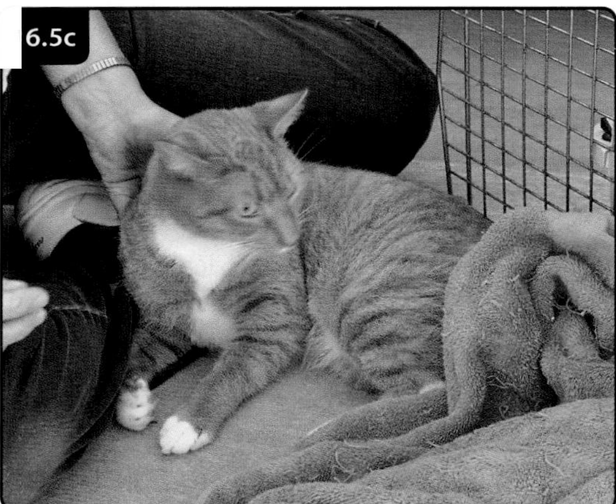
16.5c

16.5a–c. Coral snake envenomation in a cat. Coral snakes contain a venom that is neurotoxic and can cause diffuse lower motor neuron disease. Some victims experience respiratory muscle paralysis and require ventilator assistance until the effects of the venom dissipate over a 5–7-day period. This cat was found outside its house in lateral recumbency and totally unable to move, although it was able to breathe well enough to maintain its PCO_2 at a normal level (35–45 mmHg). A dead coral snake was found beside the cat. Permit approved imported antivenom was available and was administered to this cat. Shown is the cat at the time of admission with diffuse lower motor neuropathy, a dead eastern coral snake, and the same cat on day 7 of hospitalization.

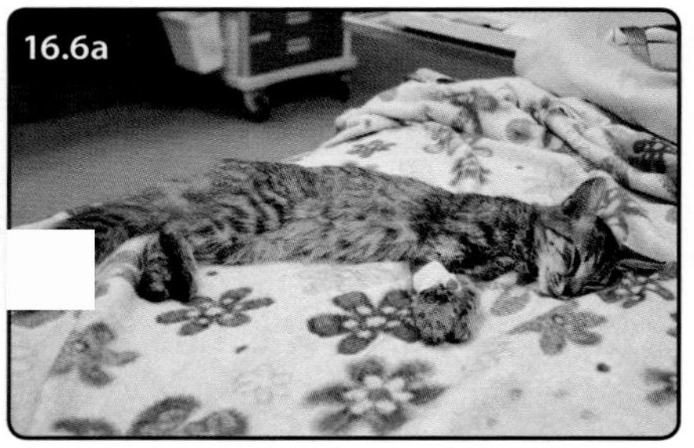
16.6a

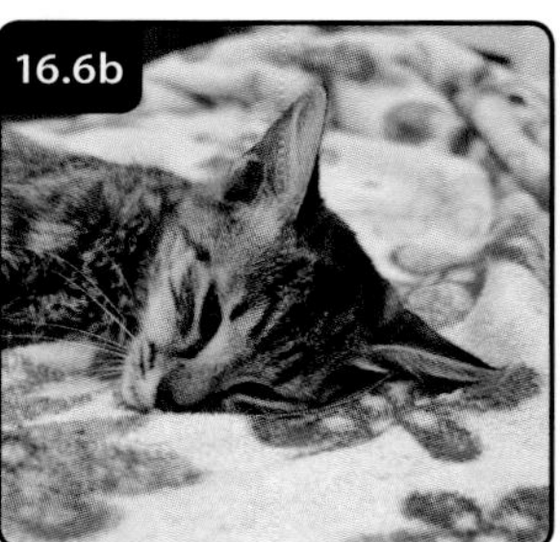
16.6b

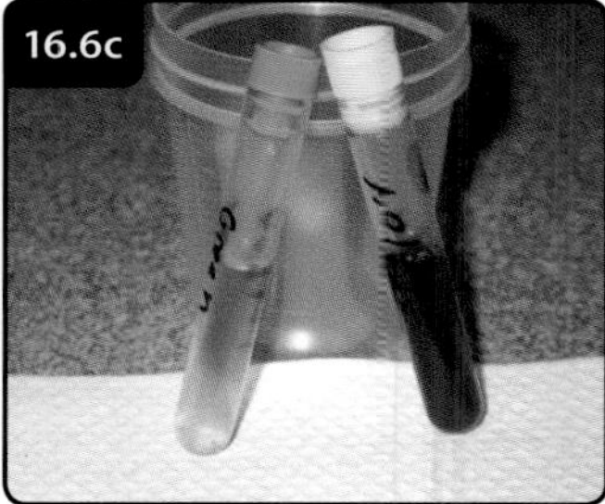
16.6c

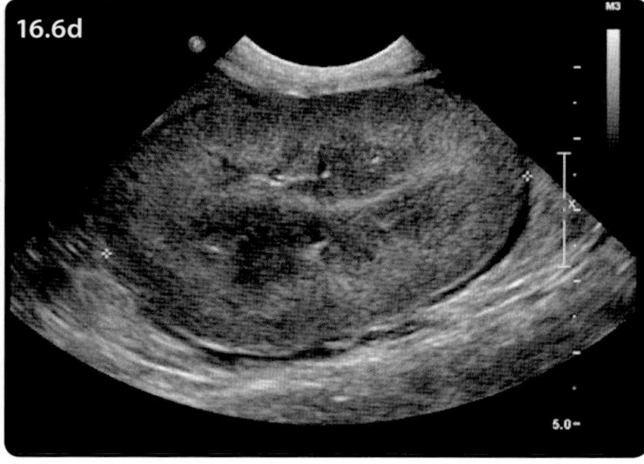
16.6d

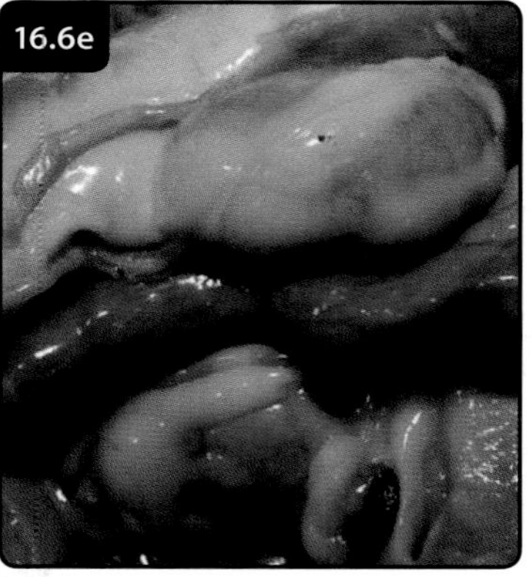
16.6e

16.6a–f. Ethylene glycol intoxication in a cat. This young cat presented to the emergency clinic in a comatose state. It was observed to be ataxic the day before. The main physical examination findings included minimal response to stimulation (Figures 16.6a, b), marked dehydration, and palpably enlarged kidneys. The serum chemistries showed a severe metabolic acidosis with a large anion gap (>30) and marked azotemia. The ethylene glycol test was positive (Figure 16.6c). Abdominal ultrasound showed diffuse hyperechogenicity (Figure 16.6d is an example taken from another patient). The cat was anuric and subsequently euthanized. Postmortem examination showed enlarged kidneys, which were attributed to subcapsular renal edema (Figure 16.6e) and other renal pathology. The histopathology of the kidney shows marked tubular damage and oxalate crystals in some of the tubular lumens (Figure 16.6f). If the cat had been presented earlier while it was ataxic and potentially more treatable, treatment would have included hemodialysis, ethanol, sodium bicarbonate, and crystalloid fluids.

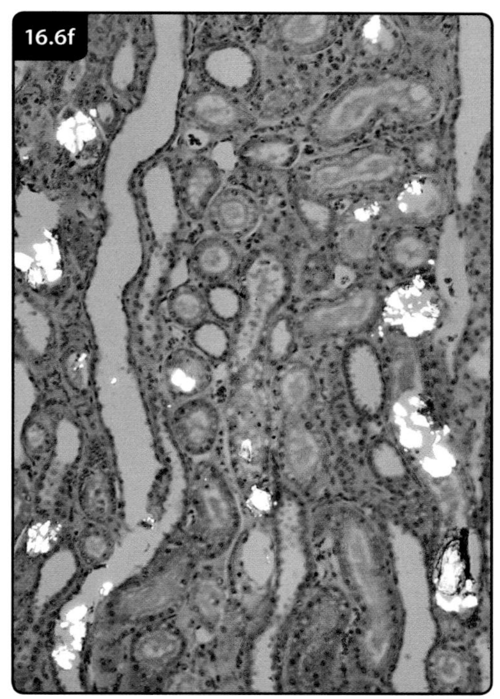
16.6f

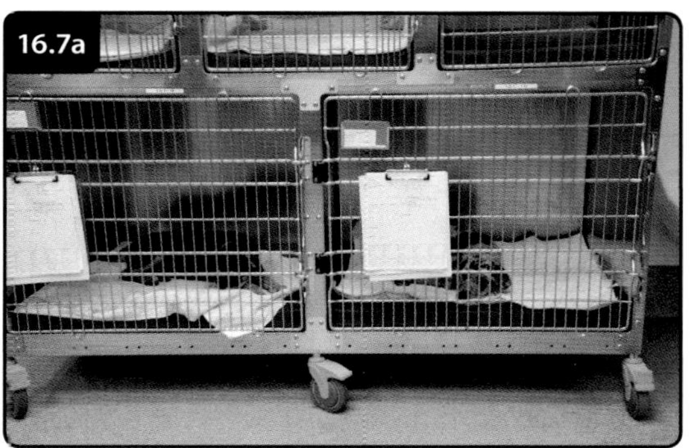
16.7a

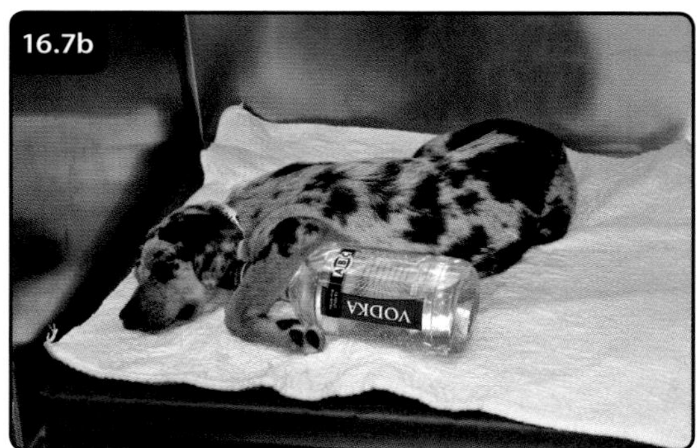

16.7b

16.7a–c. Ethylene glycol intoxication in two puppies. The owner brought his puppies to the emergency clinic shortly after they became ataxic while he was changing the antifreeze on his car. He had limited finances, so treatment was begun immediately with orally administered vodka, which was 90 proof (45% ethanol). The dose was extrapolated from the standard recommendation for 20% ethanol at a dose of 5.0 ml/kg every 6 hours. Over the next 24 hours, the inebriated puppies slept well and survived with no adverse effects from the ethylene glycol ingestion. The images show the puppies depressed at admission (Figure 16.7a) and one of the pups sleeping from the effects of the vodka (Figure 16.7b) and then normal without any renal or brain abnormalities on the following day (Figure 16.7c). The other pup also did well.

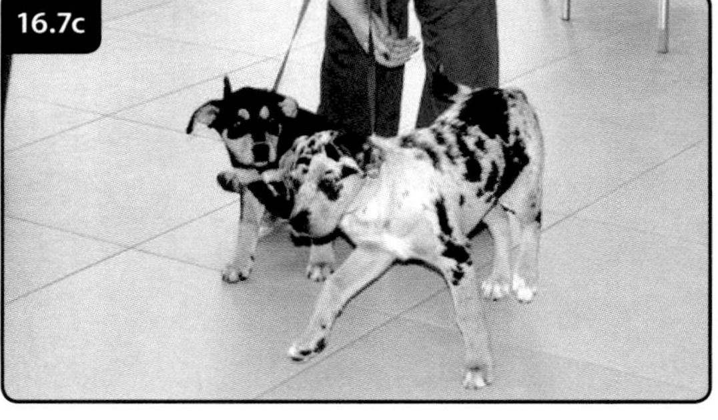
16.7c

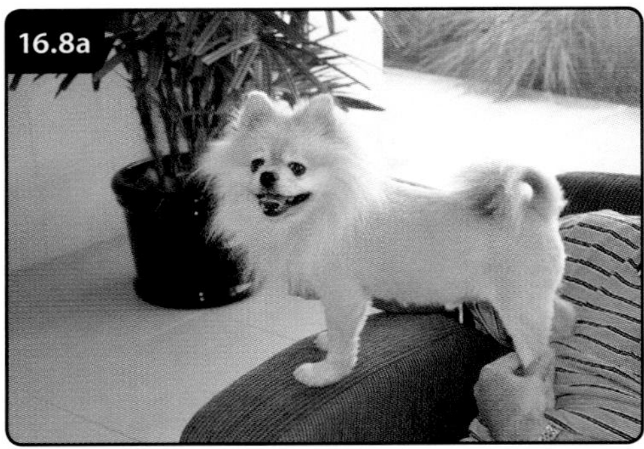

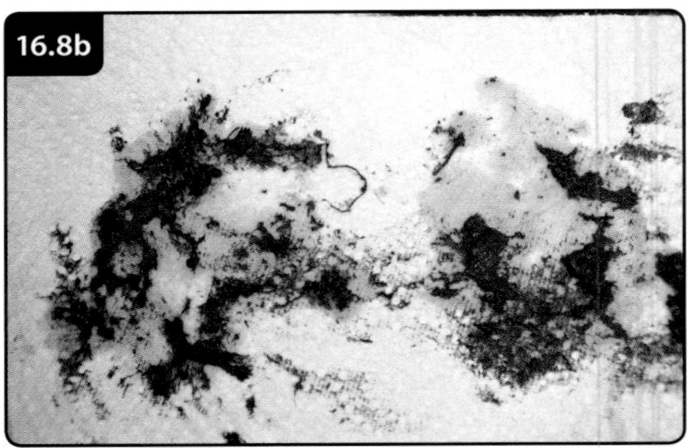

16.8a, b. Hydrogen peroxide gastritis. Hydrogen peroxide is a fairly effective emetic that is used in emergency situations to rid the patient of the potential adverse effects of an ingested toxin. The owner of this Pomeranian dog gave it hydrogen peroxide orally after he saw the dog ingest a substance that turned out to be harmless. The dog vomited, but then proceeded to have repeated vomiting and depression for the next 24 hours. The next day's stool was loose and had melena as a result of the gastritis caused by the hydrogen peroxide, but the dog eventually fared well.

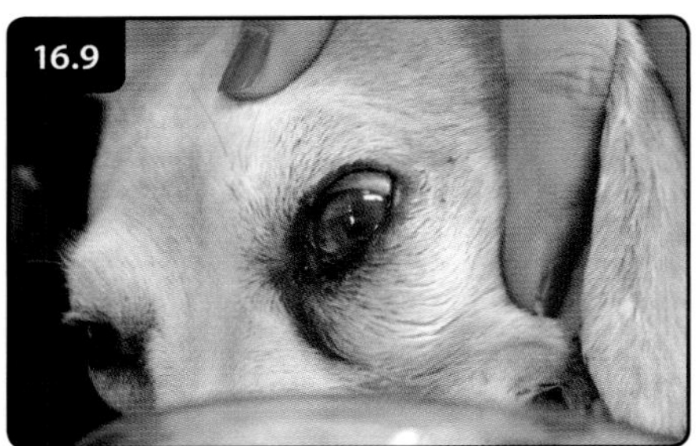

16.9. Organophosphate toxicity. This class of toxins has systemic cholinergic side-effects. Shown is miosis in such an intoxicated dog, which was accompanied by additional signs of ptyalism, vomiting, and seizure activity. Atropine and 2-PAM (pralidoxime chloride) are the antidotes.

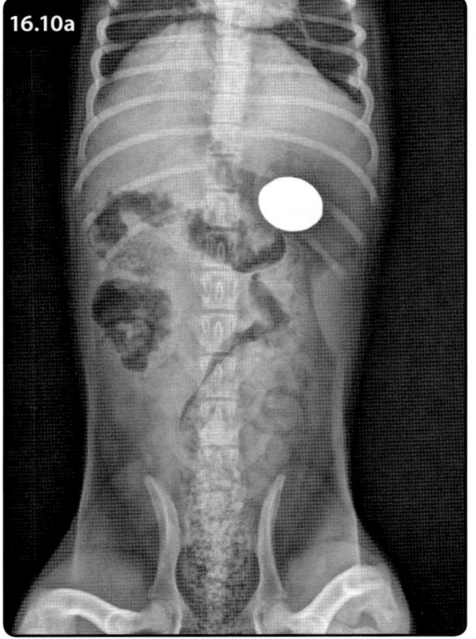

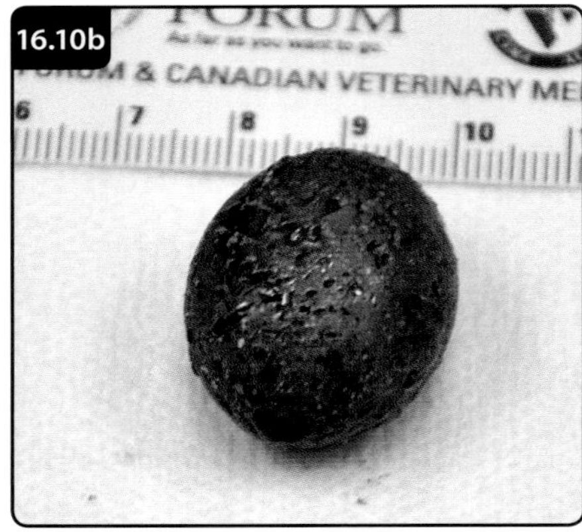

16.10a, b. Lead toxicity. Lead is a heavy metal that can interfere with several enzyme systems in the body and cause a multitude of clinical signs, especially neurologic and gastrointestinal (GI). The radiograph shows a large sized gastric foreign body that was later identified as a lead sinker. Objects such as this are usually too big to pass through the GI tract, and therefore require either surgical or endoscopic removal.

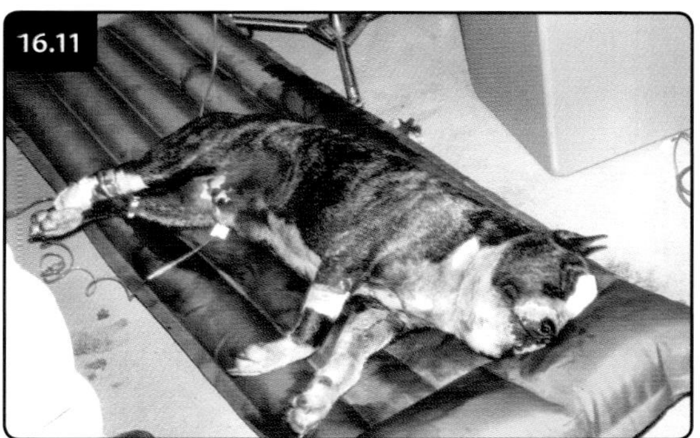

16.11. Rattlesnake envenomation in a dog. Rattlesnake envenomation is fairly common in areas indigenous to this particular reptile. In the southeastern USA, the eastern diamondback rattlesnake and the water moccasin are particularly dangerous because their venom has widespread adverse effects on several organ systems, especially coagulation, red blood cells, and the nervous system. The venom is also tissue toxic. This dog was bitten by an eastern diamondback approximately 3 days prior and the owner could not afford the much needed antivenom. The dog died from a hemorrhagic diathesis.

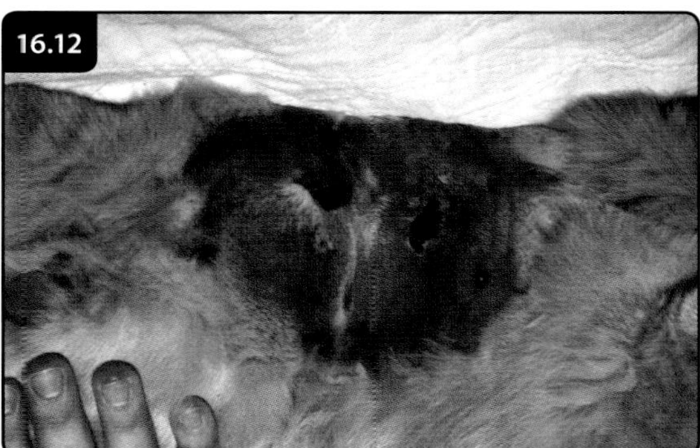

16.12. Rattlesnake bite in a cat. The lateral abdomen of this cat was the site of a bite by a rattlesnake. The cat was hypotensive and had hemorrhagic lymphedema at the bite site, as shown in Figure 16.12. The two black marks represent local necrosis at the bite sites.

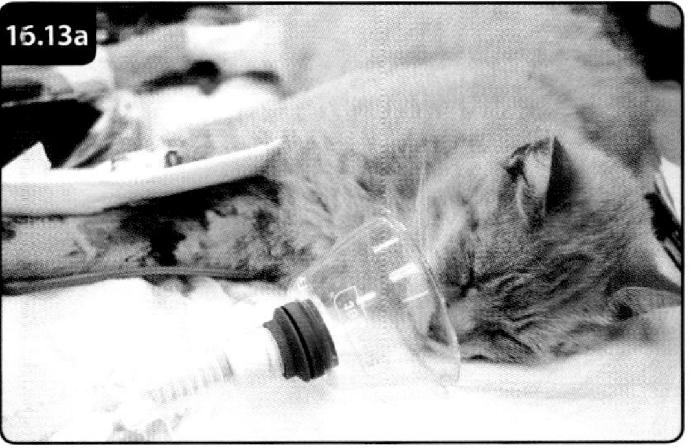

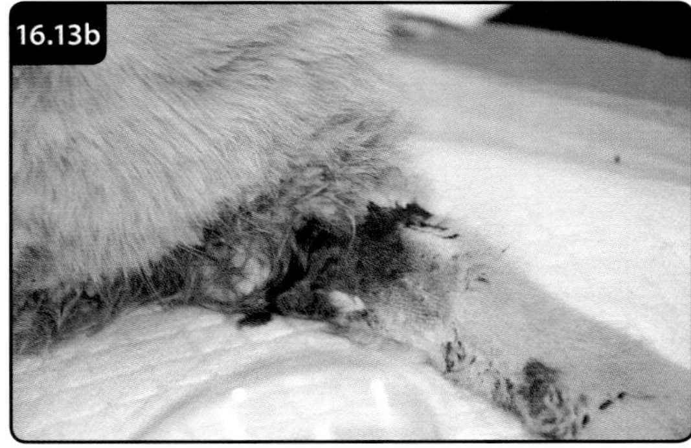

16.13a, b. Water moccasin bite in cat. This cat was envenomated by a water moccasin. The playful and teasing nature of this cat caused it to be bitten on the left forelimb. Swelling, pain, and hemorrhagic lymphedema are the typical signs. In the southeastern USA, antivenom is recommended for moderate and severe pit viper bites in dogs and cats.

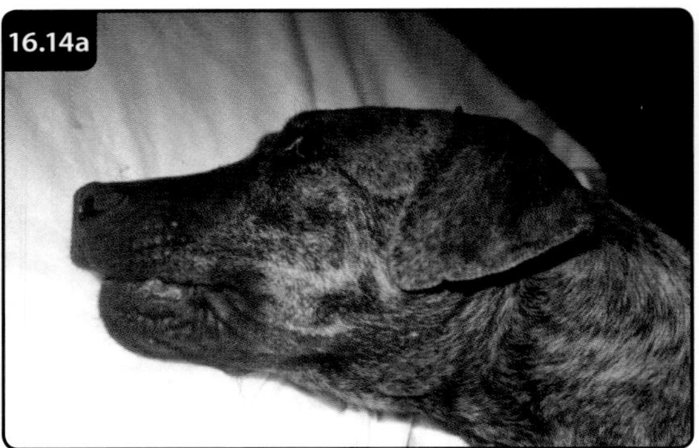

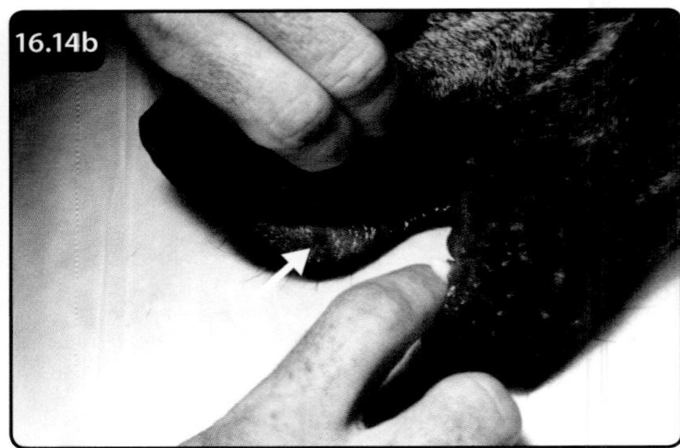

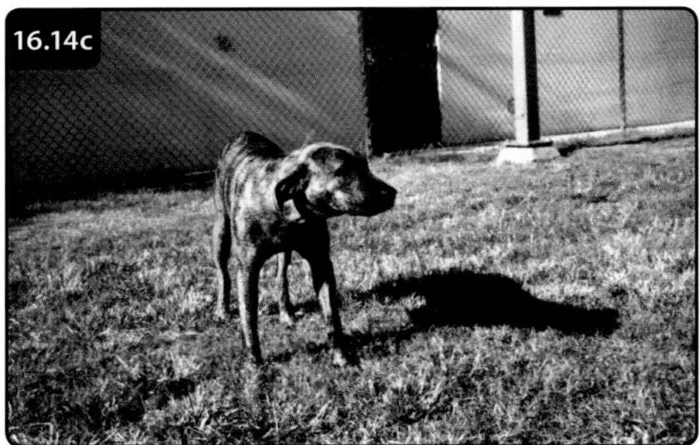

16.14a–c. Eastern coral snake envenomation in the dog. The eastern coral snake is found in the southeastern USA. It has a potent neurotoxin that can cause diffuse lower motor neuron paralysis that can involve the respiratory muscles and diaphragm. The venom does not cause necrosis. Instead, the bite site appears as a small slit or a small hematoma bleb (Figure 16.14b, arrow). This dog was found in its back yard unable to move (Figure 16.14a). A dead coral snake was seen a few feet away. On examination, the respiratory muscles were functioning and the PCO_2 level was normal. Therefore, no ventilator assistance was necessary. The dog was treated with one vial of coral snake antivenom and provided with meticulous patient support. Gradual improvement ensued over the following week (Figure 16.14c).

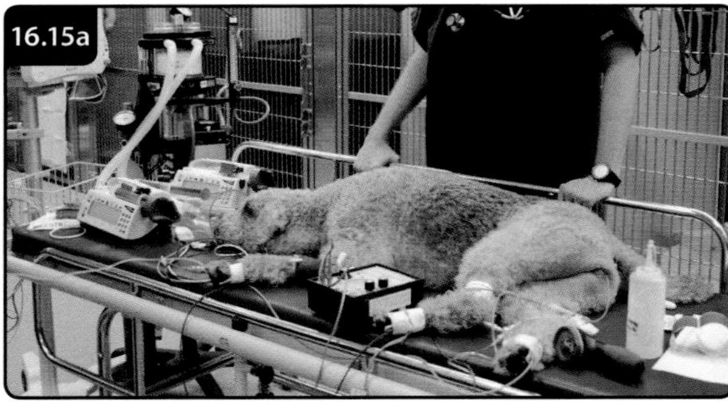

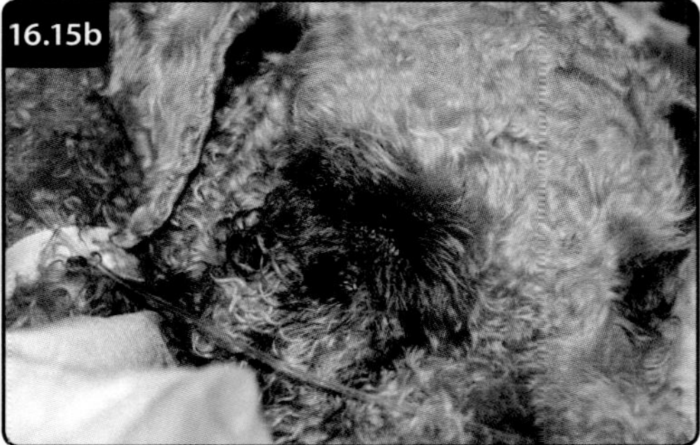

16.15a, b. Timber rattlesnake envenomation. This Airedale dog was admitted in a state of paralysis after being bitten in the face by a timber rattlesnake. The venom from this snake can have vasculotoxic, hematoxic, and neurotoxic properties. This dog suffered from all three effects and died despite receiving respectable doses of antivenom. Death can occur quickly, as it did in this dog, if the venom is inoculated directly into an artery (arteriolization).

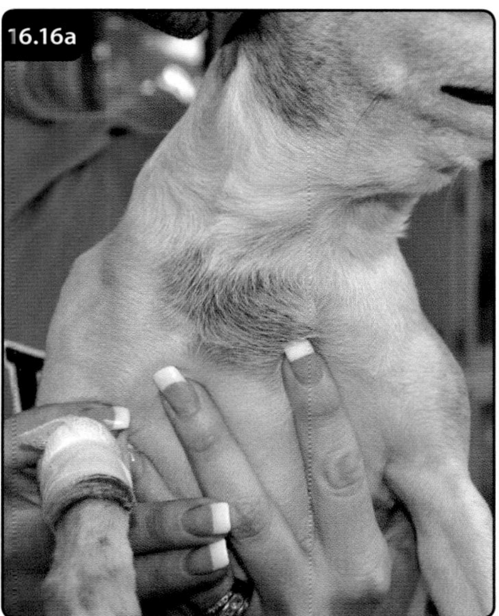

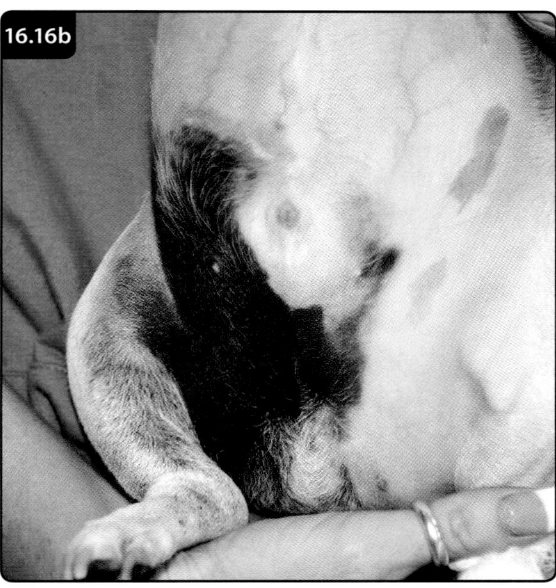

16.16a, b. Anticoagulant rodenticide poisoning. The jugular hematoma in Figure 16.16a is the exact reason why the jugular veins should never be the site of venipuncture in an animal with a suspect bleeding disorder, as shown in this dog that also had a large inguinal ecchymosis (Figure 16.16b). Attempts to establish hemostasis at this jugular vein site by applying pressure would be limited by the amount of airway compromise it could cause.

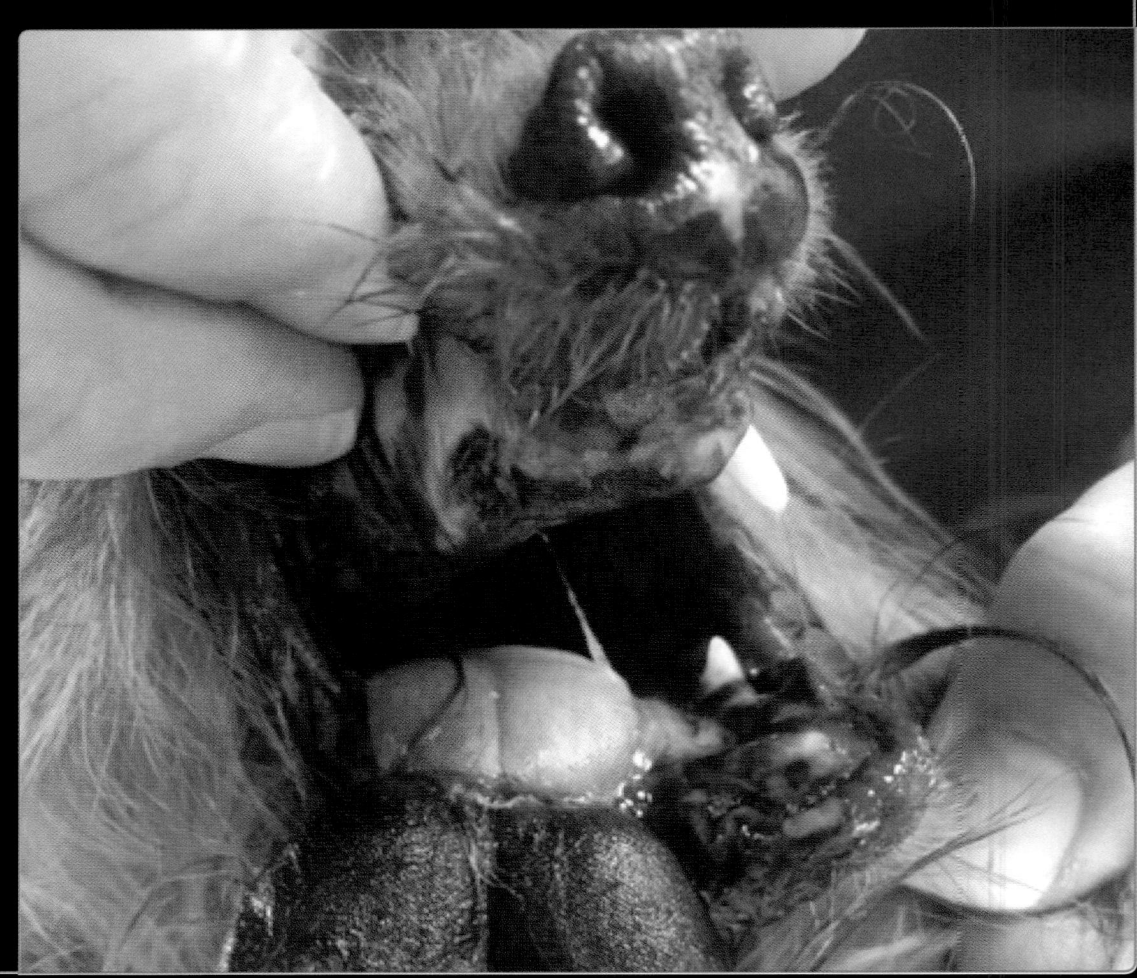

▲ This dog's own perioral hair is wrapped around its tongue cutting off its blood supply and causing one-half of the tongue to become necrotic.

17

Miscellaneous disorders

The word miscellaneous means 'consisting of diverse things or members; heterogeneous' (Merriam-Webster). In clinical medicine, many of the miscellaneous disorders are often the most interesting. The conditions described in this section do not fall into the more common organ system disorders, but many of these cases can enter the front door of any busy small animal practice at any time, and some of these conditions have distinct clinical signs that make them very diagnosable by the busy practitioner. The unique conditions or techniques provided in this section include feline cryptorchidism, calvarial hyperostosis, cartilaginous exostoses, rapid abdominocentesis, nutritional bone disease, mucopolysaccharidosis, polymyositis, thiamine deficiency, and others. Hopefully, the reader will find this section interesting mainly because of the diverse disorders included. The legends associated with each image highlight the distinguishing features of the respective disorder. Any major spark of interest generated can be fortified with additional information easily accessible in the major veterinary textbooks as well on the internet with the use of an efficient search engine such as Google.

This section concludes this illustrated presentation of clinical medicine. The 1,200 images used in the first and second editions of *Clinical Signs in Small Animal Medicine* represent only a fraction of the editor's 45 years of clinical experience. It is hoped that this graphic learning resource will benefit the reader in such a way that when one of these cases enters the door of the reader's veterinary clinic, that trigger in the memory bank will fire off with the message "I have seen this before", thus providing the information necessary toward making an accurate clinical diagnosis. With this being done, then the author will consider his mission accomplished.

17 Miscellaneous disorders

- Septic shock classic features: hypotension, hypothermia, thrombocytopenia.
- Sudden facial hemorrhagic lymphedema swelling, hemorrhagic oral mucosa, subdued mentation – think venomous pit viper snake bite (in Florida).
- Chest plus abdominal fluid accumulation commonly depicts a bad disease. Common causes: neoplasia, heart failure, diffuse inflammation, hypoproteinemia.
- Take the patient out of the cage and look at it!
- If something just 'ain't' right – think neurology.
- If the patient is eating and drinking without excess fluid losses, it doesn't need intravenous fluids.

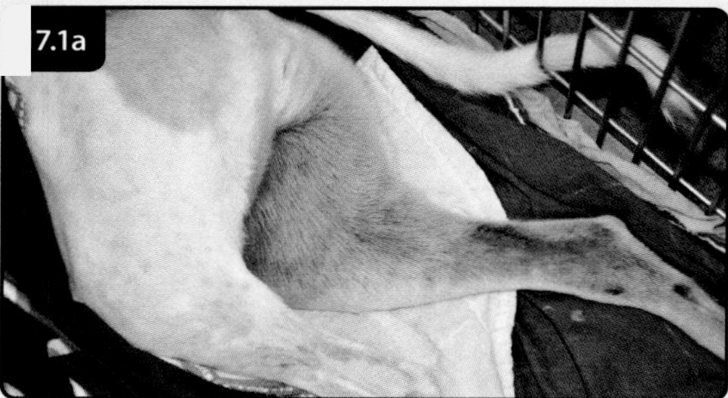

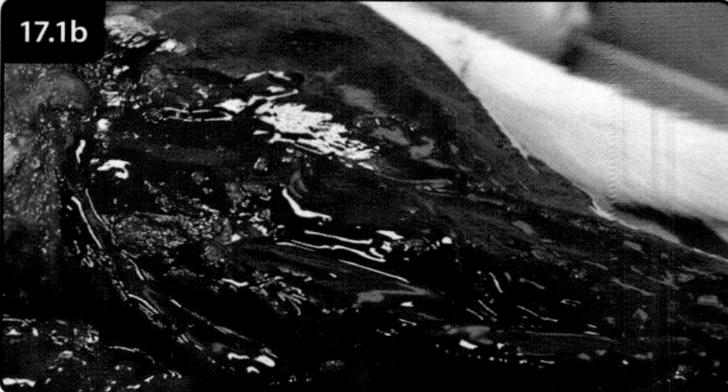

17.1a, b. Thigh hemorrhage associated with a traumatic tear of the femoral artery in a dog. This Greyhound slipped and tore its right femoral vein, causing acute blood loss. It was euthanized at the owner's request. Figure 17.1a shows the dog's right thigh swollen and discolored from the hemorrhage. Figure 17.1b shows the extreme hemorrhage at necropsy.

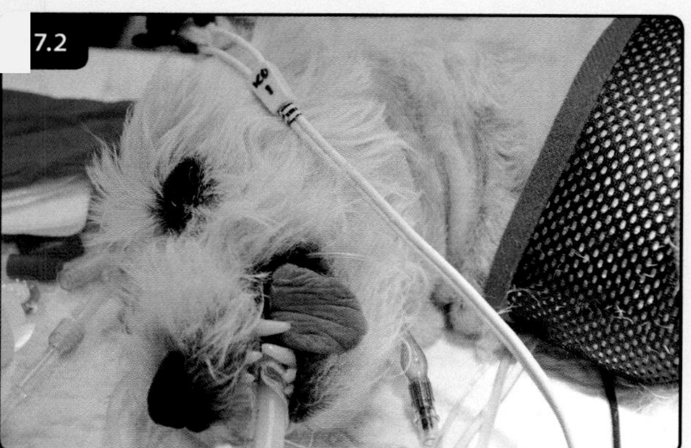

17.2. Dog with classic oral mucosa signs of hypoperfusion. The cyanotic oral mucous membranes despite intubation and oxygen supplementation indicate deficient tissue oxygen extraction at the peripheral level. This dog might require pressor treatment if hypotension occurs, or it might indicate irreversible shock.

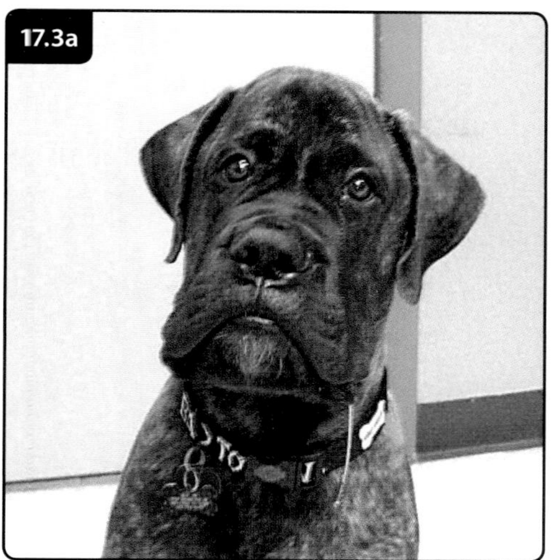

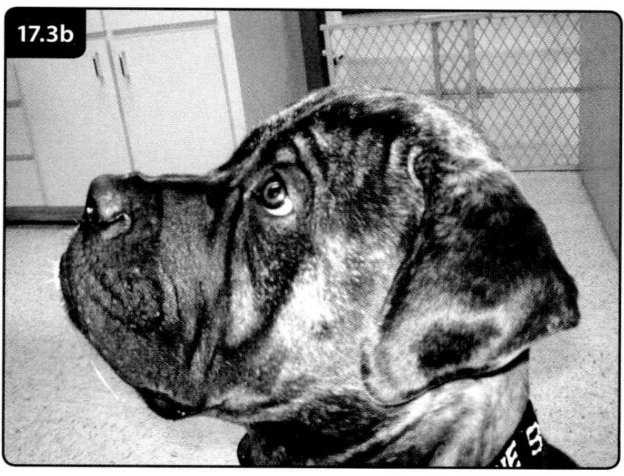

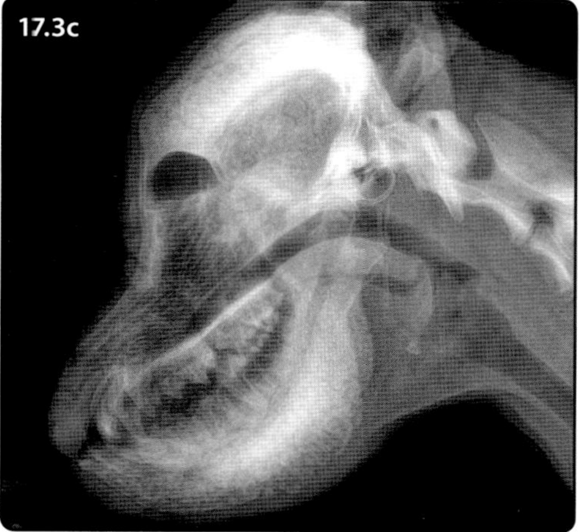

17.3a–c. Craniomandibular osteopathy (calvarial hyperostosis). Craniomandibular osteopathy is a familiar condition to most veterinarians, characterized by a periosteal proliferation of the mandible and temporomandibular joint of smaller breeds of dogs (West Highland White, Cairn, and Scottish Terriers). It can affect other breeds as well. The Bull Mastiff has a unique form of the disease that features a disproportional proliferation of the calvarium. Figures 17.3a, b show a young Bull Mastiff with the characteristic dome-like calvarium. The radiograph (Figure 17.3c) shows marked proliferation of the dome of the skull, but there is also mandibular proliferation as well. The author has successfully treated these dogs with long-term prednisone (1–2 mg/kg per day for 1–2 weeks followed by gradual taper to alternate day treatment for 4–6 months) and avoided extreme and irreversible consequences.

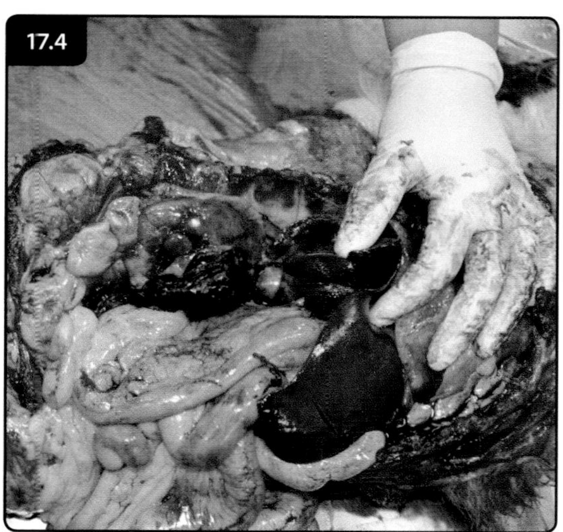

17.4. Iatrogenic liver fracture from cardiopulmonary resuscitation (CPR). Vigorous CPR was done on this dog when it arrested in the ICU. The postmortem findings included thoracic bruising and a fractured liver that bled and contributed to the dog's hypovolemia in its near terminal stages. Although a fair degree of compression is necessary to fill and empty the dysfunctional heart, too much pressure can be injurious to thoracic, abdominal, and skeletal structures.

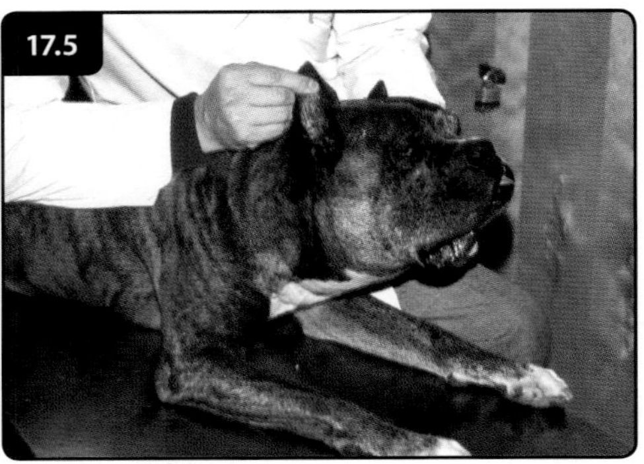

17.5. Suspect l-asparaginase-induced acute pancreatitis. This dog received l-asparaginase for a diagnosis of lymphoma. Within a day after receiving the drug, the dog acutely vomited, had vasocollapse, and succumbed to acute hemorrhagic pancreatitis. A necropsy confirmed the pancreatitis. This drug is known to cause acute pancreatitis in humans, and the signs that occurred shortly after this dog's treatment implicated l-asparaginase as the cause.

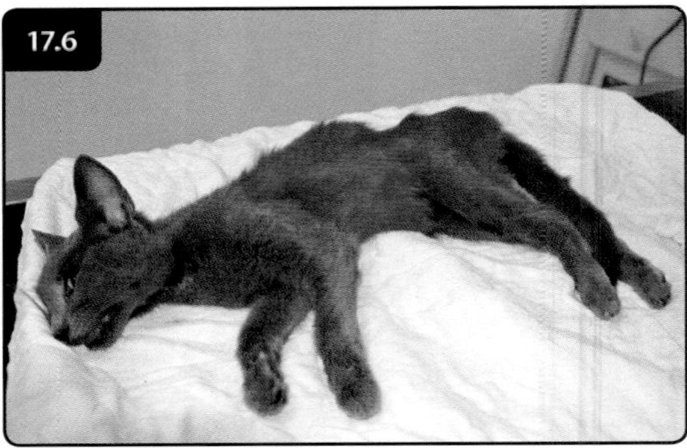

17.6. Calculating fluid requirements in the cachectic patient. It is easy to overestimate the intravenous fluid requirements to correct dehydration if skin turgor is a major criterion. Emaciation decreases the skin resiliency that would usually be present if fat were in the subcutis. Intravenous overload would have a very detrimental effect on such a debilitated animal.

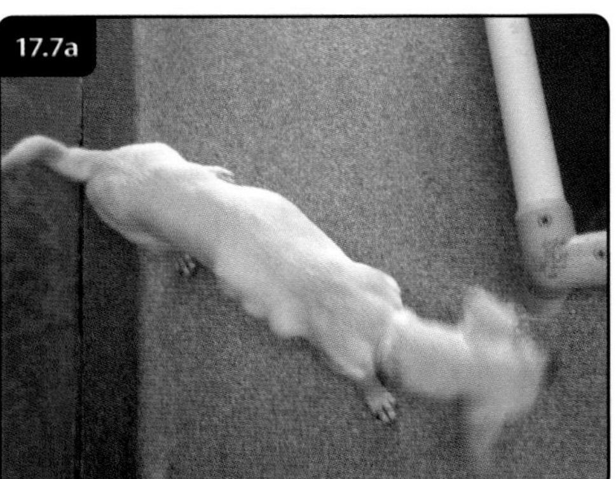

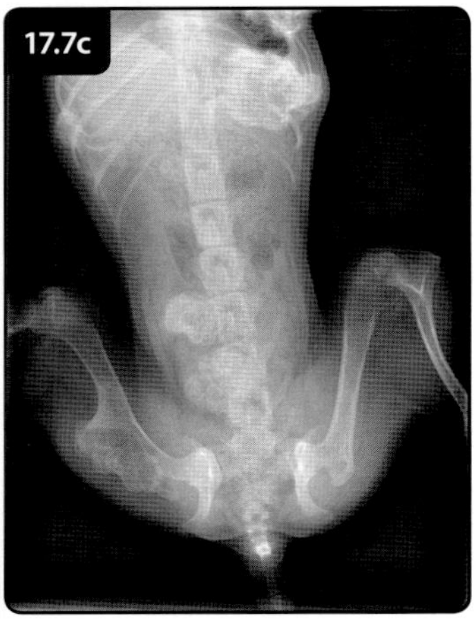

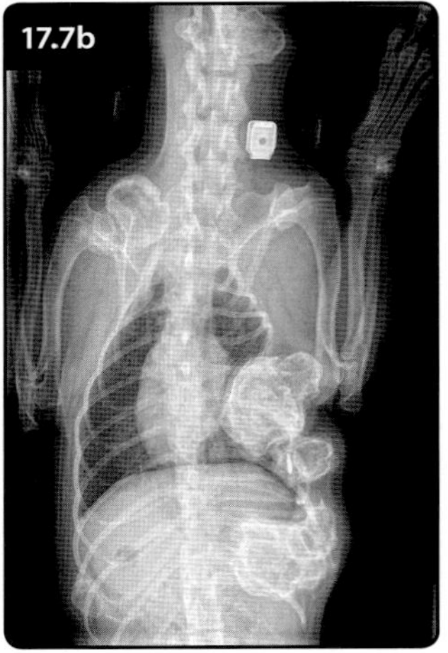

17.7a–c. Multiple cartilaginous exostoses. This young dog has very firm mineralized subcutaneous masses, which are compatible with this disorder. This condition is characterized as multiple ossified protuberances arising from metaphyseal cortical surfaces of long bones; other bones can be involved as well. Shown are the masses on the dog and as seen on the radiograph. (Courtesy Dr. Alex Alvarez and colleagues)

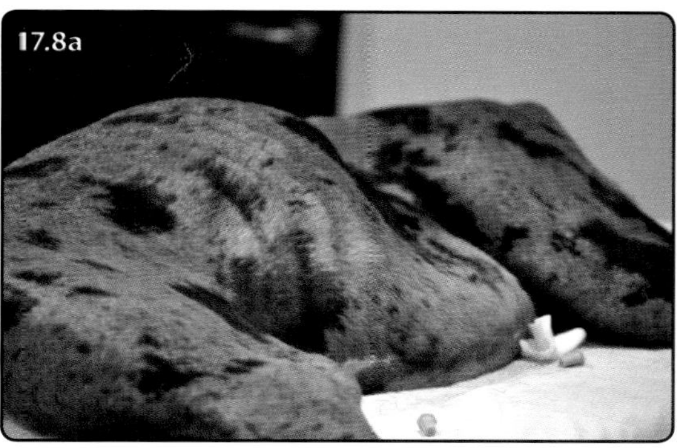

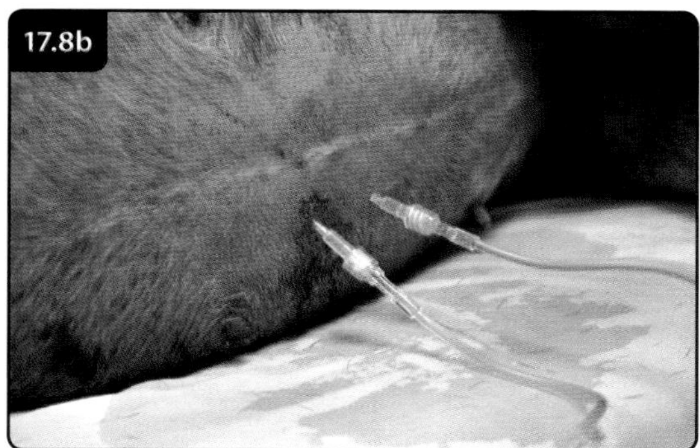

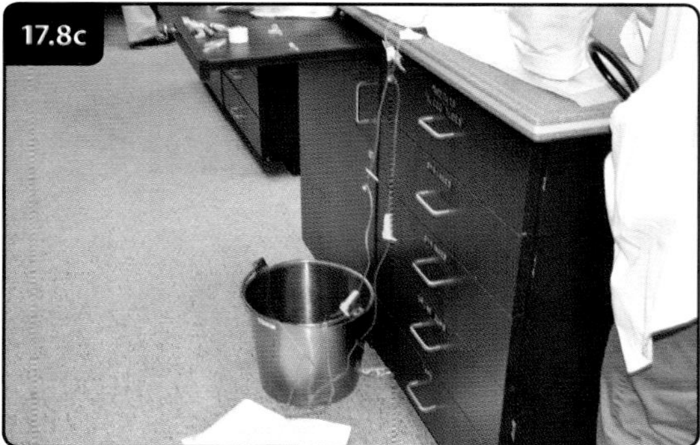

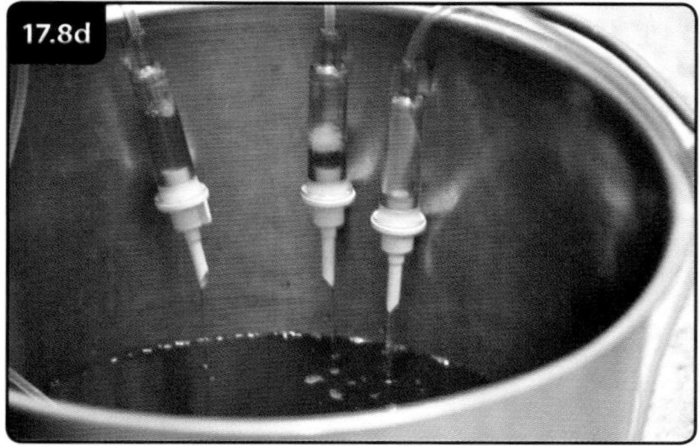

17.8a–d. Rapid abdominocentesis. Tense ascites (extreme fluid build-up) can place pressure on the diaphragm and interfere with its range of motion. The technique shown is simple and efficient. It does not require sedation; only gentle restraint on a comfortable table surface is necessary for holding down the animal. This procedure works well for right-sided congestive heart failure, tumor ascites, and hypoproteinemic ascites. When liver dysfunction is the cause of the ascites, it might help to simultaneously administer plasma or crystalloid while the ascites is being drained. The pictures show two 18 gauge needles being used to drain the abdomen. Polyethylene cannulas can also be used, but they will sometimes kink and interfere with drainage. The entire procedure should take no more than 30–45 minutes, using gravity as the only means for the drainage.

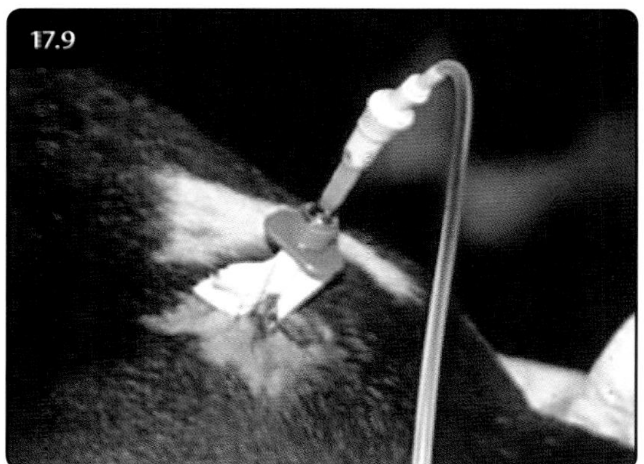

17.9. Intraosseous parenteral fluid administration. This technique is quite useful in emergency situations when an intravenous catheter cannot be placed. In the adult dog, a Jamshidi bone marrow needle can be used. In a very small animal, a smaller cannula such as an 18 gauge needle is recommended. Intraosseous fluid administration can be viewed as delivering the fluids into a great vein until the blood pressure is increased high enough to facilitate the placement of an intravenous catheter. This image is also shown in Case 6.4 where it shows the contrast compared with using a hypodermic needle in a pediatric patient.

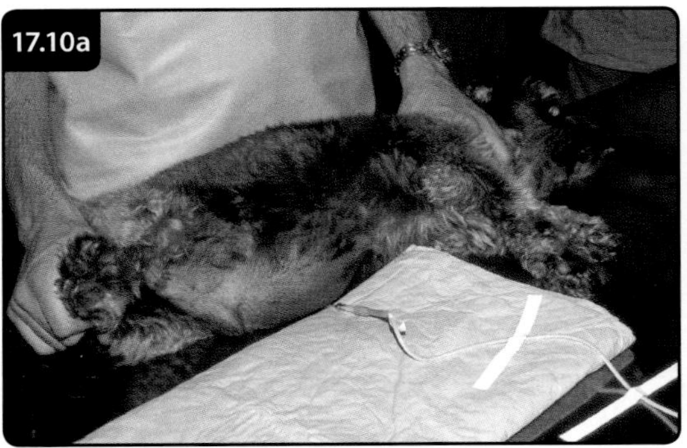

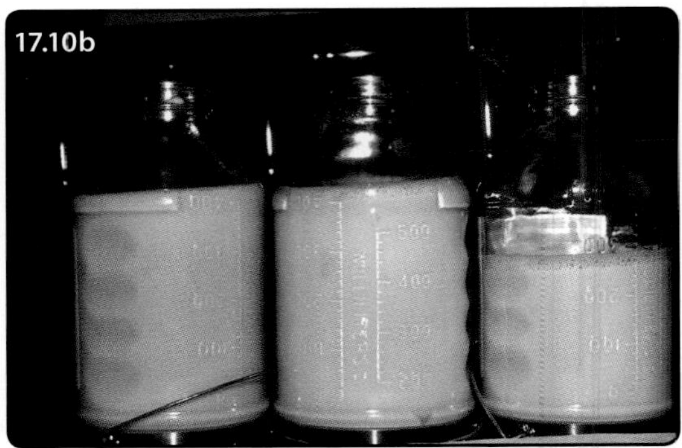

17.10a, b. Chylous ascites. This Schnauzer had recurrent chylous ascites. The condition can occur following trauma to the abdominal lymphatics or it may accompany ascites caused by certain tumors such as lymphoma. Palliative treatment consists of abdominocentesis when needed and a low fat diet, which might lessen the fluid build-up. Treating the underlying cause is certainly a main consideration where indicated.

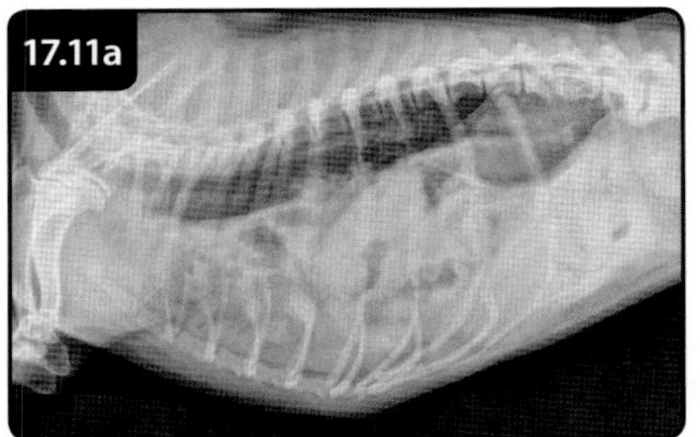

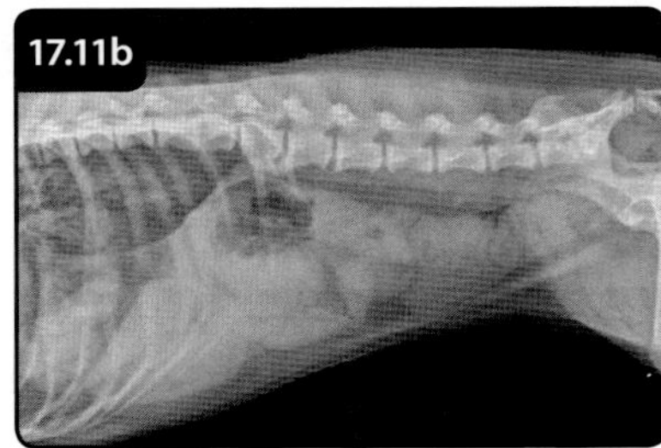

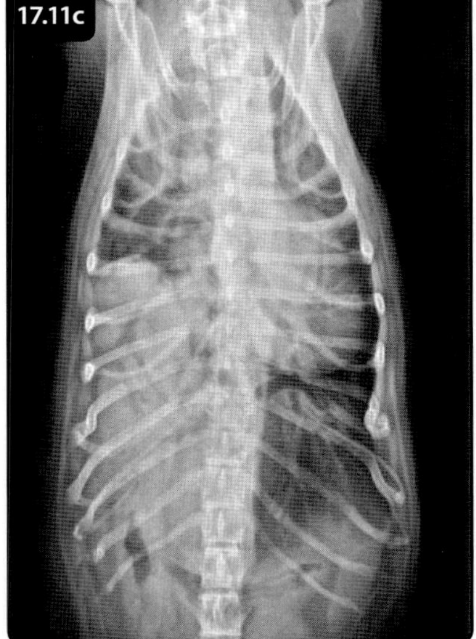

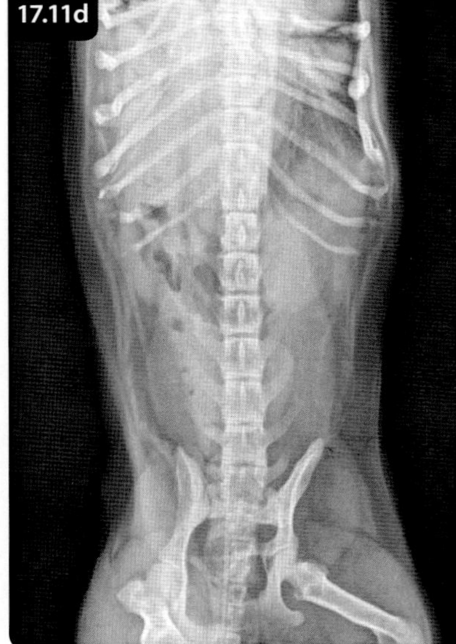

17.11a–d. Diaphragmatic hernia. The radiographic views of the chest and abdomen show that the abdominal viscera has moved into the right side of the thorax. The small bowel is visible on the chest side of the diaphragm. On physical examination, the right hemithoracic sounds would be muted, and abdominal palpation would fail to detect viscera in the usual location. This pathology is associated with blunt trauma to the abdominal cavity and will require surgical correction.

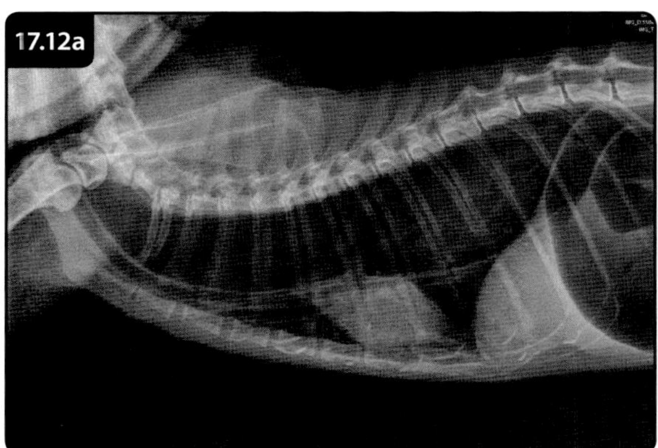

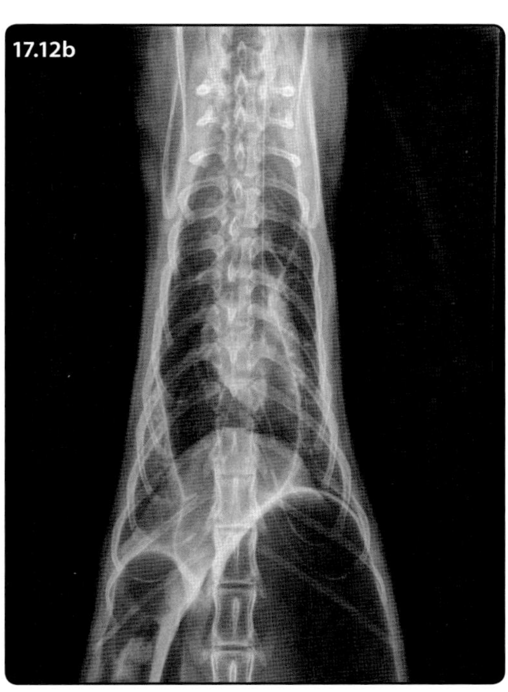

17.12a, b. Dysautonomia in a cat. Dysautonomia is a dysfunction involving the parasympathetic and/or sympathetic divisions of the autonomic nervous system. It occurs in dogs and cats and its effects are debilitating because of multiple organ involvement. The prognosis is usually grave. The radiographs shown here represent marked esophageal dysfunction (megaesophagus). Marked aerophagia is also present. Treatment is only palliative.

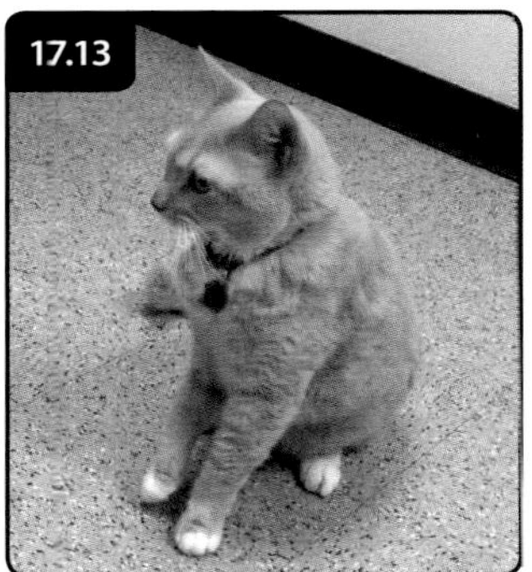

17.13. Joint pain and fever following vaccination. This young cat received its booster vaccine, which included calicivirus. It became depressed and had forelimb lameness 24 hours later. Physical examination showed that the cat had a fever (104°F [40°C]) and swelling of both carpi, more so on the right. This vaccine reaction is caused by the modified live calicivirus component, and it can spread to the joints to cause a transient polyarthropathy. The reaction is transient and normalcy returns within 24–36 hours.

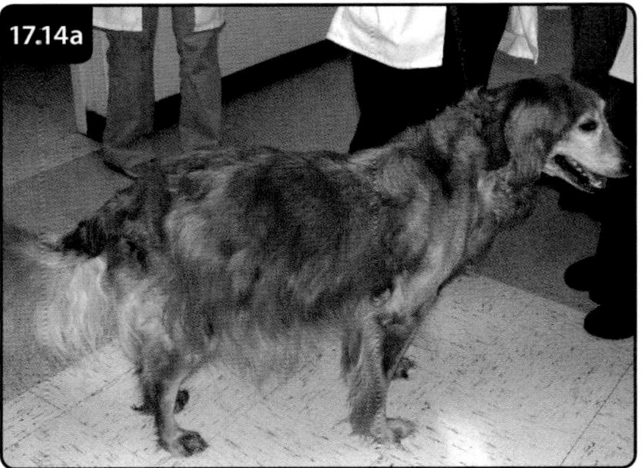

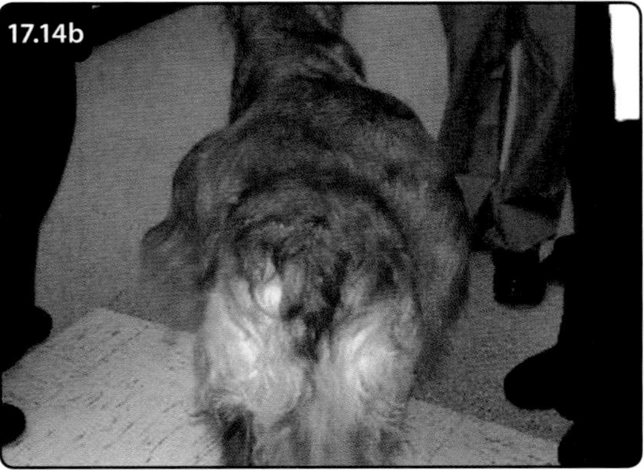

17.14a, b. Large lipomas in a dog. From the side view, this Golden Retriever's lipomas are hardly visible. A whole different perspective unveils when the dog is turned and shows its bilateral flank lipomas. The owner had finally decided to have them surgically removed, which transpired uneventfully.

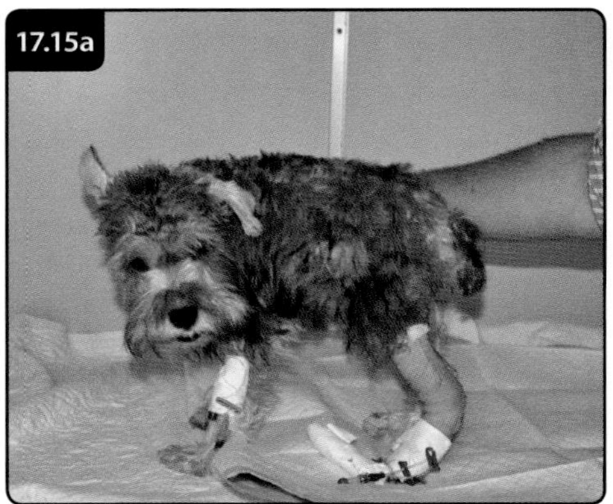
17.15a

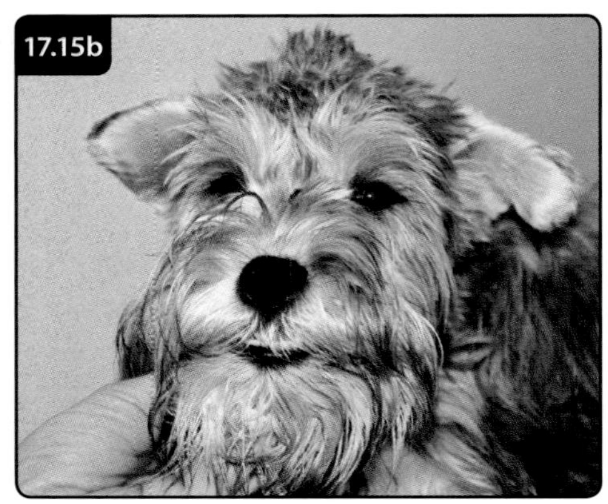
17.15b

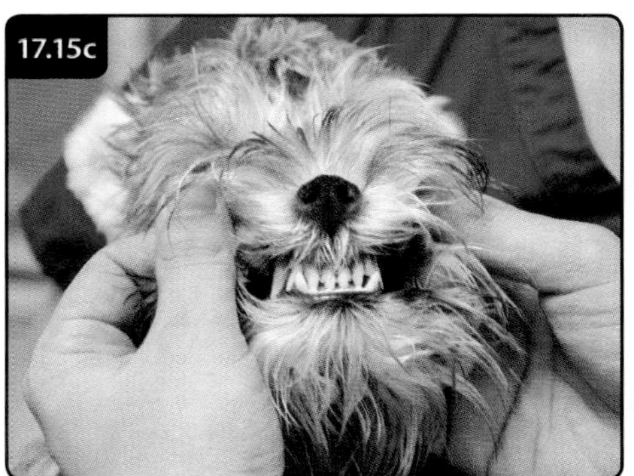
17.15c

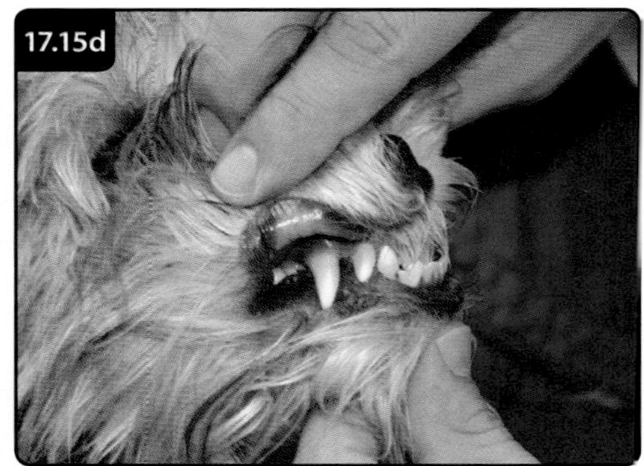
17.15d

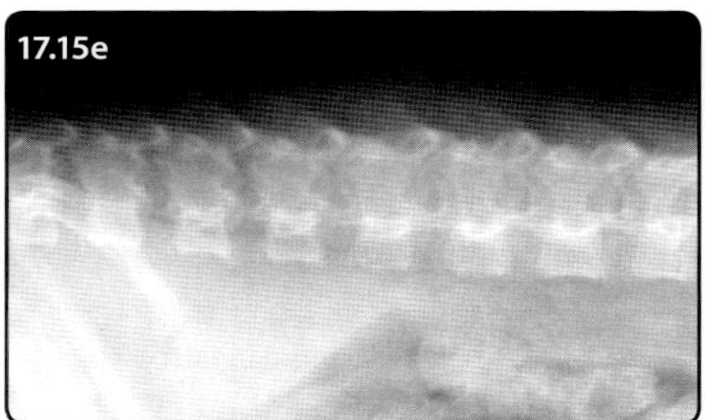
17.15e

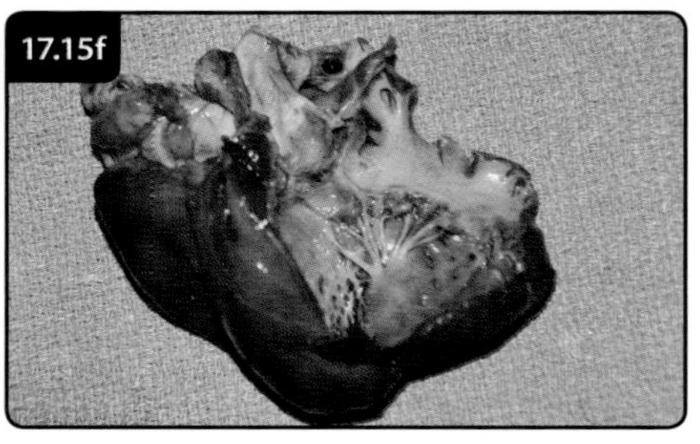
17.15f

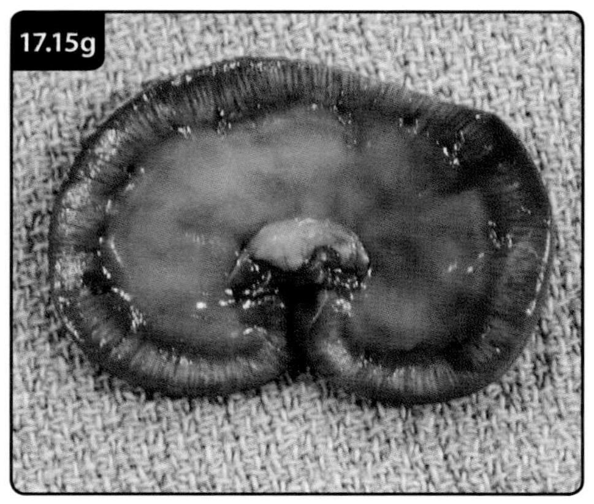
17.15g

17.15a–g. Mucopolysaccharidosis in a Miniature Schnauzer. There are several lysosomal storage diseases that are characterized as a genetic defect in the lysosomal enzymes needed to metabolize glycosaminoglycans in the cell. The defect allows chains of sugars to accumulate in various tissues, which leads to maldevelopment and organ dysfunction. The accompanying figures show the abnormal facial structure (Figures 17.15a–d), while the radiograph (Figure 17.15e) shows abnormal vertebral development. Soft tissues such as the heart and kidney are also adversely affected (Figures 17.15f, g). The prognosis is grave until gene therapy becomes available. (Courtesy Dr. Andrew Specht)

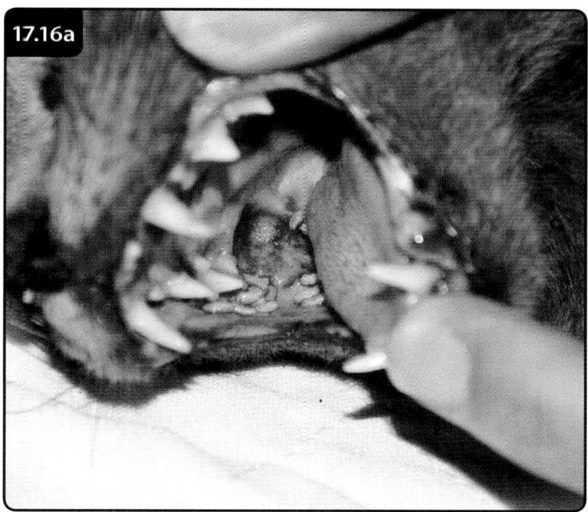

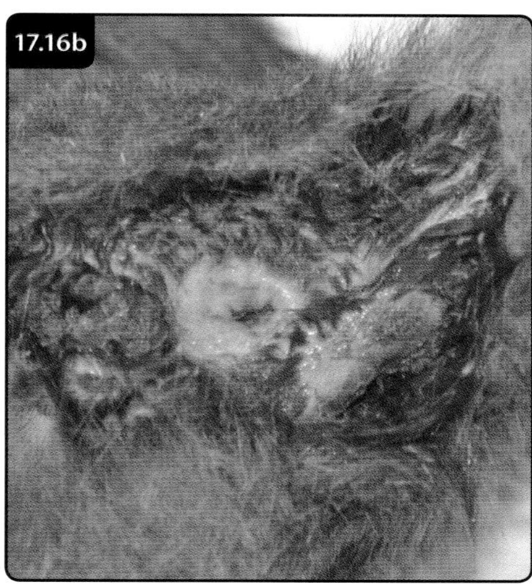

17.16a, b. Myiasis in a cat. Localized myiasis can be treated successfully in most cases, but when the fly larvae overwhelm the patient and traverse the length of the digestive tract, the prognosis is grave in most cases. In many situations, the victims will already be dealing with debilitating disease or they might have been severely traumatized, which predisposes them to the larval invasion. These figures show larvae in the oral cavity and the perineum, which signifies internal infestation. Euthanasia is indicated at this advanced stage of disease.

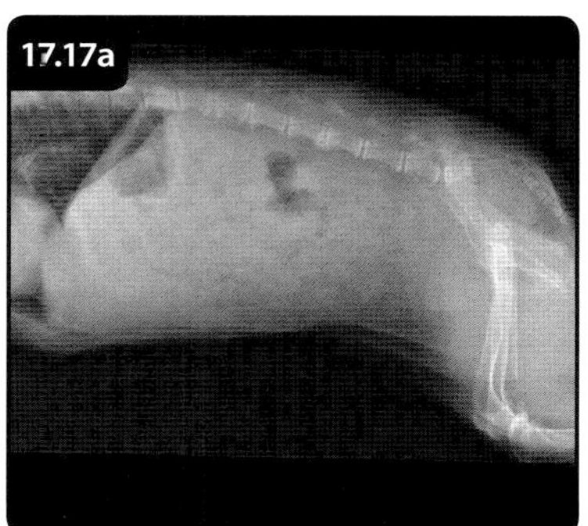

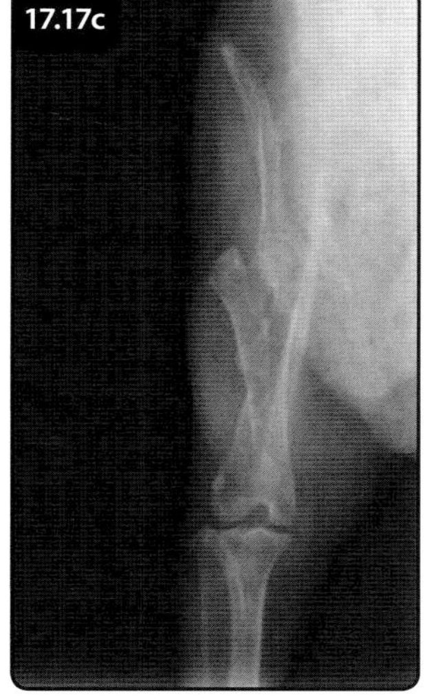

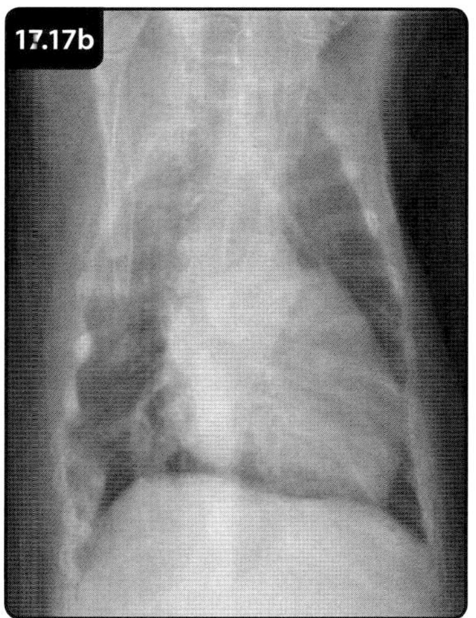

17.17a–c. Secondary nutritional hyperparathyroidism. This condition occurs when animals are fed diets that have poor calcium:phosphorus ratios, such as organ meats. The dietary calcium deficiency causes the host to produce extra parathyroid hormone (PTH) in order to achieve normal blood calcium concentrations. The increased PTH causes diffuse bone demineralization, which appears on radiographs as pale bones with thin cortices. A pathologic fracture has occurred in the right femur. Treatment is usually successful with soft comfortable bedding and a mineral balanced diet. Calcium and vitamin D supplementation is not always necessary, so long as the diet is balanced.

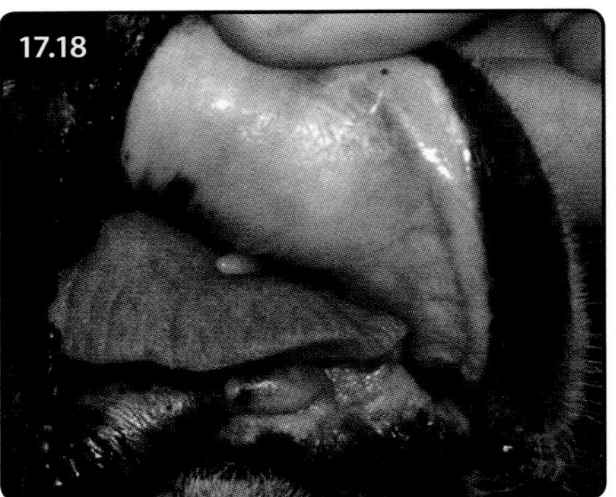

17.18 Delayed capillary refill time (CRT). Delayed CRT is a qualitative clinical tool used to detect hypotension. After compressing the oral mucosa and causing it to blanch, the pink color should return within 2 seconds. Delayed refill signifies the need for intravenous fluids in order to normalize the blood pressure.

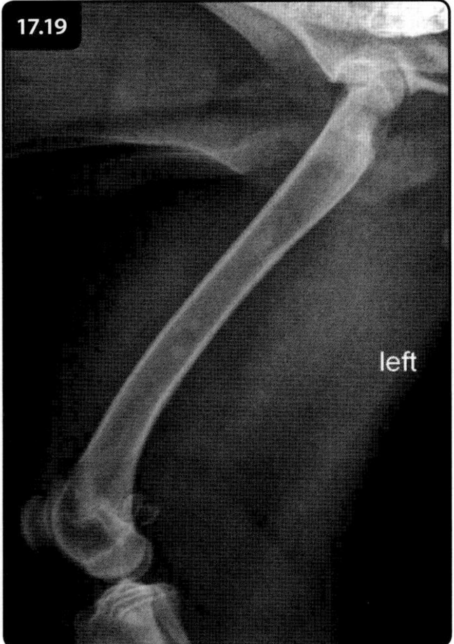

17.19. Panosteitis. This radiograph of the femur shows the hyperdense intramedullary areas characteristic of panosteitis. It usually occurs in young large-breed dogs. Pain and shifting leg lameness are common signs; fever is sometimes present. Treatment is palliative and the disease is self-limiting after several weeks.

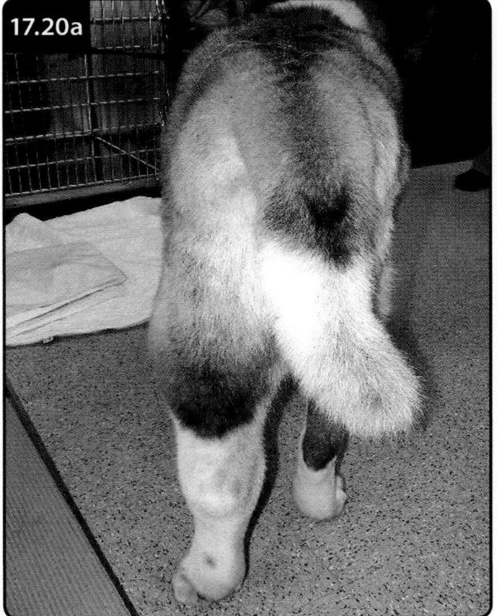

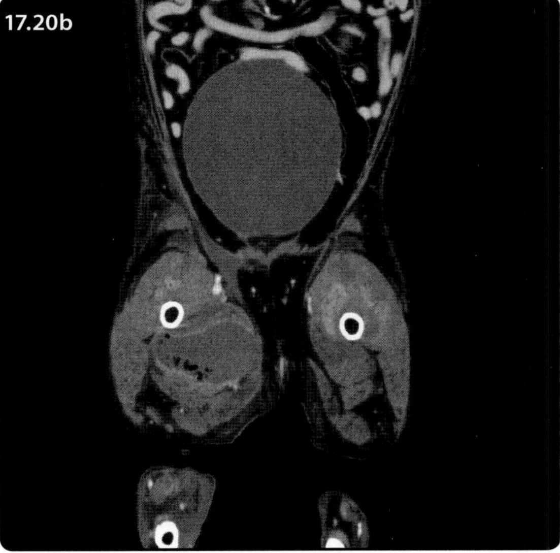

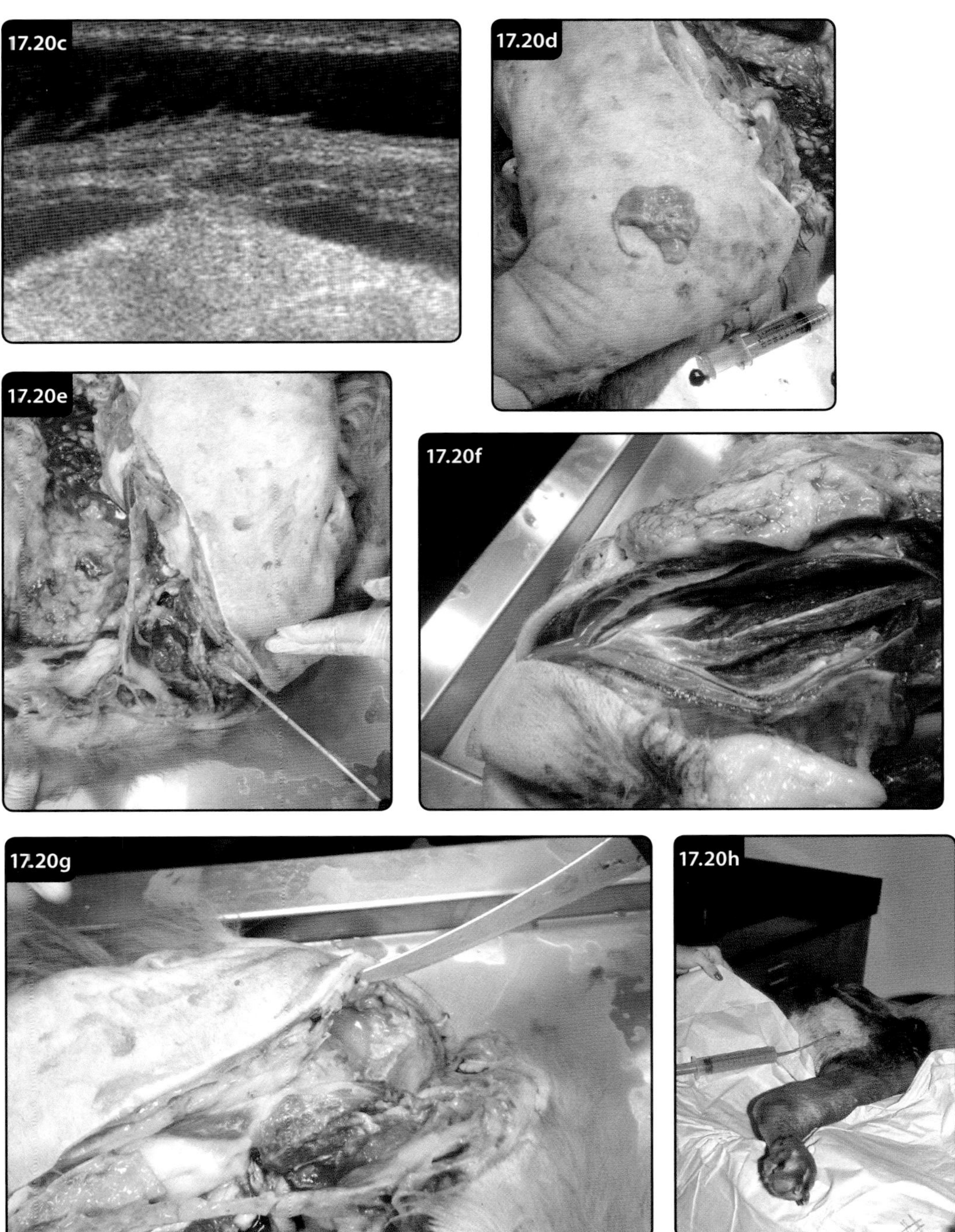

17.20a–h. Pyomyositis in a dog. This condition is characterized as a soft tissue bacterial suppurative cellulitis that involves skeletal muscle. The dog will show fever, lameness, and gross swelling in the involved muscle bellies (Figure 17.20a). A CT scan of the limb clearly shows the gas accumulated in the diseased muscle (Figure 17.20b). The ultrasonogram (Figure 17.20c) shows abnormal fluid and gas in the muscle tissues. The necropsy images (Figures 17.20d–g) are serial dissections that show the areas of suppuration involving different tissue planes. Figure 17.20h is a different dog with a drain in the proximal medial thigh that was used to drain the abscess involving the thigh muscles. Further surgical drainage might be indicated in these cases.

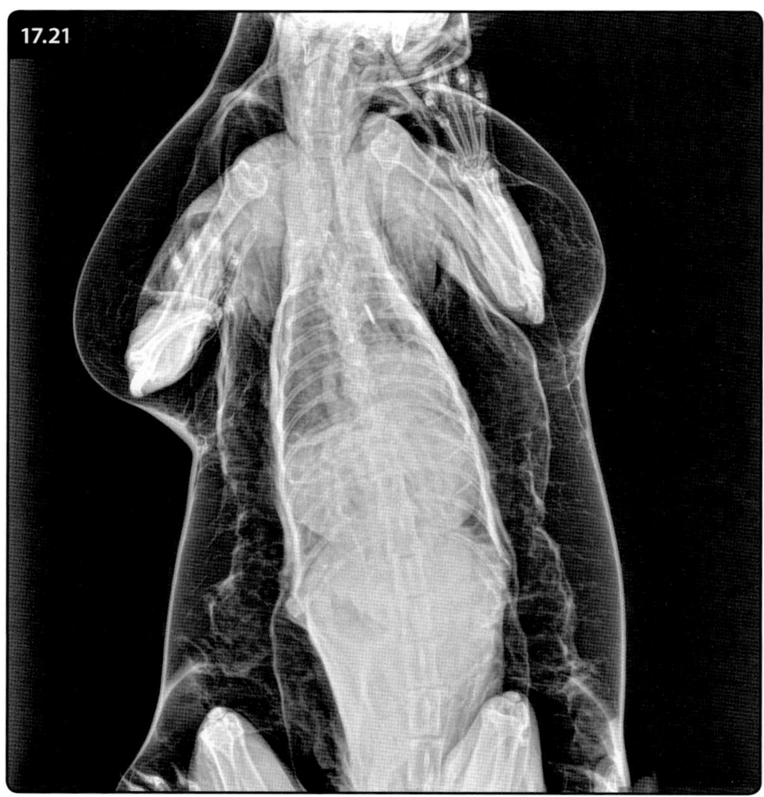

17.21. Ruptured trachea. The enormous amount of subcutaneous emphysema in this dog in addition to a pneumomediastinum are typical findings with ruptured trachea. Small tears and limited emphysema will sometimes heal without further action, but large amounts of accumulated air should prompt that a tracheoscopy be performed to assess the tear for possible surgical repair.

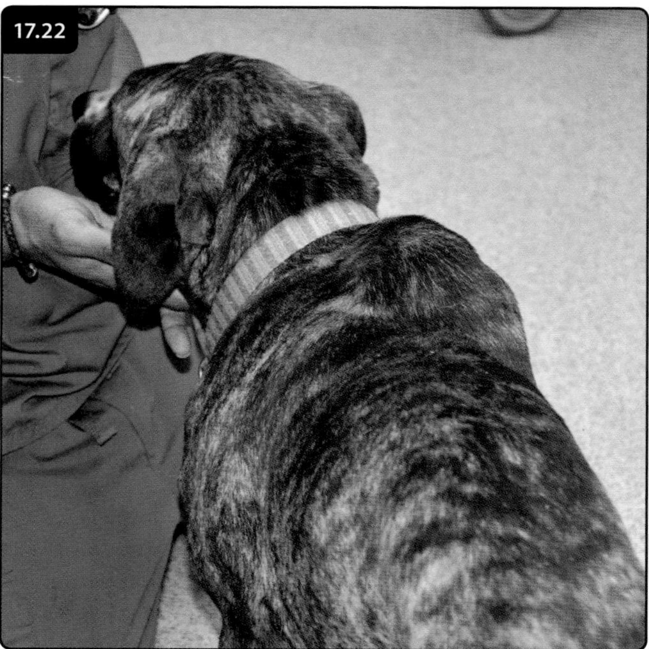

17.22. Scapula avulsion. This dog's right shoulder deformity is due to a scapular avulsion.

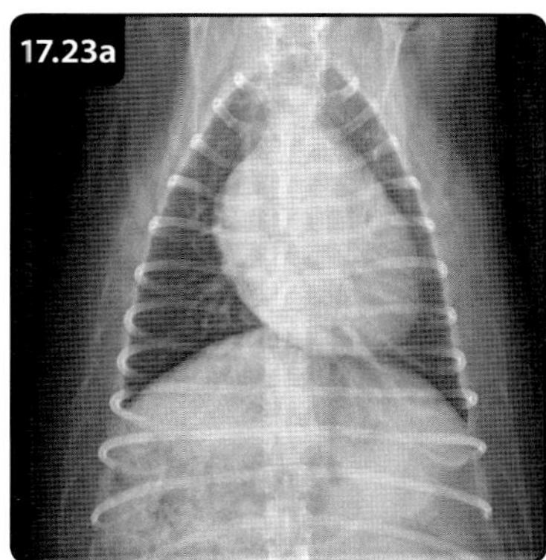

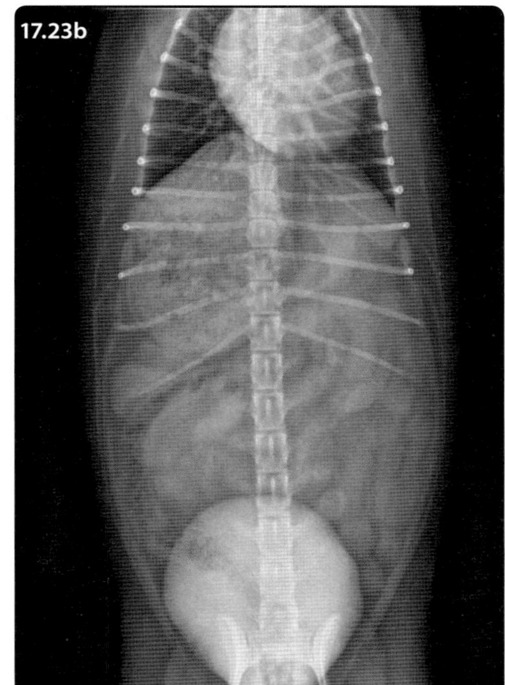

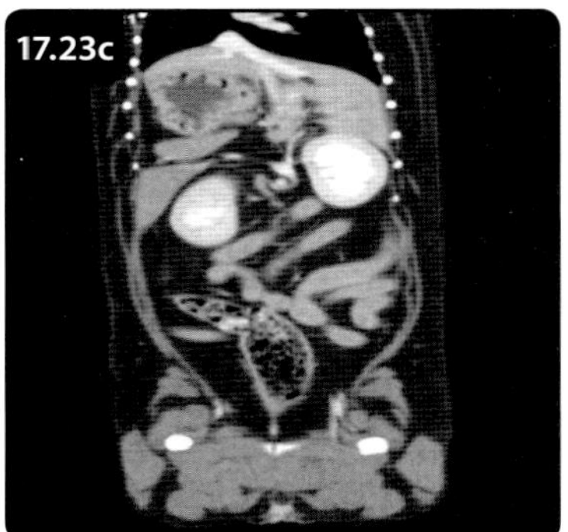

17.23a–c. Situs inversus. This is a congenital disorder where the organs in the abdomen and chest are reversed compared with their anticipated normal positions. These two dorsoventral radiographs and the CT scan show the gastric fundus on the dog's right side (in the CT the dog's right side is on the reader's right). Although the cardiac apex is pointing to the left, the chambers can be in reversed order. There are various types of this anomaly, some of which may involve the ciliary apparatus of the respiratory organs (Kartagener's syndrome). Simple organ reversal is not associated with any threat to well-being.

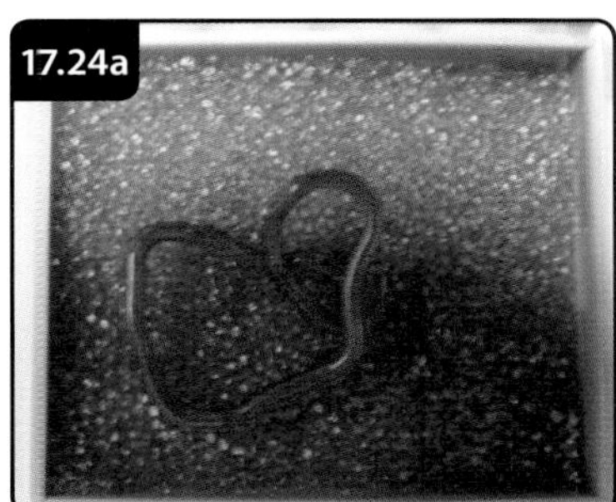

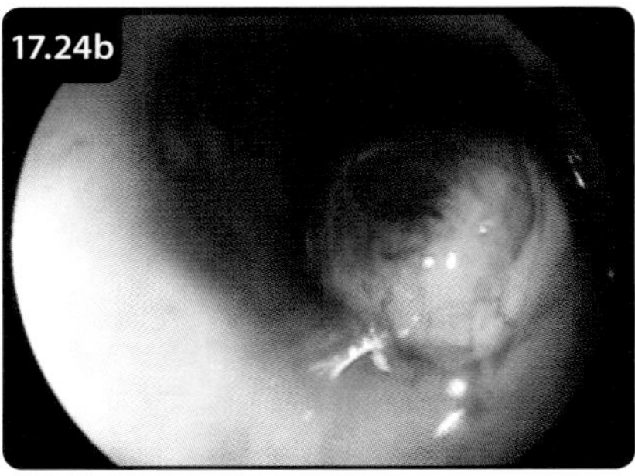

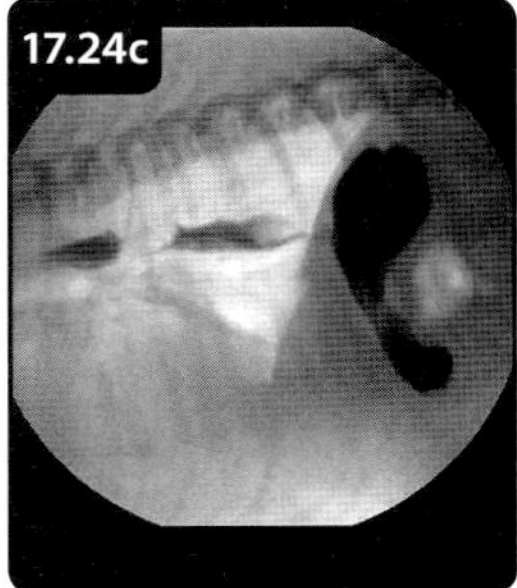

17.24a–c. *Spirocerca lupi*. This nematode infects dogs. Larvae migrate through certain organs and end up in the esophagus, where they form a large granuloma. It has been associated with the development of hypertrophic osteopathy. The figures show the parasite (Figure 17.24a), an esophascopic view of an esophageal granuloma (Figure 17.24b), and an esophageal filling defect visible during fluoroscopy (Figure 17.24c).

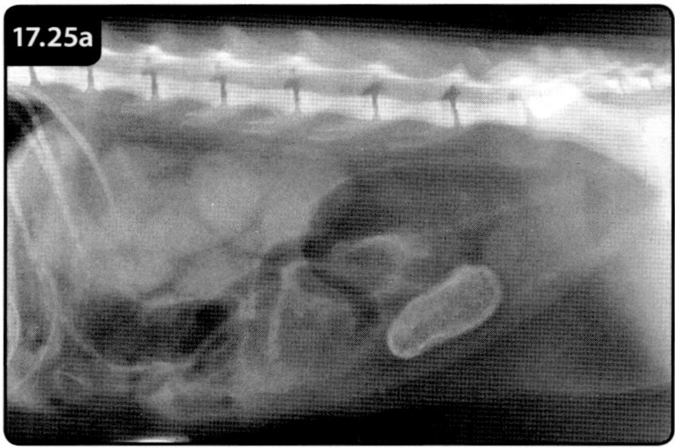

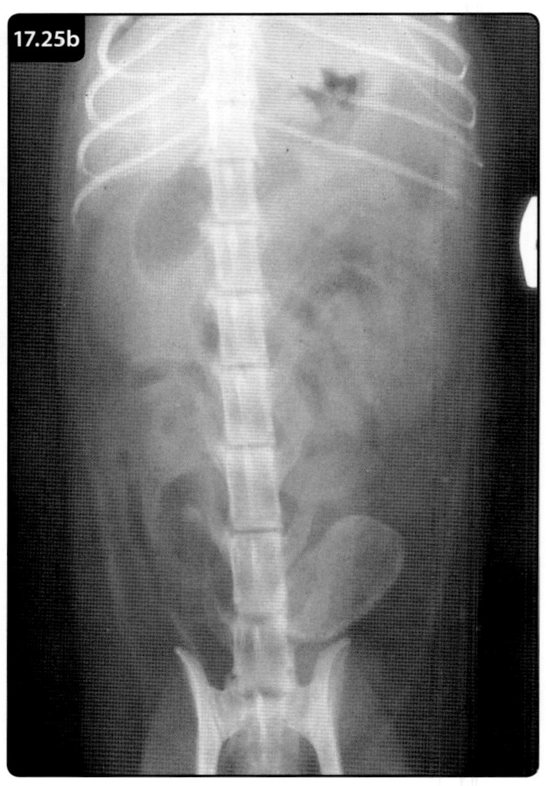

17.25a, b. Surgical sponge in abdominal cavity. These lateral and ventrodorsal abdominal radiographs were taken from a cat that was seen for vaccination without any physical problems. Examination detected an intra-abdominal mass that appeared on the radiographs as a mineralized mass lying free in the abdominal cavity. Laparotomy confirmed this finding. Biopsy showed fibers throughout the surgical specimen, thus identifying it as a retained surgical sponge left behind at the time of its spay.

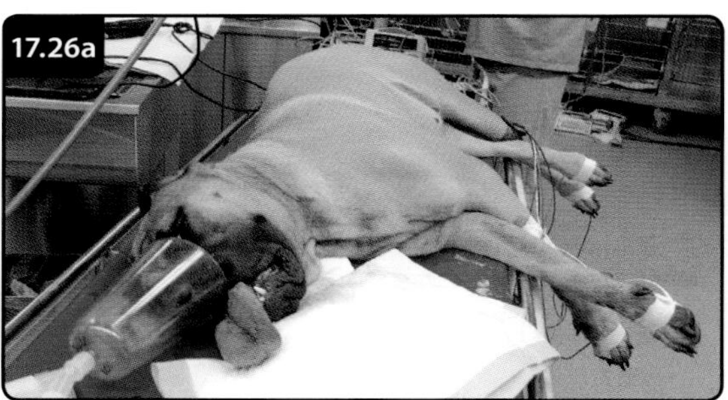

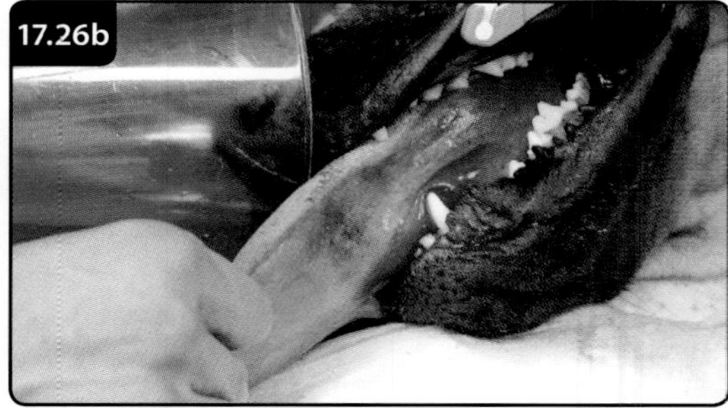

17.26a, b. Type 1 hypersensitivity involving the tongue. This Mastiff came inside from outdoors showing marked swelling of its tongue and frenulum. Some respiratory stridor was evident as well. This was diagnosed as a type 1 hypersensitivity reaction and treated with epinephrine, diphenhydramine, and glucocorticoids, which allowed for a good response. Heavy sedation was used in order to maintain the dog initially with an endotracheal tube in place until the swelling diminished, at which time oxygen was supplied by face mask. The cause was speculated to be oral contact with a venomous hymenopteran such as a bee, wasp, or yellow jacket.

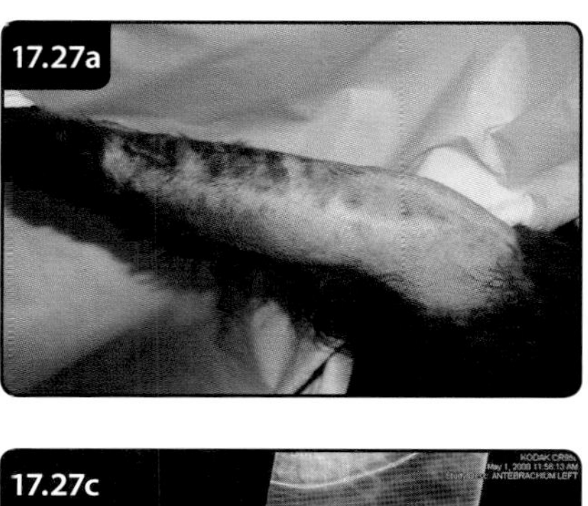

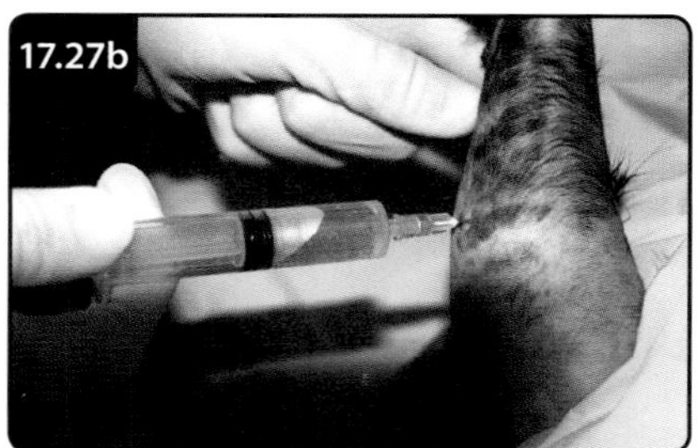

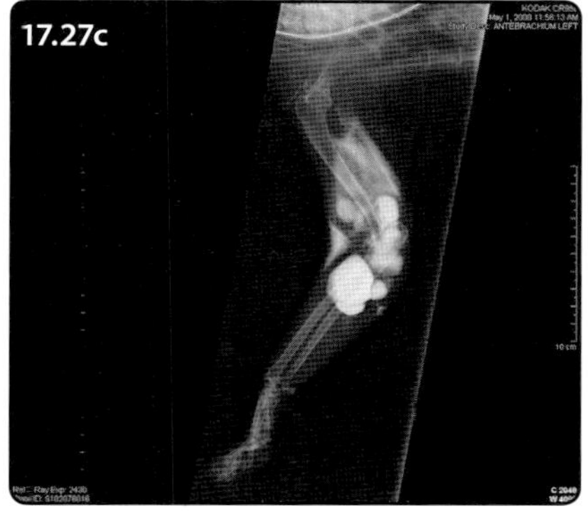

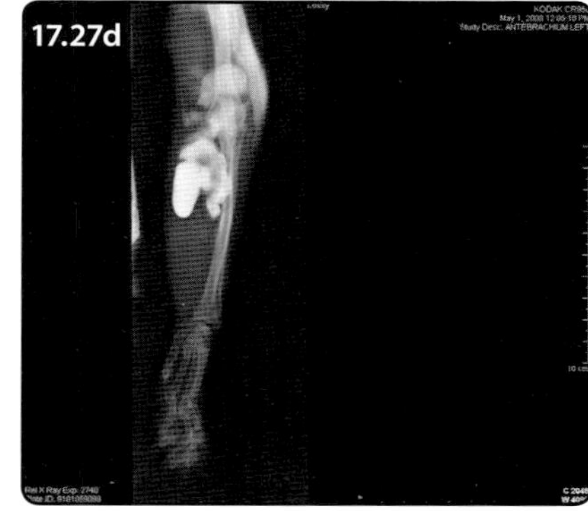

17.27a–d. Synovial cyst. This synovial cyst involving the elbow palpates as a fluctuant fluid-filled mass. The mass was aspirated, identifying the fluid as benign and compatible with synovial fluid. The contrast material that was injected into the synovial cyst denotes its boundaries, thus providing the surgeon with the necessary information for its resection.

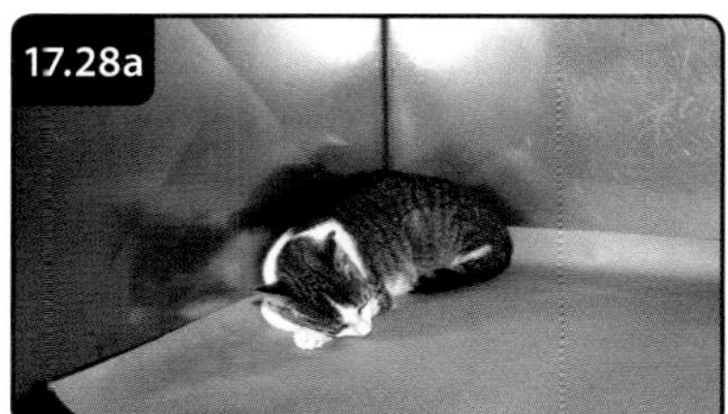

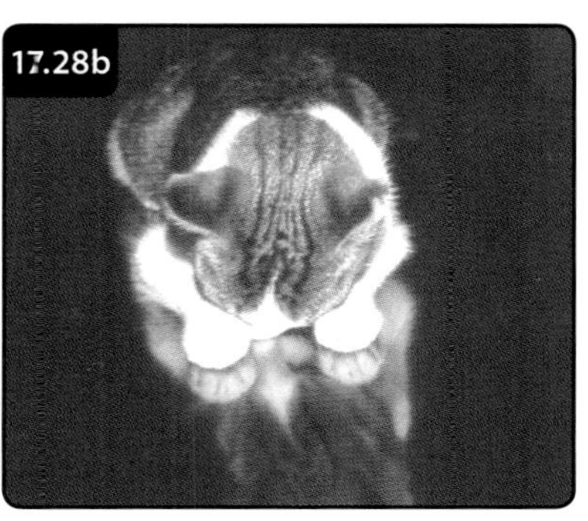

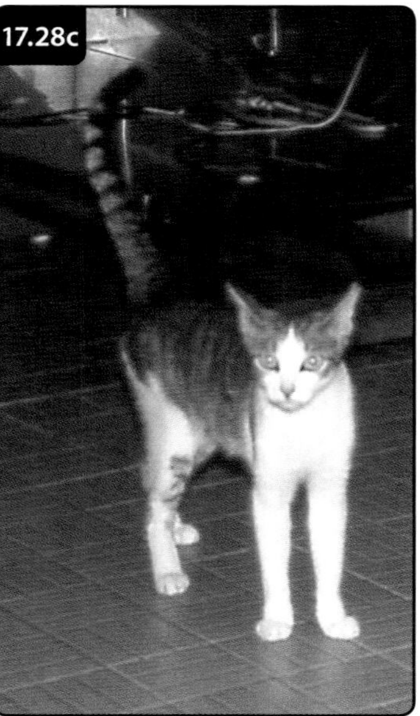

17.28a–c. Thiamine deficiency in a cat. Figures 17.28a, b show the typical posturing of a cat with thiamine deficiency. Additional clinical signs included ataxia and a 'starry' eyed facial expression. The diagnosis was based on clinical signs and the favorable response to thiamine treatment, which was apparent 24 hours after intramuscular administration of 75 mg thiamine hydrochloride (Figure 17.28c).

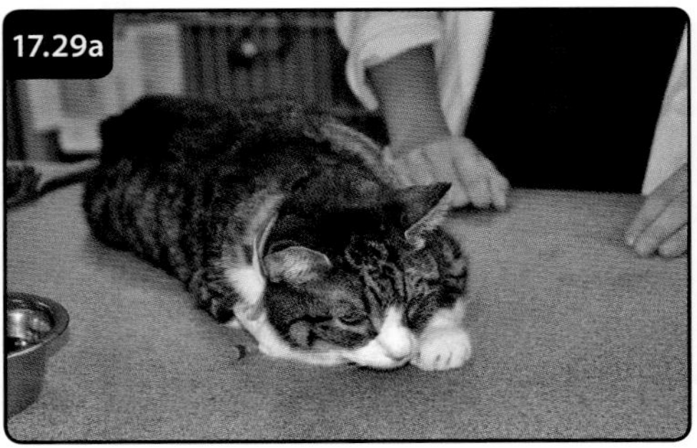

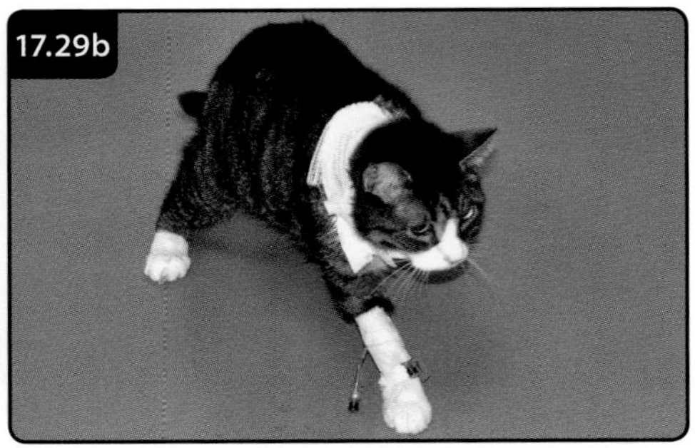

17.29a, b. Diabetic cat with thiamine deficiency. This cat had diabetes mellitus with hypokalemia. He showed muscular weakness at the time of admission. After receiving insulin and intravenous fluids supplemented with potassium chloride, the cat appeared worse on day 2. On physical examination at that time he was ataxic, had fixed medium dilated pupils, and appeared mentally dissociated. He was then tentatively diagnosed as thiamine deficient and was given 75 mg thiamine intramuscularly. The cat was normal on day 3, thus supporting the diagnosis of thiamine deficiency. This case is also described and discussed in Chapter 12 (12.55a, b).

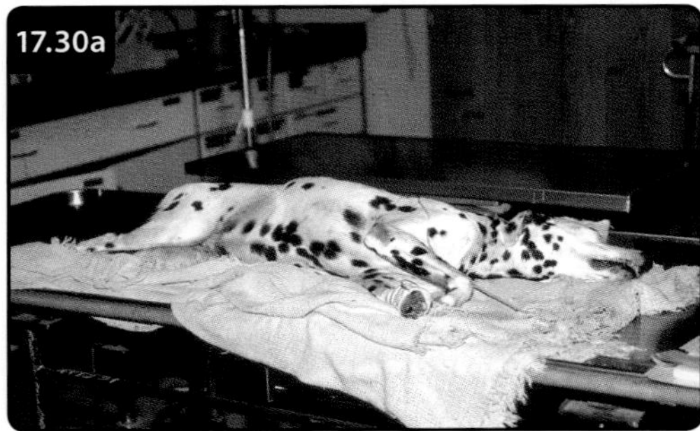

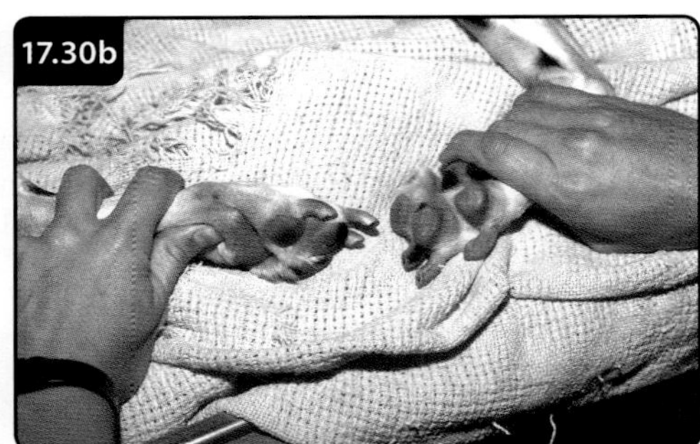

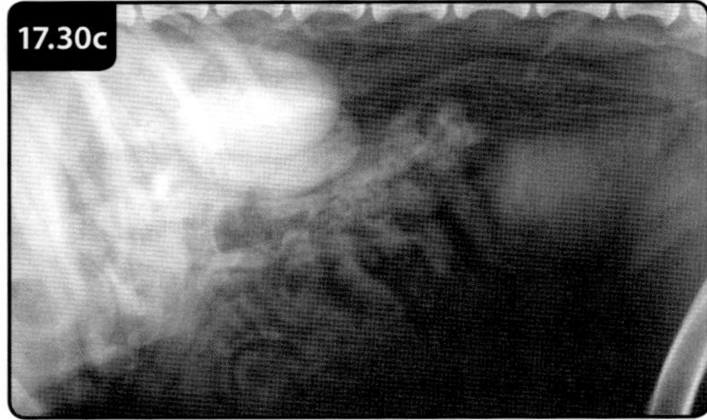

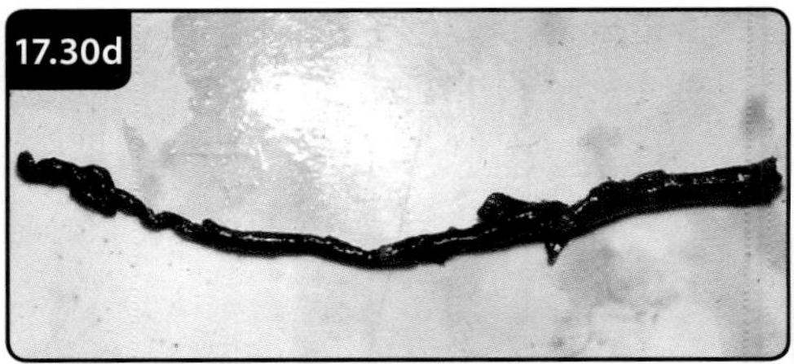

17.30a–d. Aortic saddle thrombus in a Dalmatian dog. This dog had a sudden onset of weakness involving both hindlimbs (Figure 17.30a). There were absent femoral pulses and there was noticeable acrocyanosis when comparing the perfusion of the front and rear claws (Figure 17.30b). The aortogram shows the absence of contrast media in the mid-abdominal aorta (Figure 17.30c). Surgery was able to remove only a portion of the thrombus (Figure 17.30d), and the dog went on to expire. There were no apparent causes of the saddle thrombus at necropsy in this dog.

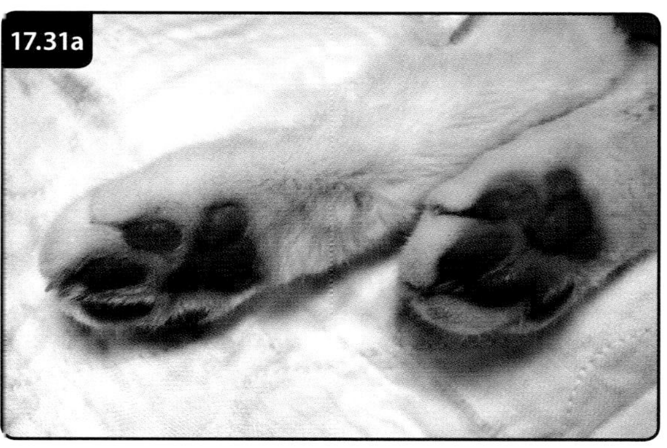

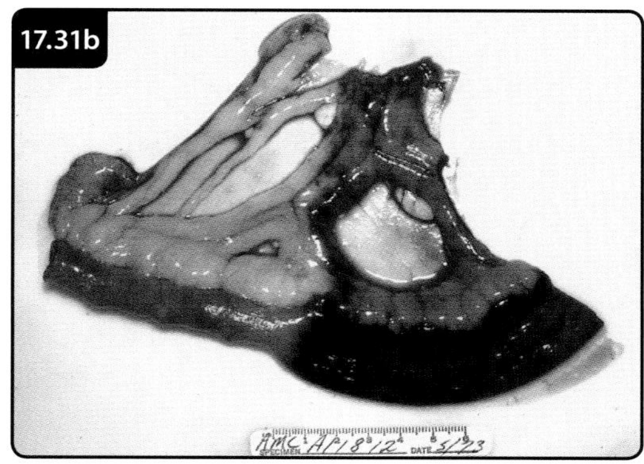

17.31a, b. Arterial thrombosis in a cat and dog. Figure 17.31a shows marked digital cyanosis (acrocyanosis) due to a saddle thrombus in a cat. As expected, the cat had underlying hypertrophic cardiomyopathy. Figure 17.31b depicts a mesenteric artery infarct with intestinal gangrene in a dog that was speculatively associated with high-dose glucocorticoid therapy for immune-mediated disease.

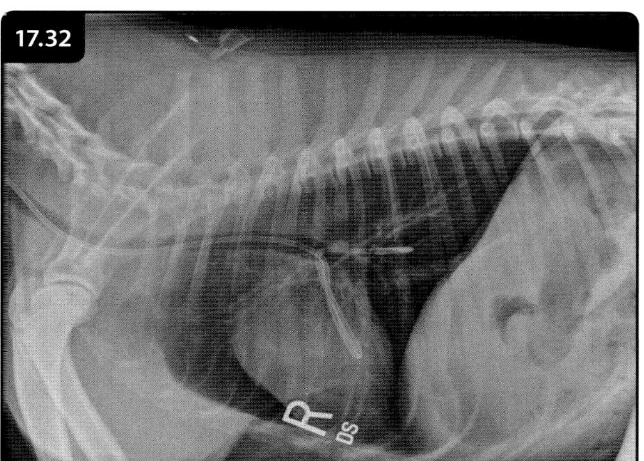

17.32. Faulty placement of a nasogastric feeding tube. The inadvertent passing of this nasogastric tube into the airway provides ample reason for doing a lateral thoracic radiograph following tube placement.

Index